Essentials of Maternal-Child Nursing

3rd Edition

By
Lynne Conrad, RNC, MSN, MHA
Maxine Karpen, RN
Linda Chitwood, RN, MS, CRNA

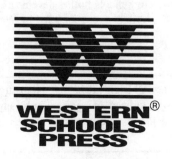

WESTERN®
SCHOOLS
PRESS

21 Bristol Drive
South Easton, MA 02375
1-800-618-1670

ABOUT THE AUTHORS

Lynne Conrad, RNC, MSN, MHA, is currently employed as Patient Progressions Coordinator at Albert Einstein Medical Center. She also is a Clinical Editor for Springhouse Corporation and has taught nursing theory at Holy Family College and worked as an instructor in the School of Nursing at Albert Einstein Medical Center.

Maxine Karpen, RN, writes extensively in the fields of nursing, medicine, health and fitness for professional as well as lay readers. She is a contributing editor to Nursing Spectrum and writes regularly for the Journal of Clinical Laser Medicine and Surgery, AIDS Patient Care and Medical Post. She was one of the contributing writers to The Complete Home Health Guide of the College of Physicians and Surgeons, Columbia University.

Linda Chitwood, RN, CRNA, MS, has been a practicing nurse for many years. She is currently president of Media Medical Inc., a health-care media service, based in Memphis, Tennessee. She has many years experience writing for the medical profession. She has published articles in Health Care News and Nursing. She has written on many subjects, such as anesthesiology, gynecology, pediatrics, and pain.

ABOUT THE SUBJECT MATTER EXPERT

Peggy Murray, RNC, MN, has worked in Maternal-Child nursing for nearly twenty years as staff nurse, head nurse, and as Perinatal Clinical Nurse Specialist at Mercy Hospital an Medical Center in San Diego, California. She has been an officer of NAACOG and is Certified as a childbirth educator, lactation educator, and Inpatient Obstetrical Nurse.

Proofreader: Jackie Bonham, RN, MSN

Indexer: Sylvia Coates

Typesetter: Kathy Johnson

Western Schools' courses are designed to provide nursing professionals with the educational information they need to enhance their career development. The information provided within these course materials is the result of research and consultation with prominent nursing and medical authorities and is, to the best of our knowledge, current and accurate. However, the courses and course materials are provided with the understanding that Western Schools is not engaged in offering legal, nursing, medical, or other professional advice.

Western Schools' courses and course materials are not meant to act as a substitute for seeking out professional advice or conducting individual research. When the information provided in the courses and course materials is applied to individual circumstances, all recommendations must be considered in light of the uniqueness pertaining to each situation.

Western Schools' course materials are intended solely for *your* use and *not* for the benefit of providing advice or recommendations to third parties. Western Schools devoids itself of any responsibility for adverse consequences resulting from the failure to seek nursing, medical, or other professional advice. Western Schools further devoids itself of any responsibility for updating or revising any programs or publications presented, published, distributed, or sponsored by Western Schools unless otherwise agreed to as part of an individual purchase contract.

ISBN: 1-57801-028-4

IMPORTANT: Read these instructions *BEFORE* proceeding!

Enclosed with your course book you will find the FasTrax® answer sheet. Use this form to answer all the final exam questions that appear in this course book. If you are completing more than one course, be sure to write your answers on the appropriate answer sheet. Full instructions and complete grading details are printed on the FasTrax instruction sheet, also enclosed with your order. Please review them before starting. *If you are mailing your answer sheet(s) to Western Schools, we recommend you make a copy as a backup.*

ABOUT THIS COURSE

A "Pretest" is provided with each course to test your current knowledge base regarding the subject matter contained within this course. Your "Final Exam" is a multiple choice examination. **You will find the exam questions at the end of each chapter.** Some smaller hour courses include the exam at the end of the book.

In the event the course has less than 100 questions, mark your answers to the questions in the course book and leave the remaining answer boxes on the FasTrax answer sheet blank. **Use a <u>black pen</u> to fill in your answer sheet.**

A PASSING SCORE

You must score 70% or better in order to pass this course and receive your Certificate of Completion. Should you fail to achieve the required score, we will send you an additional FasTrax answer sheet so that you may make a second attempt to pass the course. Western Schools will allow you three chances to pass the same course...*at no extra charge!* After three failed attempts to pass the same course, your file will be closed.

RECORDING YOUR HOURS

Please monitor the time it takes to complete this course using the handy log sheet on the other side of this page. See below for transferring study hours to the course evaluation.

COURSE EVALUATIONS

In this course book you will find a short evaluation about the course you are soon to complete. This information is vital to providing the school with feedback on this course. The course evaluation answer section is in the lower right hand corner of the FasTrax answer sheet marked "Evaluation" with answers marked 1–25. Your answers are important to us, please take five minutes to complete the evaluation.

On the back of the FasTrax instruction sheet there is additional space to make any comments about the course, the school, and suggested new curriculum. Please mail the FasTrax instruction sheet, with your comments, back to Western Schools in the envelope provided with your course order.

TRANSFERRING STUDY TIME

Upon completion of the course, transfer the total study time from your log sheet to question #25 in the Course Evaluation. The answers will be in ranges, please choose the proper hour range that best represents your study time. You MUST log your study time under question #25 on the course evaluation.

EXTENSIONS

You have 2 years from the date of enrollment to complete this course. A six (6) month extension may be purchased. If after 30 months from the original enrollment date you do not complete the course, *your file will be closed and no certificate can be issued.*

CHANGE OF ADDRESS?

In the event you have moved during the completion of this course please call our student services department at 1-800-618-1670 and we will update your file.

A GUARANTEE YOU'LL GIVE HIGH HONORS TO

If any continuing education course fails to meet your expectations or if you are not satisfied in any manner, for any reason, you may return it for an exchange or a refund (less shipping and handling) within 30 days. Software, video and audio courses must be returned unopened.

Thank you for enrolling at Western Schools!

WESTERN SCHOOLS
P.O. Box 1930
Brockton, MA 02303
(800) 618-1670

Essentials of
Maternal-Child Nursing

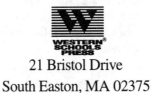

21 Bristol Drive
South Easton, MA 02375

Please use this log to total the number of hours you spend reading the text and taking the final examination (use 50-min hours).

Date	Hours Spent
_____	_____
_____	_____
_____	_____
_____	_____
_____	_____
_____	_____
_____	_____
_____	_____
_____	_____
_____	_____
_____	_____
_____	_____
_____	_____

TOTAL [   ]

Please log your study hours with submission of your final exam. To log your study time, fill in the appropriate circle under question 25 of the FasTrax® answer sheet under the "Evaluation" section.

PLEASE LOG YOUR STUDY HOURS WITH SUBMISSION OF YOUR FINAL EXAM. Please choose which best represents the total study hours it took to complete this 30 hour course.

A. less than 25 hours

B. 25–28 hours

C. 29–32 hours

D. greater than 32 hours

Essentials of Maternal-Child Nursing

WESTERN SCHOOLS
CONTINUING EDUCATION EVALUATION

Instructions: Mark your answers to the following questions with a black pen on the "Evaluation" section of your FasTrax® answer sheet provided with this course. You should not return this sheet. Please use the scale below to rate the following statements:

A Agree Strongly	**C Disagree Somewhat**
B Agree Somewhat	**D Disagree Strongly**

The course content met the following education objectives

1. Described current trends in maternal-newborn healthcare, and identified the changes in nursing practice that result from these trends.

2. Discussed the major maternal physiological and psychological changes that occur during pregnancy.

3. Discussed the key elements of the prenatal physical assessment and indicated appropriate nursing interventions based on the assessments.

4. Discussed the purpose of childbirth preparation and identified major methods and philosophies for providing effective prenatal educational support.

5. Differentiated normal labor stages and patterns and selected appropriate nursing interventions to support the laboring patient and family.

6. Discussed the causes of pain associated with labor and childbirth and indicated methods of pain relief that are most effective for women during labor and delivery.

7. Identified methods of assessing fetal well-being during the last trimester of pregnancy and during labor and delivery.

8. Identified the principles of delivery management for both vaginal and cesarean births, and specified appropriate nursing assessment and intervention strategies for the immediate care of the newborn.

9. Identified physiological and psychological changes that occur following childbirth and discussed effective nursing assessment and intervention strategies for postpartum patients.

10. Discussed the physiology of lactation, identified advantages and disadvantages of breastfeeding, and discussed effective problem-solving techniques that benefit breastfeeding women.

11. Identified normal and abnormal characteristics of the newborn and specified nursing measures for assessment of the newborn, integration into the family, and discharge planning.

12. This offering met my professional education needs.

13. The information in this offering is relevant to my professional work setting.

14. The course was generally well written and the subject matter explained thoroughly. (If no please explain on the back of the FasTrax instruction sheet.)

15. The content of this course was appropriate for home study.

16. The final examination was well written and at an appropriate level for the content of the course.

Please complete the following research questions in order to help us better meet your educational needs. Pick the ONE answer which is most appropriate.

17. What is your work status?
    A. Full-time employment
    B. Part-time employment
    C. Per diem/Temporary employment
    D. Inactive/Retired

18. For your LAST renewal did you take more Continuing Education contact hours than required by your state, if so, how many?
    A. 1–15 hours
    B. 16–30 hours
    C. 31 or more hours
    D. No, I only take the state required minimum

19. Do you usually exceed the contact hours required for your state license renewal, and if so, why?
    A. Yes, I have more than one state license
    B. Yes, to meet additional special association Continuing Education requirements
    C. Yes, for professional self-interest/cross-training
    D. No, I only take the state required minimum

20. What nursing shift do you most commonly work?
    A. Morning Shift (Any shift starting after 3:00am or before 11:00am)
    B. Day/Afternoon Shift (Any shift starting after 11:00am or before 7:00pm)
    C. Night Shift (Any shift starting after 7:00pm or before 3:00am)
    D. I work rotating shifts

21. What was the SINGLE most important reason you chose this course?
    A. Low price
    B. New or newly revised course
    C. High interest/Required course topic
    D. Number of contact hours needed

22. Where do you work? (If your place of employment is not listed below, please leave this question blank.)
    A. Hospital
    B. Medical clinic/Group practice/ HMO/Office setting
    C. Long term care/Rehabilitation facility/Nursing home
    D. Home health care agency

23. Which field do you specialize in?
    A. Medical/Surgical
    B. Geriatrics
    C. Pediatrics/Neonatal
    D. Other

24. For your last renewal, how many months BEFORE your license expiration date did you order your course materials?
    A. 1–3 months
    B. 4–6 months
    C. 7–12 months
    D. Greater than 12 months

25. **PLEASE LOG YOUR STUDY HOURS WITH SUBMISSION OF YOUR FINAL EXAM.** Please choose which best represents the total study hours it took to complete this 30 hour course.
    A. less than 25 hours
    B. 25–28 hours
    C. 29–32 hours
    D. greater than 32 hours

CONTENTS

PRETEST

Begin by taking the pretest. Compare your answers on the pretest to the answer key (located in the back of the book). Circle those test items that you missed. The pretest answer key indicates the course chapters where the content of that question is discussed.

Next, read each chapter. Focus special attention on the chapters where you made incorrect answer choices. Exam questions are provided at the end of each chapter so that you can assess your progress and understanding of the material.

1. Which of the following is a current trend in maternal-child nursing?

   a. A sharp decline in the neonatal mortality rate.

   b. Decreased lengths-of-stay after delivery.

   c. The restriction of birth participants to the father only.

   d. The leveling off of the teenage pregnancy rate.

2. The term used to describe the practice where a woman labors, delivers, recovers, and is discharged home from one room is

   a. rooming-in.

   b. LDR.

   c. single room maternity care.

   d. mother-baby couplet care.

3. Formation of major organs occurs during the _____ stage of development.

   a. embryonic

   b. zygote

   c. fetal

   d. pre-embryonic

4. Complaints of nasal stuffiness during pregnancy is most likely due to

   a. estrogen levels.

   b. progensterone levels.

   c. upper respiratory infections.

   d. prolactin levels.

5. Leg cramps can be relieved by

   a. increasing calcium intake.

   b. rubbing calves to stop cramp.

   c. wearing an ace wrap.

   d. having regular exercise and calf stretching.

6. A warning sign of a complication developing during pregnancy is

   a. weight gain of 1 lb. a week in the second or third trimester.

   b. Braxton Hicks contractions.

   c. nausea and vomiting during the first trimester.

   d. sudden increase in facial, hand/feet edema.

7. A goal of most childbirth education programs is to

    a. eliminate the need for medications during labor.

    b. provide factual information in a supportive environment.

    c. guarantee a normal, vaginal delivery.

    d. reduce the incidence of cesarean delivery.

8. The term given to the person who supports the laboring woman with care-taking activities, and who practices conditioned techniques for relaxation and breathing is a

    a. childbirth educator.

    b. "coach" or support person.

    c. physician.

    d. patient advocate.

9. Upon physical exam, the physician notes the patient's pelvic type is gynecoid. What are the implications of this finding?

    a. The patient most likely will need a cesarean delivery.

    b. This type of pelvis is seen in only 5–10% of women.

    c. This is a typical female pelvis.

    d. The use of forceps is likely.

10. Frequency of contractions is best described by which of the following statements?

    a. The time from the start of a contraction to the end of that contraction.

    b. The time from the start of a contraction to the end of the next contraction.

    c. The time between the beginning of one contraction and the beginning of the next contraction.

    d. The time between the end of one contraction and the beginning of the next contraction.

11. Pain during labor and childbirth is primarily caused by

    a. dilatation of the cervix and uterine cell hypoxia.

    b. pressure on the bladder.

    c. stretching of the pelvis.

    d. increased levels of endorphin.

12. Maternal side effects from intravenous meperidine hydrochloride (Demerol) include

    a. respiratory depression and tachycardia.

    b. hypertension and decreased pulse rate.

    c. agitation and hypertension.

    d. dehydration and neonatal hypotonia.

13. The fetal circulation consists of three circuits, the systemic, pulmonary, and

    a. cardiac.

    b. renal.

    c. placental.

    d. mesenteric.

14. The part of the fetal circulation that directs most blood flow to bypass the lungs is the

    a. aortic valve.

    b. ductus arteriosus.

    c. umbilical cord.

    d. ductus venosus.

15. The cardinal movement of labor which occurs when the fetal chin rests against the chest is called

    a. expulsion.

    b. descent.

    c. internal rotation.

    d. flexion.

16. A condition in the newborn in which a collection of blood develops between a skull bone and the periosteum without crossing suture lines is called

    a. caput succedaneum.

    b. intraventricular hemorrhage.

    c. cephalohematoma.

    d. bulging fontanelles.

17. The postpartum period generally is considered to end how long after delivery of the infant?

    a. 2 hours

    b. 2 weeks

    c. 6 weeks

    d. 6 months

18. Which of the following findings during the immediate postpartum period should be reported to the physician?

    a. Foul smelling lochia.

    b. Decreased heart rate.

    c. Constipation.

    d. Uterine cramping.

19. The discharge after childbirth is initially termed lochia rubra, which then becomes

    a. Lochia uterine.

    b. Lochia alba.

    c. Lochia sanguina.

    d. Lochia serosa.

20. The female breast is partly formed from which type of tissue?

    a. Granular

    b. Nervous

    c. Muscle

    d. Glandular

21. Lactation is *most* effectively suppressed by

    a. binding the breasts.

    b. avoidance of suckling.

    c. application of ice.

    d. injection of prolactin.

22. How many lobes are generally found in each breast?

    a. 5

    b. 10

    c. 20

    d. 50

23. The newborn period refers to the first

    a. 2 hours of life.

    b. 28 days of life.

    c. year of life.

    d. 24 hours of life.

24. With regard to vernix caseosa, the premature infant will likely

    a. not have any.

    b. be covered with it.

    c. have it only in the skin folds.

    d. have it only on the scalp.

25. A thick, sticky green or black substance found in the large intestine of the full term infant is

    a. surfactant.

    b. meconium.

    c. vernix caseosa.

    d. lanugo.

INTRODUCTION

In the entire lexicon of human experience, birth is perhaps the one most filled with wonderment, emotion, and drama (Conrad, 1988). It is no wonder that throughout the ages, poets and writers have extolled parenthood (particularly motherhood) and the miracle of life's beginning.

Throughout history, society has recognized the relationship of its generative capacity to its survival, understanding that the health of society is dependent on the reproductive health of the families that compose it (Styles, 1990). Thus, maternal-newborn nursing is not simply one of the oldest specialties but also one of the widest in scope, inextricably bound to the origins of family and to the roots of society.

The scope of maternal-newborn nursing runs the gamut from before conception through adolescence, and through the reproductive years of the parents, and covers a spectrum that ranges from epidemiology to bedside care. Therefore, the study of maternal-newborn nursing includes not only a knowledge of anatomy and physiology of the reproductive organs; and the development of a new life from conception to birth; but also an understanding of human growth and development and their relationship to society.

The future of each child depends on its heritage, its prenatal environment, and the care given to it at birth, during infancy, and throughout childhood. Consequently, the aim of maternal-newborn nursing is two-fold: to protect the health, well-being and safety of the mother, the father and the infant, and to provide for the highest possible level of wellness for every childbearing family in terms of physical, emotional, and social well-being.

This book will prepare the nurse for the general care of the normal childbearing woman and her family, from the woman's initial diagnosis of pregnancy through the antepartum period, labor, delivery, and immediate postpartum recovery to her discharge from the birthing center or hospital. Care of the low-risk newborn throughout the transition stage until discharge home will also be highlighted. Although emphasis is given to normal physiological changes occurring during pregnancy and childbirth, abnormal changes are briefly discussed in order to alert the reader to the more common obstetrical and newborn complications.

This book will provide nurses who work in a variety of settings with basic, practical and current information to enable them to be more effective and confident in caring for pregnant women, new mothers, and babies. The text can be used as a quick reference for practicing nurses and as a study guide for nurses who desire to work in this specialty.

The terms "maternal-newborn" and "maternal-child" are used interchangeably throughout the text.

CHAPTER 1

CURRENT TRENDS IN MATERNAL-NEWBORN HEALTHCARE

CHAPTER OBJECTIVE

After studying this chapter, the reader will be able to recognize current trends in maternal-newborn healthcare, and identify the changes in nursing practice that result from these trends.

LEARNING OBJECTIVES

After reading this chapter, the student will be able to

1. Select perinatal risk factors that can complicate pregnancy and childbirth.

2. Recognize the philosophy of family-centered maternity care.

3. Identify two technological advances in healthcare that have affected maternal-newborn nursing.

4. Indicate the advantages of single-room maternity care.

INTRODUCTION

Over time enormous changes have taken place in the delivery of nursing care to the mother and the newborn. Before the turn of the century, babies were born at home, frequently delivered by an untrained midwife, neighbor, relative, or friend, or for the fortunate few, by a physician. Surrounded by loved ones, with her newborn brought promptly to her bed, the new mother basked in the attention and support of her family.

All of that changed early in the 20th century when parturition moved into the hospital setting. Within the "maternity ward," priority was often given to the institutions' procedures and practices, relegating the personal needs of the mother and her infant to second place. At that point, childbearing became far from a family affair. The father (as depicted in cartoons and later in movies) traditionally "paced the floor" of a waiting room, while the mother-to-be labored alone, or worse, in a common labor room with other women. Her children, considered to be a source of probable infection, were not permitted visiting privileges during the week or more that their mother and new sibling remained isolated from them. The infant, separated from its mother, was placed in a newborn nursery and brought to its mother only at specified times. Nursing care was separated into three sub-specialties, with one nurse caring for the mother during labor and delivery, another handling postpartum patients, and a third caring for the baby in the nursery.

By the 1940s, the "rooming-in" concept was devised. Full-term infants were placed in a crib at their mothers' bedsides, where the mothers provided their care. Nursing care remained fragmented, with the nursery nurse responsible for infant care and the postpartum nurse tending to the mother. The advantages of the system included a reduction in neonatal infection from cross-contamination, increased confidence and independence for the mother, and greater breastfeeding success. The infant showed a better weight gain and cried less. But the down side was that the new mother often evidenced problems in accepting full responsibility for the baby's care.

As is now known, new mothers experience three psychological phases: taking-in, taking-hold, and letting-go. During taking-in, new mothers are passive and dependent, requiring rest and supportive nursing care to promote bonding and attachment. With rooming-in, the mother lacked that supportive care—the taking-hold phase (wherein the mother is ready to learn mothering skills) had been hoisted upon her too soon. And, unfortunately, the letting-go phase (wherein she establishes maternal role patterns and incorporates those changes into her personal and family life) was almost totally neglected. For these reasons, many mothers did not opt for rooming-in programs.

After World War II, the focus changed from the person providing care to the recipient of that care. With the change came a change in terminology, and obstetrical care became maternity care. The broadened scope includes both prenatal and postnatal care and promotes the health and well-being of the mother, the child, and the entire family.

The World Health Organization (WHO) offers this definition of maternity care:

> The object of maternity care is to ensure that every expectant and nursing mother maintains good health, learns the art of child care, has a normal delivery, and bears healthy children. Maternity care in the narrower sense consists in the care of the pregnant woman, her safe delivery, her postnatal examination, the care of her newly born infant, and the maintenance of lactation. In the wider sense, it begins much earlier in measures aimed to promote the health and well-being of the young people who are potential parents, and to help them develop the right approach to family life and to the place of the family in the community. It should also include guidance in parent-craft and in problems associated with infertility and family planning *(see figure 1-1).*

TRENDS

Overall Changes in the Healthcare Industry

The healthcare industry is in a state of transition, and the nurse's ability to adapt to change may well affect professional survival. Economic, social, and health status changes have influenced the settings for the delivery of healthcare, the practitioners who provide it, and the manner and degree of reimbursement. The "graying of America" has changed economics within society and the healthcare industry. This, compounded by a physician surplus, has caused increased competition for the healthcare dollar, constrained resources limiting the availability of prenatal and preventive sources to dependent families, and created a shift away from acute care for the young to chronic care for the elderly.

Perinatal nursing will be most affected by several demographic trends: a declining birth rate; changes in childbearing patterns; increased numbers of women working during pregnancy and childbearing years; high rates of low birth weight infants; and an increase in sexually transmitted diseases in women.

Birth Rate

The declining birth rate, more than any other factor, will have a direct effect on the practice of perinatal nurses. Between 1957 and 1976, the birth

FIGURE 1-1
The Wheel of Family-Centered Postpartum and Newborn Care

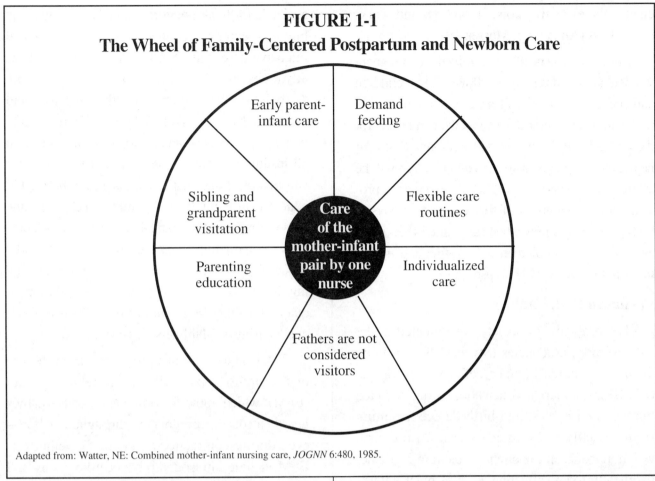

Adapted from: Watter, NE: Combined mother-infant nursing care, *JOGNN* 6:480, 1985.

rate in the U.S. steadily declined. Although a slight increase occurred in 1977 and has continued to the present time, in all probability the birth rate will decline once the "baby boomers" (those born in post-World War II days when birth rates soared) no longer produce children. With a decline in the numbers of those needing perinatal services, there will be a concomitant decline in demand for providers of these services.

Changing Patterns of Childbirth and Their Effect on Maternal-Infant Mortality Statistics

Due to medical advances and improved technology, the infant mortality rate in the United States has steadily decreased to 8.2 per 1,000 population (Pelletteri, 1995). Despite these improvements, black infants have a mortality rate of 18.9 per 1,000 population. This is associated with a higher number of younger mothers and unequal provision of health care. More and more babies are being born to women at the extremes of their child-bearing years as increasing numbers of women defer motherhood until they are in their thirties, and teenage pregnancies soar. At both ends of the spectrum, the younger and older mother face increased risks of complications during pregnancy: pre-term delivery; low birth weight babies; maternal, fetal, neonatal, and post-natal mortality.

The number of babies born to unmarried women is rising and teen pregnancy increases the chance of delivering a low-birth-infant due to inadequate prenatal care, socioeconomic status, education and nutritional status (Neff & Spray, 1996).

In addition, women, in increasing numbers, are working outside the home during pregnancy and immediately after delivery, compounding the risk (to themselves and to the fetus) of exposure to toxic chemicals, excessive noise, radiation, and workplace stress (Andreoli & Musser, 1985).

The goals for health care reform for pregnant women and children are as follows: (1) all children and pregnant women will have continuous access to health insurance or have a mechanism to pay for the basic health services, (2) personal costs for health care of pregnant women and children will be affordable for everyone, (3) health coverage is provided for a continuum of services that emphasize both primary and preventive care; and, (4) an unbiased process is implemented to refine and update the benefits package (Thompson, 1992).

Perinatal Risk Factors

The problems of society are reflected in the risks to today's neonates (Styles, 1990). Among them are acquired immune deficiency syndrome (AIDS) in mothers and newborns, drug addicted mothers and babies, and birth defects resulting from sexually transmitted diseases. Low birth weight remains an important problem in reproductive health today, affecting 12% of black infants and 5% of infants born to white and Asian women (Pelletteri, 1995). Prematurity accounts for 80–90% of infant mortality within the first year of life. In addition to maternal age and marital status, risk factors for low birth weight infants include the mother's medical history during past pregnancies, race, socioeconomic status, educational level, smoking, alcohol consumption, and the presence or absence of prenatal care. Sexually transmitted disease (STD) in the mother can result in infant death or in a baby born with pneumonia, cerebral palsy, epilepsy, deafness, blindness, or mental retardation.

Technological Advances

Advances in technology have revolutionized the diagnoses and treatment of many health conditions. Increasingly sophisticated computers have made swifter diagnosis and continuous monitoring possible. Among those with the greatest effect on maternal and newborn nursing are the instruments available for fetal monitoring and the care given by highly specialized professionals in the neonatal intensive care unit (NICU). As a result of these advances, the Committee on Practice in The Association of Women's Health, Obstetric, and Neonatal Nurses (AWHONN) recommends that policies, procedures, and protocols be developed in all institutions for the use of advanced equipment and treatment and that nursing staff be thoroughly educated in them. The Committee recognizes the value of these technological advances but discourages the temptation that they replace the "hands-on-care" of the patient that nurses provide. The nursing process must remain the foundation of quality nursing care (Committee on Practice, 1991, cited in May & Mahlmeister, 1994, pg. 10).

Fetal monitoring has progressed from the use of the stethoscope to electronic fetal monitors (EFM), which allow for observation of the baby's heartbeat during pregnancy, throughout labor—even during contractions. "Indirect" methods of EFM include ultrasound, phonocardiography and abdominal fetal electrocardiography. "Direct" (internal) fetal monitoring, used during labor and delivery, is done with a spiral electrode attached to the baby's scalp. The strength of labor contractions can now be measured by means of an internally-placed catheter attached to a monitor. Telemetry, utilizing radio transmission, now makes it possible to monitor contractions and fetal heartbeat even when the mother is not in the same room as the monitor. This new development allows for more comfort and mobility during labor *(see figure 1-2)*.

Amnioinfusion

In order to prevent or minimize the effects of meconium aspiration syndrome (MAS), sterile saline may be introduced, via catheter, into the uterus while the woman is in labor. The technique, first introduced in the mid 1980s, has been shown to alleviate variable decelerations due to umbilical cord compression after rupture of membranes. The

FIGURE 1-2
Electronic Fetal Monitoring

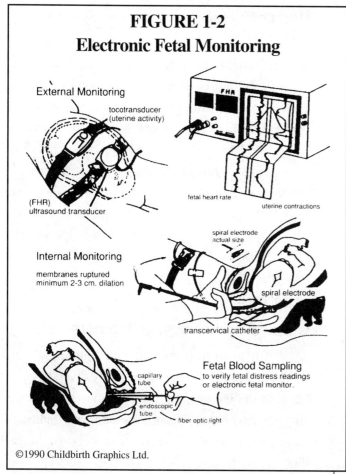

External Monitoring

tocotransducer
(uterine activity)

FHR

fetal heart rate

uterine contractions

(FHR)
ultrasound transducer

Internal Monitoring

membranes ruptured
minimum 2-3 cm. dilation

spiral electrode
actual size

spiral electrode

transcervical catheter

Fetal Blood Sampling
to verify fetal distress readings
or electronic fetal monitor.

capillary
tube

endoscopic
tube

fiber optic light

©1990 Childbirth Graphics Ltd.

fluid also dilutes the amniotic fluid which has become thick from meconium passed in utero. Nursing actions include assisting the physicians with intrauterine catheter placement, assessment of maternal/fetal vital signs and contraction pattern, and regulation of the infusion to 100–250 ml/hr until the fluid is clear.

Experts predict that in the future even normal births will utilize "high tech" innovations, with the result of lowering perinatal mortality and morbidity. Risk assessment and genetic counseling will begin well before pregnancy—even before mate selection and during pregnancy; risk situations will be monitored on a 24-hour-a-day basis, allowing for more active obstetrical intervention (McKenzie & Vestal, 1983). Fetal assessment tools will become more sophisticated, and new corrective techniques will become increasingly available, including in-utero surgical correction and medical

management of defects, direct fetal blood transfusion and drug injection, and genetic diagnosis.

Many of today's common obstetrical problems, such as pregnancy-induced hypertension and diabetes, will be curable, and treatment for infertility will abound. The challenges for nurses will be enormous, as they will have to provide humanistic, family-oriented care in a world of high technology.

CURRENT PROBLEMS

Decreased Lengths of Stay

Our grandmothers endured a "confinement" of two weeks following childbirth (Lemmer, 1987). By the time our mothers had their babies, the average postpartum hospital stay had declined to one week. As healthcare becomes increasingly ambulatory-dominant, today's new mother is up and out of the hospital or birthing center in one to two days at the most. "Keep 'em vertical" has become the byword of third-party insurers, both private and government, who are intent on keeping down the ever-escalating costs of in-hospital stays.

Early discharge poses a challenge to the nurse, who must provide nursing intervention during a brief time frame and disseminate information, reinforce learning, and affirm the mother's role in hours, rather than days. Since early discharge often precludes extensive patient teaching, the nurse will have to become adept at individualizing teaching based on the unique needs of each patient (Styles, 1990).

Budgetary Constraints

With fiscal austerity increasing and hospitals employing accounting systems that "cost out" nursing care, perinatal nurses will have to demonstrate a consciousness of cost as well as quality of care (McKenzie & Vestal, 1983). The future will, in all probability, also bring increased restrictions on the purchase of equipment, along with constraints on the development of new perinatal technology. And as childbirth moves into birthing centers and homes, new nursing skills will have to be developed to permit the transition without a loss in quality of care and without compromising patient safety.

An ever increasing number of individuals are joining managed care companies. Their main goal is to coordinate for a particular patient and family all of their health care activities prescribed by the health professionals in an effective and cost-efficient manner (May & Mahlmeister, 1994). To accomplish this goal, the team uses clinical pathways and case management. Managed care paths, which are similar to standardized care plans for particular patient groups, specify the expected progress and outcomes that the patient should make from the start of health care delivery to its completion. In addition, a case manager is responsible for ensuring that the patient's progress is within the scope and time frame indicated on the managed care path. The managed care system, therefore, promotes the appropriate use of resources, facilitates collaborative practice, coordinates patient care, and ensures continuity of quality health care.

Currently, 16% of American women in their childbearing years have no insurance coverage. That figure will escalate as healthcare costs rise, as more cost-containment programs are instituted, and as governmental support of social and health programs diminishes. More and more children will be removed from Medicaid rolls, guidelines for Aid to Families with Dependent Children (AFDC) will become tighter, and supplemental food programs for women infants and children (WIC) will suffer increased budget cuts. This trend will have a negative effect on the use of perinatal services and on the health of women and their children.

Higher Patient Acuities

In addition to facing budget constraints and shorter patient stays, today's maternal-newborn nurse is finding an increased case load of higher acuity patients. Multiple socioeconomic problems coupled with lack of available prenatal care has contributed to the increasing census of patients who smoke, abuse alcohol or drugs, who lack proper nutrition during pregnancy, and who have neglected their health. Many have STDs, anemia, Rh sensitization, hypertension, excessive weight gain or loss, or chronic diseases. Large numbers go into premature labor, delivering at-risk, low-birthweight babies.

Cultural and Language Barriers

A further challenge to maternal-newborn nurses is adapting to the increasingly diverse population in the United States. Each group has its own customs and mores, deeply rooted in its traditions and history, many of which relate to body image, illness, childbearing, and infant care.

In dealing with cultures that differ from their own, nurses will have to reach a compromise between their own beliefs, value systems and technical knowledge and the values of the patient. Language barriers will have to be anticipated and dealt with, and in instances where interpreters are not available, nurses may have to develop a working vocabulary of terms important to their specialty.

Along with population changes, family structures are in a state of transition. A wide variety already exists, among them the nuclear family, the extended family, the single-parent family, and the aggregate family (those with parents who bring children of previous marriages into their new relationship). In addition, the number of women working outside the home is increasing. As family roles change, the stability of the family may be threatened, leading to increased stress and mental health problems. Working with families will become more complex and a greater challenge for the nurse.

Legal and Ethical Dilemmas

As technology burgeons, new ethical dilemmas associated with their use arise (Styles, 1990). The ethical considerations affecting reproductive rights, and those that have a direct effect on the health of the mother and infant, are particularly complex and emotional (Andreoli & Musser, 1985). Among the issues that have surfaced are the following:

• Should treatment be withheld for newborns with life-threatening conditions.

• Should the fetus be considered a patient separate from the mother, and, if so, what rights does it have and how do these rights affect the mother's rights?

• When the mother's rights and interests conflict with the fetus's rights, how are the conflicts resolved?

• Does the mother have a right to refuse treatment for the fetus?

• When does life begin?

• What are the rights of a surrogate mother, a sperm-donor father, and a mother who carries a fetus that resulted from in-vitro fertilization of another woman's ovum (Styles, 1990)?

Many of these issues have been addressed in courts and are the subject of legislation and ongoing debate. Maternal-newborn nurses, in particular, will have to play a major role in the ongoing debates, examining the moral, ethical, scientific, and social issues involved, and will have to demand that a balance be maintained between technology and personal care.

CHANGES IN MATERNAL-NEWBORN NURSING

Social, economic, political, and technological factors have contributed to the many changes that have occurred in maternal-newborn nursing within recent years. The focus is now on childbirth as a social and familial process, with less technical interference, greater humanism, a wider range of choices and options, and a reaffirmation of the natural birth process. In addition, recognition of the importance of maternal-infant bonding in the first hours and days of the newborn's life has led to the encouragement of maximal mother-infant contact (Cohen, 1991).

Family-Centered Care

Based on the philosophy that health includes physical, social, economic, and psychological dimensions, the family centered approach assumes that the family is the basic unit of society and should be viewed as a total unit, with consideration given to each member. Since childbearing and the rearing of children are functions of the family, it is therefore appropriate to share this experience as a unit, with each member enjoying recognition and consideration (Cohen, 1991).

Thus, in family-centered care the emphasis is on the delivery of professional healthcare that fosters family unity while maintaining the physical safety of the childbearing unit—the mother, father, and infant. It is unique in that the nurse attends, educates, and counsels all age groups. Integration and bonding take high priority, and much anticipatory counseling is offered. In family centered care, the nursery and postpartum staffs are combined to form one mother-baby unit.

Labor, Delivery, Recovery, and Postpartum Care (LDRP)

LDRP, also called single-room maternity care, was devised as a replacement for the traditional maternity unit or alternative birth center, and is found in hospitals serving both low-risk and high-risk parturients. In it the woman labors, delivers, and recovers in the same room and in the same bed, and in most cases the baby remains with its mother during her stay. From the time of the mother's admission until her discharge, a primary care nurse is assigned to the family. The LDRP system has the advantage of providing comprehensive medical care within a single setting, in a more homelike environment, while maintaining all of the advantages of hospitalization.

Mother-Baby Couplet Care

Couplet care, also known as dyad care, is a system in which one nurse cares for the postpartum mother and her infant as a single unit. It focuses on and adapts to both the physical and psychosocial needs of the mother, the family, and the neonate, and fosters family unity while maintaining physical safety and providing a secure environment in which nurses are available for consultation, reinforcement, and individualized education. While nurses help both parents to assume responsibility for their baby's care, they can also assess the family's adaptation and attachment. This system facilitates parental-infant attachment, neonatal transition, lactogenesis, lactation, and involution, while supporting the taking-in and taking-hold phases of the postpartum period.

Certified Nurse Midwife (CNMW)

Certified nurse-midwives are licensed health care practitioners educated in the two disciplines of nursing and midwifery. They provide primary care to women of childbearing age including: prenatal care, labor and delivery care, family planning decisions, preconception care, menopausal management and counseling in health maintenance and disease prevention.

Consumer Demands, Hospital Marketing, and Competition

In the past, consumer demands caused many changes in obstetrical practice. ASPO/Lamaze and the International Childbirth Association formed coalitions as consumers advocated change through patient education and demanded family-centered care.

In the future, the term "health" will probably have a broader connotation. As the trend shifts from a medical perspective to a "wellness" orientation, the consumer will demand an emphasis on maintenance of health and the consideration of the total person. As this occurs, holistic medicine may well become the model for the healthcare system.

Consumers will take more responsibility for their own health, reducing the number of visits to physicians and tending to treat their own problems. Alternative healthcare services (such as birthing centers and hospices) will become increasingly popular, care will proliferate. As a result, competition for the hospital patient will become more acute, and the public will be deluged, even to a greater degree than at present, with TV, radio, and print commercials selling hospital services—birthing rooms, sibling visitation, and other inducements for new parents.

Consumers of maternity care will have particular demands as they become more vocal in their opposition to the routinized and standardized care in settings that cater to the needs of the provider rather than those of the patient. Parents are demanding full participation in all phases of childbearing, the right to be involved in decisions affecting their bodies and their health, and the right to employ practices they believe to be important for their babies' and their own happiness. (See Appendix, "The Pregnant Patient's Bill of Rights.") Their demands will become even stronger as time goes on.

EXAM QUESTIONS

CHAPTER 1
Questions 1–5

1. The factor most associated with the increased risk for perinatal complications is
   a. heredity.
   b. extremes in maternal age.
   c. geographic location.
   d. multiparity.

2. Which of the following is a current trend in maternal-child nursing?
   a. Decreased lengths-of-stay after delivery.
   b. A sharp decline in the neonatal mortality rate.
   c. The restriction of birth participants to the father only.
   d. The leveling off of the teenage pregnancy rate.

3. Which of the following behaviors best describes a newly delivered woman in the "taking-in" phase?
   a. receptive to teaching
   b. depressed
   c. dependent
   d. able to perform self-care activities

4. The maternity care delivery system that emphasizes professional quality health care of the total family unit is called
   a. childbearing-centered care.
   b. traditional obstetrical care.
   c. family-centered care.
   d. alternative birthing center.

5. The term used to describe the practice where a woman labors, delivers, recovers, and is discharged home from one room is
   a. rooming-in.
   b. LDR.
   c. single-room maternity care.
   d. mother-baby couplet care.

CHAPTER 2

PREGNANCY: DIAGNOSIS, SYSTEMIC CHANGES, PSYCHOLOGY

CHAPTER OBJECTIVE

After studying this chapter, the reader will be able to recognize the major maternal physiological and psychological changes that occur during pregnancy.

LEARNING OBJECTIVES

After reading this chapter, the student will be able to

1. Identify the signs of pregnancy.
2. Recognize major stressors on the childbearing family that may affect adaptation to pregnancy and parenting.
3. Indicate major changes in maternal systems as a result of pregnancy.

DIAGNOSIS

It is important that the nurse distinguish between signs and symptoms that are presumptive of pregnancy, those that are probable, and those that are positive. Presumptive signs are those based on reasonable evidence of pregnancy; probable signs show that pregnancy is likely; positive signs confirm, without a doubt, that pregnancy has occurred.

Signs and Symptoms—Presumptive Signs

Amenorrhea: If a woman in good health ceases to menstruate during her reproductive life, she may well presume that she is pregnant. Cessation of menses is often the woman's first indication of pregnancy, but it is only a tentative and highly presumptive sign of pregnancy, and insufficient for diagnosis, since it may be caused by a number of other factors.

Breast changes: Early in pregnancy, the breasts begin to enlarge, become nodular and progressively fuller and firmer, with increased pigmentation of the areolae. Along with increased vascularity, the superficial veins become more apparent and there is frequently a feeling of throbbing, tingling, or prickling and/or sore nipples.

Chadwick's sign: Due to increased vascularity and increased edema of the cervix combined with hypertrophy and hyperplasia of the cervical glands, the vagina and cervix often appear purple or dark bluish in color. This is often demonstrable soon after the first missed menstrual period.

Changes in skin pigmentation: Because of increases in hormones and in vascularity, several skin changes may be noted during pregnancy. Vascular "spiders" and palmar erythema may result from capillary dilatation and proliferation, and any hematomas present may increase in size, while new ones may develop, particularly on the face and hands. In 50% of all pregnancies, areas of the body that are subject to stretching—the abdomen, breasts or thighs—may become striated. These blue or pink streaks are called striae gravidarum. The linea alba (the whitish line extending from the symphysis pubis to the umbilicus) darkens and becomes the linea nigra. The vulva, nipples, areola, and umbilicus may also darken and chloasma ("the mask of pregnancy") may appear as irregular-shaped, brownish colorations around the eyes, cheekbones, and nose.

Nausea, with or without vomiting: Nausea and vomiting, commonly called "morning sickness," occur in less than half of pregnant women. Nausea usually comes on within two weeks after the missed period, and generally subsides before the third missed period. It is rarely pathological, except when excessive or prolonged. (Refer to hyperemesis gravidarum, page 45.)

Urinary symptoms: The desire to void may be felt frequently during early pregnancy due to bladder compression caused by the enlarging uterus. This symptom usually disappears after the third month when the uterus rises up above the brim of the pelvis and ceases to produce bladder pressure.

Fatigue: Some women experience fatigue during the first trimester, but its cause is undetermined. Possible causes of fatigue include strain on the sacroiliac joint as the uterus enlarges, iron deficiency, the action of progesterone, and stress. Women with poor posture before pregnancy are particularly prone to fatigue.

Quickening: Also known as "feeling life," quickening is a sensation of fetal movement that usually occurs during the sixteenth to eighteenth week. It may occur earlier in multiparas. Intestinal movements often simulate quickening.

Signs and Symptoms—Probable Signs

Abdominal enlargement: Mechanical distention of the abdomen occurs due to increasing uterine size and to the rising of the uterus from the pelvis at approximately 13 to 14 weeks gestation.

Uterine changes: The uterus grows from approximately 2 ounces to 2 pounds (at term), and changes from a solid organ with an approximate capacity of 2 cc to a thin-walled muscular sac capable of holding a fetus. It assumes an oval configuration while increasing in contractile ability as it rises out of the pelvic cavity. Both the endometrium and the myometrium increase in thickness and vascularity up to the third month, then begin to thin. The shape of the fundus changes from spherical to cylindrical as the pregnancy progresses. In early pregnancy, the amount of elastic connective tissue increases along with the size and number of blood vessels.

Cervical changes: With increasing vascularization, the cervix becomes softer (Goodell's sign) and cyanotic in color (Hegar's sign) and there is a proliferation of cervical glands that secrete thick, white mucus.

Braxton Hicks contractions: Intermittent contractions of the uterus may occur irregularly and may be palpated after the first three months. Though they are usually painless earlier in pergnancy, they may increase in intensity during the last 6–8 weeks of pregnancy. Braxton Hicks contractions are differentiated from true labor by their irregularity, and by the fact that they do not increase in strength, duration, or frequency. They are usually confined to the groin and lower segment of the abdomen.

Ballottement: The diagnosis of pregnancy may probably be confirmed by ballottement—pushing of the uterus with the finger inserted into the vagina, causing the embryo to rise and fall.

Outline of fetus: Palpation of the fetus to determine its size and position is rarely elicited before the fourth month, at which time the fundus is midway between the symphysis and the umbilicus.

Endocrine tests: Protein hormones—human chorionic gonadotropin (HCG), human chorionic somatomammotropin (HCS), and human chorionic thyrotropin (HCT)—are present only during pregnancy. Detection of HCG in blood or urine is the basis for modern pregnancy tests. Testing can be done by agglutination, radioreceptor assay, or radioimmunoassay.

Agglutination testing, when done by slide, takes two minutes. When done by test tube it takes two hours, but this method is more sensitive. Testing is usually done six weeks after the last menstrual period. Radioreceptor assays take one hour and are highly sensitive and accurate. Testing can be done two weeks after conception. Radioimunoassays, which take one to three hours, are very accurate and can be used eight to nine days after conception.

Home pregnancy tests are used 15 days after a missed period, and claim 95% reliability when used correctly. However, the risk of false positives or negatives is always present.

Signs and Symptoms—Positive Signs

Fetal heart action: The fetal heart rate (FHR) may be heard by Doppler scanning (ultrasonic monitoring) at 12 weeks, and by fetoscope at 16–20 weeks. The normal rate is 120 to 160 beats per minute with regular rhythm. In obese women, or in those with pendulous abdomens, auscultation may be more difficult.

Fetal movement: By the end of the third lunar month the fetus moves, but this movement is not felt by the mother (Raff & Freisner, 1989). By the end of the fifth lunar month "quickening" occurs and the mother can feel movement. The movements of an active fetus can be heard by doppler when the examiner is listening to the fetal heart tones.

Fetal outline: Between the fourth and fifth lunar month, enormous changes in the fetus occur, as it grows from an average of 6.5 inches long, with a weight of 4 ounces, to 10 inches in length, weighing 8 ounces. As it grows, the fetal outline becomes more apparent. The sizes and weights of the average fetus are as follows:

End lunar month	Inches	Pounds
6	12	1.5
7	15	2.5
8	16.5	4
9	19	6
10	20	7

Adapted from: Ladewig, London & Olds, 1990.

Calculating Expected Date of Delivery (EDD)

a. From the date of the first day of the last menstrual period (LMP), add nine months and seven days OR count back three months and add seven days (Nägele's rule).

b. Length of pregnancy varies, making calculation difficult. The average length is 266 days from time of conception or 280 days from the first day of the LMP, a total of 10 lunar months or 40 weeks.

Fetal Growth and Development

Weeks one to three are called the pre-embryonic or zygote stage, in which the ovum is fertilized and the three layers of embryonic disk form.

Weeks four to eight are called the embryonic stage, characterized by extremely rapid growth and tissue differentiation and the formation of major organic systems (organogenesis). The embryo changes in shape and the major features of the external body become recognizable by eight weeks (morphogenesis).

Weeks 9 to 40 are called the fetal stage, during which there is growth and development of the major body organs and differentiation of tissues and organs. At this time the fetus becomes recognizable as a human being. The body proportions change and the organs begin to function and supply a portion of the fetus's metabolic needs (Neeson, 1987).

MATERNAL SYSTEMIC CHANGES

Cardiovascular: Blood volume increases about 30% to 40% (hydremia) causing an additional workload for the heart. The erythrocyte count declines due to hemodilution. Blood pressure drops in the second trimester, then rises in the third trimester. Some women experience supine hypotension syndrome in the second half of pregnancy (a drop in blood pressure when they lie on their backs) caused by compression of the inferior vena cava and characterized by faintness. Cardiac volume increases by 10%, and as the diaphragm elevates, the heart is displaced left and upward. The heart rate and cardiac output (the amount of blood pumped by the heart each minute) increase. Cardiovascular changes can cause hemorrhoids, varicosities of the legs and vulva, edema of the legs and fainting (Neeson, 1987).

Respiratory: Swelling of nasal tissue, nasopharynx, larynx, trachea and bronchi may occur due to estrogen-induced capillary engorgement. Nose breathing becomes difficult, epistaxis may occur, and the voice may change. Tidal volume (the amount of air inhaled or exhaled with each breath) increases along with the respiratory rate, often resulting in hyperventilation. Dyspnea, in early pregnancy, often results from low carbon dioxide levels, and in the last trimester may be caused by the uterus pushing up against the diaphragm. The chest cavity expands laterally (Raff & Freisner, 1989).

Urinary: Several urinary changes predispose the pregnant woman to urinary infection. The renal plasma flow increases, causing increased urinary output. Pressure causes dilation of the ureters. As the uterus enlarges, it exerts increasing pressure on the bladder, causing additional frequency (Raff & Freisner, 1989).

Gastrointestinal: Mechanical distention of the abdomen causes striae gravidarum. Decreased peristalsis and muscle tone reduce gastric motility, contribute to nausea, and can lead to constipation. Hemorrhoids can appear. Hormonal and metabolism changes can also lead to nausea and "morning sickness" and reverse peristalsis can cause heartburn. Flatulence may also occur (Raff & Freisner, 1989).

Musculoskeletal: There is relaxation of the ligaments and joints due to an increase in relaxin. Leg cramps (in late pregnancy) result from decrease in calcium or increase in phosphorus. As the body alignment changes, postural imbalance can occur, which often leads to lordosis, backaches, a tendency to fall, and a waddling gait (Raff & Freisner, 1989).

Reproductive: The greatest degree of change occurs in the reproductive system. As the uterus grows, its weight, capacity, the amount of its elastic tissue, and the number of its blood vessels increase. (Its blood supply increases from 20 to 40 times during pregnancy.) The cervix becomes more vascular and edematous, and hypertrophy and hyperplasia of the cervical glands cause its softening (Heger's sign). Its glands secrete thick white mucus. The vaginal blood vessels grow larger and the mucosa becomes bluish (Chadwick's sign). Sexual interest may heighten during the second trimester. The breasts enlarge and become nodular, fuller, and firmer, and the nipples and areolae become pigmented. Superficial veins in the breast become prominent, and there are feelings of tenderness, tingling, and heaviness. In the third trimester, colostrum, a pre-milk fluid, is secreted (Raff & Freisner, 1989).

Metabolic: Pregnancy usually produces a "diabetic" state with three conditions normally occurring as pregnancy progresses. There is a glucose drain from the mother as the fetus develops and uses more maternal glucose for growth. Maternal fasting blood glucose also normally decreases to 60 to 90 mg/dl even though there is an increase in the production of glucose from the liver postprandially. Secondly, an accelerated starvation state may develop as a result of an increased need by the mother and fetus for carbohydrates and calories with the growing pregnancy. Finally, there is an increasing resistance to insulin as the pregnancy progresses due to the higher levels of maternal hormones (estrogen, progesterone, human placental lactogen). There is, therefore, a persisting increased need for insulin. Overall, insulin production often increases about two to three times prepregnant levels to maintain euglycemia (normal blood glucose). In some women, the pancreas cannot meet this challenge and blood glucose will increase beyond desirable levels. Two to three percent of all pregnant women will develop a temporary problem with carbohydrate metabolism called gestational diabetes mellitus (Pelletteri, 1995). (Refer to gestational diabetes on page 43.)

PSYCHOLOGY OF PREGNANCY

Definitions

- *Adaptation or successful adjustment* is a continually changing process to provide the most satisfactory balance between all of an individual's internal and external demands and situations.

- *Developmental tasks* are those personal adaptations made at specific periods of one's life. Successful completion of each task forms a basis for the accomplishment of future tasks. Conversely, failure to accomplish tasks leads to difficulty with future tasks.

- *Psychosocial* refers to the multiple aspects of one's thoughts, emotions, behaviors, and all the interpersonal behaviors and classifications within one's society (Pohodich, Ramer & Sasmor, 1981).

Psychosocial readiness for childbearing is manifested by the ability to cope with demands and to complete the tasks of pregnancy, childbearing, and parenthood. It has been achieved when the parent has

- The capacity to establish and maintain intimate relationships

- The ability to give to and care for another human being

- The ability to learn and to adjust patterns of daily life

- The ability to communicate effectively with others

- An established sexual identity (Neeson, 1987)

The objectives of nurses' roles in psychosocial care are manifold. They must assess those psychosocial factors that affect a person's readiness for parenthood; identify risk factors associated with early or delayed childbearing and implement supportive care as necessary; assess the patient's cultural perspective in relation to childbearing and determine how that perspective will affect nursing care during pregnancy, labor, birth, and the postpartum period; recognize areas in which cultural variations are likely to occur in birth practices; and incorporate patient and family practices into the plan of nursing care whenever possible (Neeson, 1987).

Developmental Tasks of Pregnancy

Since pregnancy usually occurs within a family context, the health and stability of the family will influence the course of the pregnancy, and, conversely, the pregnancy will affect the family (Raff & Freisner, 1989). In order to make the necessary adjustments for good mental health both for herself and her family, the pregnant woman must work through a series of developmental tasks. Four tasks must be accomplished in sequence for the mother-to-be to prepare for the phases of pregnancy and motherhood. These phases are pregnancy validation, fetal embodiment, fetal distinction, and role transition. If she is unable to complete these tasks and shows signs of maladjustment to pregnancy, a referral for mental healthcare is the most appropriate nursing action (Neeson, 1987).

- **Pregnancy validation** is also called incorporation. Psychological changes start when the mother begins to think she is pregnant (Perez, 1988). As she commences to make pregnancy part of her life, she views the embryo or fetus as a part of herself. However, surprise, disbelief, and ambivalence are often felt, and one of the emotional tasks of the first trimester is to resolve ambivalent feelings. (This is usually accomplished by the fourth month.) While feeling ambivalent, the mother needs reassurance that her feelings are normal, and she should be encouraged to express all of her feelings, both negative and positive (Pohodich, Ramer & Sasmor, 1981). The nurse's role at this time is to assess the woman's coping abilities and identify risk factors so that proper

intervention can be planned if necessary. The woman's support systems must also be assessed, both emotional and financial (Perez, 1988). Emotional support is critical during pregnancy, and in many instances the nurse may be the woman's sole source of emotional support. The nurse must also help the patient determine her motivation for childbearing, since it will affect her adjustment to pregnancy, her relationship with her child, and her family's future development. If her motivations are not positive, if she denies pregnancy beyond the first trimester, or if she evidences excessive anxiety, her adjustment to pregnancy may be difficult and she may require counseling.

- **Fetal embodiment** is also called differentiation. As the pregnant woman begins to realize that the fetus is present within her body and is a separate person, she thinks about the baby, pictures it, and contemplates her future role as a mother. At this time she restructures her relationship with her partner and her own mother (or a mother substitute) and becomes more serious about preparations for birth. She may start buying maternity clothes and eating larger amounts of food, and she may evidence mood swings and changes in sexuality (Pohodich, Ramer & Sasmor, 1981). The nurse should allow the woman to listen to the fetal heartbeat to help enhance the feeling of fetal embodiment, and should explain to her why her emotions are changing, reassuring her that these changes are normal and temporary. In addition, nurses should encourage open communication and support among family members, and discuss mothering and the life changes that accompany it. A high degree of anxiety during this period indicates poor adjustment and the need for counseling (Perez, 1988).

- **Fetal distinction,** also called separation, is a time of great introspection. The mother-to-be will start preparing a physical space in her home for her baby, gather clothing and equipment, and make plans for the birth as she begins to let go of her "fantasy child" and accept her "reality child." She may choose names, read about parenting, attend childbirth classes, and encourage the father-to-be to participate in these activities. To nurture her unborn child she must feel nurtured herself, and she becomes more dependent upon those around her. This dependency may cause stress in her partner, and the nurse must help the woman and her family cope with it. By the end of her pregnancy, she should be ready to let the baby out, at which time separation has been accomplished. The nurse must now provide information on child care and assess the woman's developing mothering behavior while determining if her expectations are realistic. If they are not, the patient should be referred for counseling.

STRESSORS ON THE CHILDBEARING FAMILY

Stressors abound in today's world. They are an inevitable part of life and have been studied in great detail by scores of social scientists. Glass and Singer have identified urban stressors that include frustrations over noise, air pollution, litter, and overcrowding. Rural dwellers are not exempt, either. A study by Coward and Jackson shows that rural stressors include substandard housing, social isolation, contaminated water supplies, unemployment, and multigenerational housing arrangements. Dr. Bruno Bettelheim blames the national educational system, which prolongs a physically matured person's financial dependency beyond puberty, as a family stressor. Other studies show that problems related to racism, economics, employment, housing, and healthcare are the greatest stressors for minorities (Avant, 1988).

Beyond those that affect society, the childbearing family faces additional stressors. Researchers Malloy, Miller, and Myers-Walls have found that pregnancy itself is a stressor, while others have reported associations between stress and high-anxiety in pregnancy, citing as causative factors fears about labor and delivery and concerns about the well-being of the unborn child. Miller and Myers-Walls have identified three major categories of stressors in new parents: physical, psychological, and financial. Physical stressors include the physical changes and discomforts of pregnancy, changes in sexual activity, relocation to new places or remodeling of current homes, fatigue and exhaustion, time management, direct caregiving, and housekeeping tasks. Psychological stressors include worries about children (safety, school progress, comparison with peers), adults' concerns about their adequacy as parents, feelings about responsibility for their children's behavior, decreases in marital satisfaction, and role changes needed as their children develop. Financial stressors include the costs of raising and educating children and disagreements about money (Avant, 1988).

Family relationships that are stress-producing may physically affect the course of the pregnancy, leading to nausea, vomiting, hypertension, preeclampsia, difficult labor, and postpartum psychosis (Raff & Freisner, 1989). Some of these may be symptoms of a mother's unhealthy relationship with her own mother, the couple's changing expectations, and changing demands on each other's skills. Failure to receive spousal assistance is also a significant cause of stress, as the household's division of labor often falls into more traditional male-female models after the birth of the first child.

The nurse can play a strong part in fostering families' coping skills (Avant, 1988). Using the three classifications of stressors, potential interventions can be organized. Physical stress can be dealt with by utilizing patient education resources or anticipatory guidance to help prevent the discomforts of pregnancy. Schedules can be planned to include rest and prevent fatigue. Time management strategies can be taught. If the stressors are psychological, the nurse may focus on parent-child or parent-parent interactions to determine strengths and deficiencies. Effective techniques include demonstrating the newborn's capabilities to the parents, teaching them to read the newborn's cues, organizing infant care, and counseling parents about their marital relationship. In dealing with financial stress, a referral to a family agency, social services agency, or a financial counselor may be indicated. In assisting families to make use of social support systems, the nurse helps build the family's strength and internal resources. And sometimes, reassuring the mother or father that they are good parents is the best intervention of all.

Role Changes

Interpersonal relationships change when a couple becomes a family (Pohodich, Ramer & Sasmor, 1981). By offering support and guidance, the nurse can promote personal growth for the woman and her family and help them to prepare for successful bonding with their baby.

Role transition is the final task of pregnancy. Concerns over labor and delivery often cause anxiety, and the woman may fear loss of control (Pohodich et al., 1981). She may be concerned about the baby's or the father's health and may become impatient and uncomfortable with her large size. Nurses must determine what kind of childbirth experience is wanted and to what degree the mother wishes to participate consciously in it. This is the time to teach about labor and birth and help make preparations in the home for the baby's arrival. Of great importance is a discussion of the partner's role in childbirth and child care. Teaching relaxation and controlled breathing techniques and demonstrating alternative sleeping or resting positions may alleviate discomforts.

The father may be faced with ambiguity about his role, as well as with increased financial pressures and a drastic change in his social life with his partner (Avant, 1988). Often he may be lacking in social support networks. His reactions to impending fatherhood can range from joy to anxiety, jealousy, or depression, and will depend on his relationship with his mate and his parents (especially his father). As he prepares for fatherhood he may become introspective, reassessing his life, his beliefs, and his relationships (Pohodich et al., 1981). He must deal with his mate's emotional changes, her worries, her dependency, and her mood swings while wondering if he is needed or wanted in the process of pregnancy. He may feel jealous of the mother or the fetus (Pohodich et al., 1981). Open communication between expectant parents should be encouraged and information on baby and child care should also be given to the father, including encouragement to attend prenatal classes. When possible, the nurse should help the father explore his feelings about the pregnancy, help him understand the changes in his mate's sexual needs, and reassure him that sexual activity will not harm the mother or the fetus. The basics of labor and delivery should be explained to him, and his desired role in that process and in childrearing should be explored. Extreme jealousy, lack of support, and the refusal or inability to accept the role of father indicate the need for referral and counseling (Pohodich et al., 1981).

Children undergo a change in position and status when a new baby is born, and if they are insecure about their parents' love they may be threatened by the new infant (Raff & Freisner, 1989). Siblings of all ages require education and support from both parents during their mother's pregnancy. Those between 18 months and 3 years may experience particular difficulty, since they are still in the process of resolving their own separation anxieties. The nurse should help involve them in the pregnancy and in preparing for their new sibling. A pediatric nurse can be a valuable resource person in providing information on the preparation of children and on what kinds of problems may be anticipated. A sibling class can also be helpful.

Expectations

The mother-to-be may have an unrealistic concept of what it is to be a parent. She may fantasize about the baby, and her unrealistic expectations may include perceptions of her newborn as a grown child, a "perfect child," or as someone who will protect and love her and who will "save" her marriage (Pohodich et al., 1981). She should be assisted in understanding that her newborn will be tiny, helpless, demanding, and dependent, and that it cannot meet her romantic fantasies nor cement a fragmented relationship.

Preparation

Parental readiness for their new role is related to their understanding of the parental role and their willingness to adapt to it, their recognition of the uniqueness of children as individuals, their level of knowledge of the basic stages of growth and development, their emotional maturity, and the family's interpersonal and communications skills. Various community organizations can assist in preparation for parenthood, ideally covering the psychological as well as the physical aspects of parenthood in their approaches. There are counseling services in maternity centers, classes for expectant parents, organizations such as La Leche League, community nurses, and private physicians. Nursing intervention's goal in preparing the family includes assisting the parents to verbalize freely about any possible or potential problem, allowing sufficient time for developing a therapeutic nurse-client relationship, providing assistance to the client in the identification problems and the setting of goals, and providing reassurance to the couple concerning the normality of the changes accompanying pregnancy. The severity of any detected problem will

determine the scope of intervention necessary (Raff & Freisner, 1989).

Cultural Implications

Throughout the world and throughout history, ceremonial rituals surround life's important events (Ladewig, London & Olds, 1990). Pregnancy and childbirth rituals have been passed from generation to generation via folk tales and teaching and reflect a group's values. To understand a family's reaction to pregnancy, the nurse must become familiar with that family's cultural perception of male/female roles, family life styles, health values, and beliefs, and the meaning of children in the society.

In some cultures pregnancy is viewed as an illness, and in others as a natural occurrence. In the latter (sometimes found among African-Americans, Mexican-Americans, Native Americans, and Asian-Americans), prenatal care may not assume a high priority (Ladewig et al., 1990). Rules and expectations will also be defined by each society's norms, and variations will be found in attitudes toward attachment, techniques for giving birth, feeding, infant care, toileting, cleansing, and parenting (Johnston, 1980). Health practices are influenced by home remedies, by folk beliefs, and by the cult's indigenous healers. In the Mexican-American culture, the healer is called a curandero, and in some Native American tribes, the medicine man fulfills a healing role. In some cultures, pregnancy is seen as a time of vulnerability, and women who believe in evil spirits will take precautionary measures against spirits. Mexican-Americans may believe that "mal aire" (bad air) at night is related to evil spirits, and many Southeast Asians believe wind may enter the body of a vulnerable person (Ladewig et al., 1990). In Latin America and the Near Eastern and Asian cultures, the equilibrium model of health is based on a balance between light and dark, heat and cold. Imbalances are often corrected by foods, medications, or herbs classified as hot or cold. For instance, Vietnamese consider pregnancy a cold state, and will avoid cold drinks and food after delivery. Some Asians may turn to herbalists and some blacks may turn to faith healers, root doctors, or spiritualists.

In dealing with cultural variations, nurses must become aware of their own cultural biases and values, and must be sufficiently flexible in order to provide care that is culturally relevant to those receiving it. Ethnocentrism, the belief that one's own values and practices are the best and only ones, is a detriment to the nurse-patient relationship, since without cultural awareness the nurse cannot intervene properly and receive cooperation (Johnston, 1980).

The nurse must thoroughly assess the patient's values and practices and identify the main beliefs, values, and behaviors that relate to her pregnancy and childbirth. If discrepancies exist between the woman's beliefs and that of the healthcare system, the nurse must consider whether the woman's system is supportive, neutral, or harmful in relation to the possible intervention. When it is supportive or neutral, it can be incorporated into the nursing plan. If detrimental, the nurse will have to identify ways to persuade the woman to accept the proposed therapy or accept her rationale in refusing, remembering that ultimately it is each woman's right to make her own healthcare choices (Johnston, 1980).

EXAM QUESTIONS

CHAPTER 2
Questions 6–10

6. A presumptive sign of pregnancy is
   a. fetal outline.
   b. amenorrhea.
   c. fetal heart action.
   d. abdominal enlargement.

7. Complaints of nasal stuffiness during pregnancy is most likely due to
   a. upper respiratory infections.
   b. progesterone levels.
   c. prolactin levels.
   d. estrogen levels.

8. Mrs. Jones's first day of her last menstrual period was January 2. Using Nägele's rule, her expected date of delivery is
   a. October 9.
   b. October 20.
   c. September 9.
   d. November 2.

9. Formation of major organs occurs during the _____ stage of development.
   a. zygote
   b. embryonic
   c. fetal
   d. pre-embryonic

10. A patient who is 8 weeks pregnant complains of urinary frequency. How should the nurse advise her?
   a. It is due to pressure from the uterus on the bladder.
   b. Inquire how much she normally drinks.
   c. Encourage her to decrease her fluid intake.
   d. Mention it to the doctor; she may have an infection.

CHAPTER 3

THE ANTEPARTUM PERIOD

CHAPTER OBJECTIVE

After studying this chapter, the reader will be able to recognize the key elements of the prenatal physical assessment and indicate appropriate nursing interventions based on the assessments.

LEARNING OBJECTIVES

After reading this chapter, the student will be able to

1. Select appropriate educational interventions that may help to alleviate some of the discomforts of pregnancy.

2. Specify socioeconomic factors that may negatively affect the outcome of pregnancy.

3. Recognize methods for assessing fetal well-being during pregnancy.

4. Identify warning signs of antepartum complications.

MATERNAL PHYSICAL ASSESSMENT

Nurses are assuming a more important role in prenatal care, particularly in assessment, and often they have the first contact with a pregnant woman (Ladewig, London & Olds, 1990). The nurse's attitude in establishing an environment of comfort and open communication will convey concern and support for the patient and facilitate the nurse-patient relationship throughout pregnancy.

History

The course of a woman's pregnancy depends largely on her past health care, her emotional status, and the presence or absence of disease (Ladewig, London & Olds, 1990). The history is a screening tool for determining these factors and for identifying those that may negatively affect a pregnancy (Raff & Freisner, 1989). Ideally, the history should be taken at the first prenatal assessment and should include an obstetrical exam to determine the condition of the reproductive organs. Information about previous pregnancies and outcomes, such as gravidity, parity, term and pre-term births, abortions (spontaneous and elective), stillbirths, and the number of living children is very important to help anticipate potential problems that may develop in the current pregnancy. After a complete obstetrical and medical history is elicited, the physical exam should be performed. The pelvis is evaluated for shape and size, and its measurements taken. There is a vaginal exam to confirm pregnancy, to obtain a Pap smear, and to take internal pelvic measurements. The breast exam includes evaluation for lactation. Finally, the EDD is calculated.

Subsequent monitoring allows for the detection of change in mother or fetus and should include the following: abdominal palpation and auscultation; checking of fundal height; checking fetal heart rate; Leopold's maneuvers; urine testing; weight determination; blood pressure reading; nutritional, sleep, hygiene, rest, and elimination patterns; and exercise assessments and assessment of common conditions that cause discomfort.

Not to be neglected is an assessment of the woman's personal belief system and life-style—her beliefs about pregnancy, childbirth, the father's role, and the needs of the fetus; her use of tobacco or drugs; her occupational or recreational pursuits (Becker, 1982). The following aspects of support must be assessed: housing, marital status, family composition and communication patterns, the woman's education and knowledge about infant care, her self-concept, her ability to cope, and the social services or community agencies she is involved with. Her mate's feelings about pregnancy and parenting should not be overlooked.

When the nursing diagnosis is based on a comprehensive assessment, it will provide the basis for a healthier outcome for mother, baby, and family.

Normal Physical Changes: Assessment of Systems

Vital signs

Blood pressure is within normal range at 90 to 140 mm Hg systolic and 60 to 90 mm Hg diastolic. Establishing a baseline at the first prenatal visit is necessary for future comparisons. It will drop in the second trimester, then rise in the third. After establishing the patient's blood pressure (and referring her to a physician if it's out of range), assess the patient's knowledge about hypertension and counsel her on self-care and medical management (Ladewig, London & Olds, 1990).

The normal pulse rate of 60 to 90 beats per minute may increase during pregnancy. Be alert for irregularities.

The normal respiration rate is 16 to 24 breaths per minute. Pregnancy may induce hyperventilation, and thoracic breathing will be noted. Assess for respiratory disease.

Temperature should range from 98° to 99.6° F. Assess for infection or disease if it is out of range, and refer the patient to a physician.

Weight

Note initial weight to establish a baseline for gain during pregnancy. Evaluate eating habits, cooking practices, income status, abnormal habits (including pica), and refer for nutritional counseling if necessary.

Skin

Slight edema of the lower extremities is normal. Pigmentation changes may include spider nevi, linea nigra, *striae gravidarum,* and chloasma. Assure the patient that these are normal changes and explain their physiological basis. Counsel on relief measures for slight edema.

Nose

Nasal mucosa may be edematous, resulting in stuffiness and epistaxis. Counsel on relief measures.

Mouth

Gingival tissue may undergo hypertrophy, and excessive secretion of saliva (ptyalism) may occur. Counsel on good dental hygiene. Remind the patient to visit a dentist at six-month intervals.

Neck

Small, mobile, nontender nodes may appear. The thyroid may develop small, smooth, lateral lobes on both sides of the trachea. Slight thyroid hyperplasia may occur by the end of the first trimester. Basal metabolic rate may decrease in the first trimester and increase in the third. Ascertain iodine intake.

Chest and lungs

The chest wall increases in circumference. There is lateral movement of the heart's apex with exaggerated splitting of the first heart sound and a loud third sound (Neeson, 1987). A systolic murmur is found in 90% of pregnant women. Brachial blood pressure will be highest when the patient sits. Spider angiomas may appear. Blood volume increases. Reassure the patient, explaining that these pregnancy-related changes are normal.

Breasts

Engorgement occurs, nodes may appear, and tingling may be felt. The areolae darken and the nipples may become pigmented and erect (Ladewig, London & Olds, 1990). Superficial veins dilate and become more prominent. Striae may be seen in multiparas. The tubercles of Montgomery enlarge, and colostrum may be present after the 10th week (Neeson, 1987). Demonstrate the proper method of checking the breasts and encourage the patient to do this monthly. Discuss what constitutes normal changes, teach and institute relief measures, and encourage the use of a supportive brassiere.

Abdomen and gastrointestinal system

Purple striae (silver on a multipara) may occur. Diastasis of the rectus muscles may occur late in pregnancy. As the uterus grows, there is progressive enlargement of the abdomen *(see figure 3-1)*. Muscle tone and peristalsis decrease. Hemorrhoids may be present. Teach self-help techniques and provide information about exercising *(refer to table 3-1)* (Neeson, 1987).

Extremities

Varicose veins may be more evident. Late in pregnancy, edema of the hands and ankles may occur. Discuss prevention and self-help measures (Raff & Freisner, 1989; Ladewig, London & Olds, 1990).

Spine

The lumbar spinal curve may be accentuated, leading to balance problems. Discuss proper footwear and exercise.

FIGURE 3-1
Uterine Growth During Pregnancy

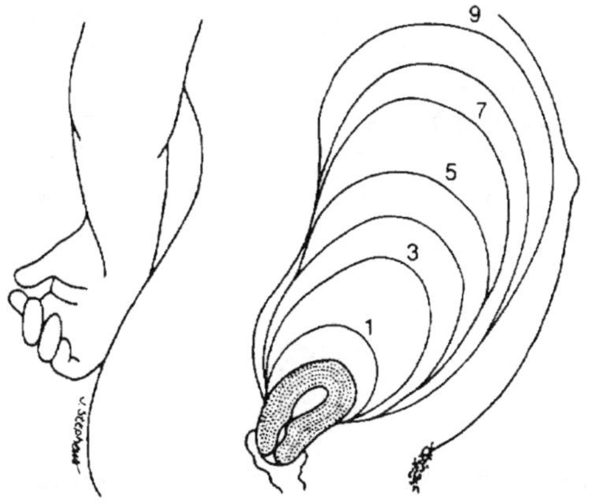

Uterine growth during successive months of pregnancy (Childbirth Graphics).

Source: May, K. & Mahimeister, L., *Maternal & Neonatal Nursing, Family-Centered Care,* 1994. Philadelphia, PA: Lipponcott

Pelvic area

The uterus grows and gains contractile ability, and rises out of the pelvic cavity. There may be increased white vaginal discharge and decreased bladder tone. The cervix enlarges at four weeks, softens at six weeks and takes on a bluish coloring, and the isthmus of the uterus softens. At 8 to 12 weeks the vagina appears bluish. The perineum increases in vascularity. Recommend frequent emptying of the bladder, and discuss hygiene and self-help techniques.

Urinary system

Renal plasma flow increases, the ureters may dilate, and there is increased pressure on the bladder.

Musculoskeletal system

The ligaments and joints relax and body alignment may change.

TABLE 3-1 *(1 of 2)*
Self-Care Measures for Common Discomforts of Pregnancy

Discomfort	Influencing factors	Self-care measures
FIRST TRIMESTER Nausea and vomiting	Increased levels of hCG Changes in carbohydrate metabolism Emotional factors Fatigue	Avoid odors or causative factors. Eat dry crackers or toast before arising in morning. Have small but frequent meals. Avoid greasy or highly seasoned foods. Take dry meals with fluids between meals. Drink carbonated beverages.
Urinary frequency	Pressure of uterus on bladder in both first and third trimester	Void when urge is felt. Increase fluid intake during the day. Decrease fluid intake *only* in the evening to decrease nocturia.
Breast tenderness	Increased levels of estrogen and progesterone	Wear well-fitting supportive bra.
Increased vaginal discharge	Hyperplasia of vaginal mucosa and increased production of mucus by the endocervical glands due to the increase in estrogen levels	Promote cleanliness by daily bathing. Avoid douching, nylon underpants, and pantyhose; cotton underpants are more absorbent: powder can be used to maintain dryness if not allowed to cake.
Nasal stuffiness and epistaxis	Elevated estrogen levels	May be unresponsive but cool air vaporizer may help; avoid use of nasal sprays and decongestants.
Ptyalism	Specific causative factors unknown	Use astringent mouthwashes, chew gum, or suck hard candy.

DISCOMFORTS OF PREGNANCY AND NURSING INTERVENTION

The many physical and anatomical changes that occur during pregnancy may result in discomforts that can cause anxiety if not understood, anticipated, and dealt with (Ladewig, London & Olds, 1990). These must not be shrugged off as "minor." The nurse must assess and anticipate discomforts, offer interventions and self-care measures, and monitor their effectiveness (Lyall & Wheeler, 1983) (see *figure 3-2* and *table 3-1).*

Nausea and vomiting: These are common and troublesome but rarely pathological unless they result in weight loss or persist beyond the first trimester. Reassure the patient that nausea will usually resolve itself spontaneously; suggest the use of a kitchen fan to dispel odors while cooking; recommend an increase in protein snacks, foods high in carbohydrates, fluids between meals (but not at mealtime). Fruit-flavored tea may help. Iron and vitamins should be taken after meals, and medication should be

TABLE 3-1 *(2 of 2)*
Self-Care Measures for Common Discomforts of Pregnancy

Discomfort	Influencing factors	Self-care measures
SECOND AND THIRD TRIMESTERS		
Heartburn (pyrosis)	Increased production of progesterone; decreasing gastrointestinal motility and increasing relaxation of cardiac sphincter; displacement of stomach by enlarging uterus; thus regurgitation of gastric contents into esophagus	Eat small and more frequent meals. Use low-sodium antacids. Avoid overeating, fatty and fried foods, lying down after eating, and sodium bicarbonate.
Ankle edema	Prolonged standing or sitting Increased levels of sodium due to hormonal influences Circulatory congestion of lower extremities Increased capillary permeability Varicose veins	Practice frequent dorsiflexion of feet when prolonged sitting or standing is necessary. Elevate legs when sitting or resting. Avoid tight garters or restrictive bands around the legs.
Varicose veins	Venous congestion in the lower veins that increases with pregnancy Hereditary factors (weakening of walls of veins, faulty valves) Increased age and weight gain	Elevate legs frequently. Wear supportive hose. Avoid crossing legs at the knees. standing for long periods, garters, and hosiery with constrictive bands.
Hemorrhoids	Constipation (see following discussion) Increased pressure from gravid uterus on hemorrhoidal veins	Avoid constipation. Apply ice packs, topical ointments, anesthetic agents, warm soaks, or sitz baths; gently reinsert into rectum as necessary.
Constipation	Increased levels of progesterone, which cause general bowel sluggishness Pressure of enlarging uterus on intestine Iron supplements Diet, lack of exercise, and decreased fluids	Increase fluid intake, fiber in the diet, exercise. Develop regular bowel habits. Use stool softeners as recommended by physician.
Backache	Increased curvature of the lumbosacral vertebras as the uterus enlarges Increased levels of hormones, which cause softening of cartilage in body joints Fatigue Poor body mechanics	Use proper body mechanics. Practice the pelvic tilt exercise. Avoid uncomfortable working heights, high-heeled shoes, lifting heavy loads, and fatigue.
Leg cramps	Imbalance of calcium/phosphorus ratio Increased pressure of uteres on nerves Fatigue Poor circulation to lower extremities Pointing the toes	Practice dorsiflexion of feet in order to stretch affected muscle. Evaluate diet. Apply heat to affected muscles.
Faintness	Postural hypotension Sudden change of position causing venous pooling in dependent veins Standing for long periods in one place; especially if area is warm Anemia	Arise slowly from resting position. Avoid prolonged standing in warm or stuffy environments. Refer to physician for possible elevation of hematocrit/hemoglobin.
Dyspnea	Decreased vital capacity from pressure of enlarging uterus on the diaphragm	Use proper posture when sitting and standing. Sleep propped up with pillows for relief if problem occurs at night.

Source: *Essentials of Maternal-Newborn Nursing,* Ladewig, P. W., London, M. L. & Olds, S. B., 1990, Addison-Wesley, New York.

FIGURE 3-2
Abdominal Changes During Pregnancy

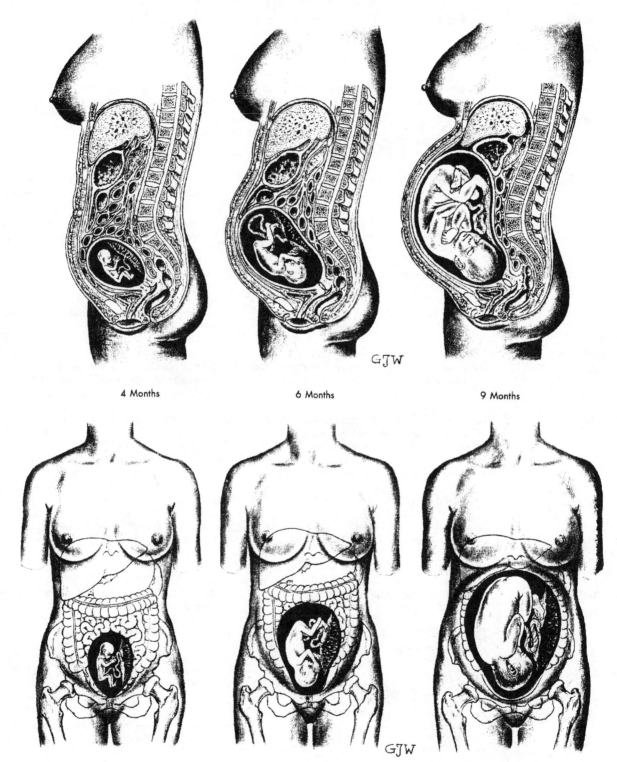

4 Months   6 Months   9 Months

Displacement of internal abdominal structures and diaphragm by the enlarging uterus at 4, 6, and 9 months of gestation.

Source: Bobak, I. & Jensen, M.D., *Maternity & Gynecologic Care: The Nurse and the Family,* 5th Ed., 1993. St. Louis: MO. Mosby-YearBook, Inc.

avoided if possible. Advise good posture, frequent fresh-air walks, and avoiding sudden movements. To decrease morning nausea, advise yogurt, cottage cheese, and juice or milk if the patient awakens at night to void.

Fatigue, backache, fainting: Reassure the patient that fatigue is normal and temporary, and recommend frequent rest periods, adequate exercise, increased social stimulation, and avoiding overexertion. Demonstrate deep breathing and relaxation exercises. Encourage her to explore opportunities to participate in enjoyable activities and to get assistance with child care, if possible (Neeson, 1987).

Backache self-help techniques include sleeping on a firm mattress, heat applications for pain relief and supporting the upper leg with a pillow when sleeping (Raff & Freisner, 1989). Teach the patient to squat instead of bending, to avoid stretching or bending awkwardly, and suggest a maternity girdle if she is obese or has a postural problem (Neeson, 1987). Advise her to avoid overexertion, rest frequently in a recumbent position, and wear comfortable, low-heeled shoes. Encourage daily exercise, including total body relaxation exercise. Suggest elevating one leg on a stool or box while standing, sitting in cross-legged fashion (i.e., tailor position), and having toddlers climb onto her lap to avoid lifting them (Raff & Freisner, 1989).

Fainting, when due to hypoglycemia, can be avoided by eating frequent small snacks. Caffeine should be avoided. Hyperventilation can be prevented by taking slow breaths when lightheaded. Recommend avoiding sudden movements and lying down in a flat, supine position (Neeson, 1987).

Dyspnea: Advise the patient to sit and stand up straight, to avoid overexertion, and to rest following exercise (Neeson, 1987). Suggest sleeping or resting in left lateral or semi-Fowler's position, with the head elevated.

Edema: Recommend the use of support hose and leg elevation when sitting. Suggest limiting (but not cutting out) salt intake and carbohydrates and increasing protein intake (Neeson, 1987). Six to eight glasses of fluid daily will increase natural diuresis. A sudden increase in edema of hands, feet, and face needs immediate medical attention.

Urinary frequency: The patient should avoid bladder distention by voiding when the urge occurs. Teach Kegel exercises to strengthen the pelvic floor muscles. Advise cutting caffeine intake (Neeson, 1987).

Constipation: Advise the patient to take time for bowel movements, to defecate when she feels the urge, and not to strain. Raising feet on a box while toileting may help. Caution her to avoid mineral oil which can interfere with the absorption of fat-soluble vitamins (A, D, K, E).

Hemorrhoids: Advise the patient to cleanse the anus carefully and place petroleum jelly in the rectum after defecation. Suggest a knee-chest position for up to 15 minutes daily and Kegel exercises (Neeson, 1987).

Vaginal discharge: Discuss good perineal hygiene and suggest a vinegar and water rinse, drying thoroughly, then dusting with corn starch (Neeson, 1987).

Breast tenderness: Recommend avoiding pressure on the breasts and soap on the nipples. Apply skin cream to soften crusts (Neeson, 1987).

Bleeding gums (epulis): Discuss maintenance of good oral hygiene, warm saline mouthwashes, flossing, and using a soft toothbrush. Remind the patient of regular dental checkups and a balanced diet. Suggest cutting hard foods into small pieces before chewing (Neeson, 1987).

TABLE 3-2 *(1 of 2)*
Daily Food Plan for Pregnancy and Lactation

Food group	Nutrients provided	Food source	Recommended daily amount during pregnancy	Recommended daily amount during lactation
Dairy products	Protein; riboflavin; vitamins A, D, and others; calcium; phosphorus; zinc; magnesium	Milk—whole, 2%, skim, dry, butter-milk Cheeses—hard, semi-soft, cottage Yogurt—plain, low-fat Soybean milk—canned, dry	Four 8oz cups (five for teenagers): used plain or with fla-voring in shakes, soups, cocoa Calcium in 1c milk equivalent to $1\frac{1}{2}$c cottage cheese, $1\frac{1}{2}$ oz hard or semisoft cheese, 1c yogurt, $1\frac{1}{2}$c ice cream (high in fat and sugar)	Four 8-oz cups (five for teenagers); equivalent amount of cheese; yogurt, etc.
Meat group	Protein; iron; thi-amine, niacin, and other vitamins; minerals	Beef, pork, veal, lamb, poultry, ani-mal organ meats, fish, eggs; legumes; nuts, seeds, peanut butter, grains in proper vegetarian combi-nation (vitamin B_{12} supplement needed)	Three servings (one serving = 2oz): Combination in amounts necessary for same nutrient equivalent (varies greatly)	Two servings
Grain products, whole grain or enriched	B vitamins; iron; whole grain also has zinc, magne-sium, and other trace elements; provides fiber	Breads and bread products such as cornbread, muffins, waffles, hot cakes, biscuits, dumplings, cere-als, pastas, rice	Four servings daily: one serving = one slice bread, $\frac{3}{4}$c or 1oz dry cereal, $\frac{1}{2}$c rice or pasta	Four servings
Fruits and fruit juices	Vitamins A and C; minerals; raw fruits for roughage	Citrus fruits and juices, melons, berries, all other fruits and juices	Two to three servings (one serving for vitamin C): one serving = one medium fruit, $\frac{1}{2}$-1c fruit, 4oz orange or grape-fruit juice	Same as for pregnancy

* The pregnant woman should eat regularly, three meals a day, with nutritious snacks of fruits, cheese, milk or other foods between meals if desired. (More frequent but smaller meals are also recommended.) Four to six glasses (8 oz) of water and a total of eight to ten cups (8oz) total fluid should be consumed daily. Water is an essential nutrient.

TABLE 3-2 *(2 of 2)*
Daily Food Plan for Pregnancy and Lactation

Food group	Nutrients provided	Food source	Recommended daily amount during pregnancy	Recommended daily amount during lactation
Vegetables and vegetable juices	Vitamins A and C; minerals; provides roughage	Leafy green vegetables; deep yellow or orange vegetables such as carrots, sweet potatoes, squash, tomatoes; green vegetables such as peas, green beans, broccoli; other vegetables such as beets, cabbage, potatoes, corn, lima beans	Two to three servings (one serving of dark green or deep yellow vegetable for vitamin A): one serving = 1/2-1c vegetable, two tomatoes, one medium potato	Same as for pregnancy
Fats	Vitamins A and D; linoleic acid	Butter, cream cheese, fortified table spreads; cream, whipped cream, whipped toppings; avocado, mayonnaise, oil, nuts	As desired in moderation (high in calories): one serving = 1 Tbsp butter or margarine	Same as for pregnancy
Sugar and sweets		Sugar, brown sugar, honey, molasses	Occasionally, if desired	Same as for pregnancy
Desserts		Nutritious desserts such as puddings, custards, fruit whips, and crisps; other rich, sweet desserts and pastries	Occasionally, if desired (high in calories)	Same as for pregnancy
Beverages		Decaffeinated beverages, including coffee and tea; bouillon; carbonated drinks	As desired, in moderation	Same as for pregnancy
Miscellaneous		Iodized salt, herbs, spices, condiments	As desired	Same as for pregnancy

Source: *Essentials of Maternal-Newborn Nursing,* Ladewig, P. W., London, M. L. & Olds, S. B., 1990, Addison-Wesley, New York.

Leg cramps: Advise limiting dairy products to 4 servings daily and decreasing phosphorus intake. The legs should be kept warm, the calf muscles stretched, and a warm bath taken before bedtime. Heavy covers should be loosened on the bed and the legs elevated at night. When cramps occur, caution the patient not to massage the calf but to stand on the affected leg to straighten the muscle. Strongly advise regular exercise (Neeson, 1987).

Nutritional Needs

The woman's nutritional status before and during pregnancy influences her health as well as her baby's. The growth of fetal and maternal tissues requires increased amounts of essential nutrients, most of which can be obtained by eating a balanced diet (Ladewig, London & Olds, 1990) (*see table 3-2*). A nutritional assessment should include the following:

- Physical factors: age; weight and height; type of body frame; prepregnancy weight; activity level; nutritional status as determined by color, nails, hair, skin turgor; lab values, including hemoglobin, hematocrit, and serum folate; nausea and vomiting; lactose intolerance; food allergies (Raff & Freisner, 1989).

- Conditions requiring special diets, such as heart disease or diabetes mellitus (Neeson, 1987).

- Sociocultural factors, including ethnic group, economic status, educational level, and food practices (such as vegetarianism).

- A diet history and log of food intake.

Nutritional adjustments must be made to cover the needs of the adolescent mother and her fetus. The 11 to 14-year-old pregnant teenager requires 2,500 calories per day, the 15 to 18-year-old requires 2,400 calories, and the 19 to 50-year-old woman requires 2,300 calories.

Predisposing factors for nutrition risk include adolescence, a history of three or more pregnancies within the past two years, poverty, food faddism, a history of unusual or restrictive diets, heavy use of tobacco, alcohol, or drugs, maintenance of a therapeutic diet for chronic illness, and prepregnancy weight less than 85% or more than 120% of standard weight for height.

As pregnancy progresses, watch for risk factors such as low or deficient hemoglobin/hematocrit, inadequate or excessive weight gain, breastfeeding plans in women with anorexia, and inadequate weight gain or poor health.

In implementing dietary changes, the nurse must motivate the patient to assume responsibility and participate actively in the change; the nurse must also respect the patient's individual dietary habits and educate the patient to the extent of her understanding. The financially distressed woman should be referred to nutritional programs (such as WIC) for supplementation of necessary foods (Raff & Freisner, 1989).

Nutritional needs during pregnancy:

- Caloric intake should he increased approximately 300 kcal daily in the second and third trimester.

- Minerals: **Calcium** to be increased by 0.4 g daily to a total daily intake of 1.2 g (adolescents 1.6 g) in the last half of the pregnancy. **Iron** supplements of 30 to 60 mg daily (ferrous sulfate or fumarate) are recommended. This should be given as a separate pill and taken several hours before or after meals.

- **Protein** to be increased by 30 g daily to a total intake of 75 g/day (82 g/day for adolescents).

- **Vitamin A:** A daily increase of 1,000 IU is recommended to supply a daily intake of 6,000 IU in the last half of pregnancy.

- **B-complex vitamins: Thiamine:** to be increased by 0.1 mg to a total daily intake of

1.4 mg (adolescents 1.5 mg). **Riboflavin:** to be increased by 0.3 mg to a total daily intake of 1.5 mg (adolescents 1.6 mg). **Niacin:** to be increased to 15 mg (adolescents 16 mg). **Vitamin B$_6$:** increase of 5 mg. **Vitamin B$_{12}$:** increase of 1 mcg. **Folic acid:** increase to 800 mg/day.

- **Vitamin C:** increase of 5 to 10 mg to a total daily intake of 80 mg.
- **Vitamin D:** 400 IU daily (Raff & Freisner, 1989).

All other nutrients should remain at nonpregnant levels.

Exercise

For the pregnant woman, exercise provides many benefits. It helps prevent constipation and conditions both the body and the mind (Ladewig, London & Olds, 1990; De Santo & Hassid, 1983). However, exercise should not be overdone during pregnancy and should be substantially reduced during the final four weeks of gestation. During an uncomplicated pregnancy, a woman can and should continue participation in exercise. In many cases, a skilled sportswoman may even continue strenuous sports, assuming she has the consent of her health care provider. Swimming and walking are generally safe for all pregnant women. The pregnant woman should warm up and cool down before and after exercise, and in general she should exercise for shorter intervals—10 to 15 minutes at a time, resting for a short period, then exercising for another 10 to 15 minutes. She should decrease physical intensity as her pregnancy progresses, avoid lengthy overheating as well as high-risk activities, wear proper exercise shoes and a brassiere, and lie down or rest on her left side for 10 minutes following exercise. ACOG guidelines recommend that a woman maintain her pulse rate at below 140 beats/minute, that she drink sufficient fluids before and after exercise, and that after the fourth month she should avoid exercising while flat on her back. A pregnant woman should also avoid any exercise that requires bending and twisting from the hips while standing (White, 1992).

The pelvic tilt helps prevent and reduce back strain and strengthens abdominal tone (Laff & Freisner, 1989). The woman should be instructed to stand two feet away from the back of a chair or a sink, bend forward at the hip joints, place her hands on the edge of the support with her arms straight, raise her hips and inhale, round her back; tuck her buttocks under, and then exhale with the knees slightly flexed. The above should be done three times, then she should drop her hands and stand erect by raising her breastbone straight up. Shoulders should be relaxed, knees flexed, buttocks tucked underneath, weight evenly balanced on the back of her feet. Pelvic tilt exercises should be done 12 times a day (Ladewig, London & Olds, 1990).

Weight Gain

The average weight gain during a normal pregnancy is 25 to 30 pounds (11 to 13.6 kg), with an average increase of 3 pounds in the first trimester, 12 in the second trimester, and 12 in the third. The weight is distributed among the fetus, placenta and membrane, amniotic fluid, uterus, breasts, increased blood volume and extravascular fluid, and fat reserves (Ladewig, London & Olds, 1990). The pattern of gain is important, since a sharp increase may be due to excess fluid retention. However, pregnancy is not a time for dieting, since severe weight restriction can lead to ketosis and can harm both mother and baby.

The appropriate gain must be determined on an individual basis, considering weight deficits or excesses and maternal growth needs. In determining the appropriate gain, the nutritional adequacy of the diet must be considered. For example, if the woman's food choices are poor, if her basal needs are low, or if she must compensate for earlier illness or poor diet, a larger weight gain may be the only way to provide adequate nutrients.

Nutritional counseling is of great importance, and the caloric intake should focus on RDA guidelines. This is of special importance to the obese woman, who runs the risk of hypertension. The underweight pregnant woman risks preeclampsia and a low-birth-weight baby, and needs particular intervention to assist her to increase her caloric and protein intake. Her ideal weight gain will be the amount she is underweight plus 25 pounds. In cases of severe obesity or underweight, a consultation with a nutritionist is advisable.

IDENTIFYING RISK FACTORS

Risk factors are findings that may signal a negative outcome for the pregnant woman or her baby (Ladewig, London & Olds, 1990). Thus, screening for them is a vital part of the prenatal assessment. It is important to identify high-risk pregnancy early in order to institute appropriate interventions. An ongoing assessment is also essential, since a pregnancy that begins as low-risk may change with time.

When a woman begins pregnancy with a pre-existing condition, the nurse must assess the course of the pregnancy, the influence of the condition on the pregnancy, and the effects of the pregnancy on the condition (Ladewig, London & Olds, 1990). A holistic view of the pregnancy must be taken, incorporating the patient's physical condition and psychosocial response, and her family's as well. Following the assessment, data must be analyzed and conclusions drawn. The nursing diagnoses formulated will then guide the nurse in developing a care plan.

Medical factors that may affect a healthy pregnancy include the following (Ladewig, London & Olds, 1990):

- Pre-existing maternal disease: cardiac, pulmonary, gastrointestinal, endocrine, diabetes mellitus, hyperthyroidism, moderate to severe renal disease, seizure disorder, venereal or infectious diseases, psychiatric disorders, Diethylstilbestrol (DES) exposure.

- Chronic hypertension

- Maternal hemoglobinopathies

- Malignancy within the past five years

- Surgery during pregnancy

- Major congenital anomalies of the reproductive tract

- Maternal mental retardation

Obstetrical factors (history) that affect pregnancy:

- History of infertility

- Previous pregnancy loss (ectopic, habitual spontaneous abortion, stillbirth, neonatal death)

- Grandmultiparity (seven or more deliveries)

- Previous multiple gestation

- Previous premature labor/delivery

- Previous prolonged labor

- Previous mid forceps delivery

- Previous cesarean delivery

- Previous low-birth-weight infant

- Previous placenta previa

- Previous macrosomic infant (over 4000 grams)

- Previous baby with neurologic deficit, birth injury or malformation

- Previous hydatiform mole or choriocarcinoma

Current pregnancy factors:

- Late or no prenatal care

- Rh/ABO sensitization

- Fetus inappropriately large or small for gestation

- Premature labor

- Pregnancy-induced hypertension

- Multiple gestation

- Premature rupture of membranes

- Polyhydramnios

- Antepartal bleeding (placenta previa, abruptio placenta)

- Abnormal presentation

- Postmaturity

- Abnormality in tests for fetal well-being

- Maternal anemia

- Abdominal x-rays during pregnancy

- Substance use during pregnancy (alcohol, smoking, drugs)

- Conception less than three months after last delivery

- Sexually transmitted diseases

- Gestational diabetes mellitus

- More than five years since last delivery

- TORCH syndrome (toxoplasmosis; others; rubella virus; cytomegalovirus; herpes simplex virus)

- Elevated hematocrit

- Preeclampsia/eclampsia

Demographic factors

Demographic factors that may affect a healthy pregnancy include the following (Ladewig, London & Olds, 1990):

- A maternal age of under 16 or over 35.

- A paternal age of under 18 or over 40.

- Weight under 100 pounds, height under 5 feet before pregnancy.

- Weight 20% above standard.

- A family history of severe inherited disease.

- Membership in ethnic groups predisposed to inherited disease.

Socioeconomic Factors

In identifying risk factors, in addition to the physical assessment the nurse must take into con-

sideration several other aspects of the patient's life (Ladewig, London & Olds, 1990). The socioeconomic factors affecting the mother's and baby's health, which form an integral part of the assessment, include the following:

- The presence or absence of severe social problems, such as inadequate housing or finances.

- Her marital status: Is she single, separated, divorced, widowed? Is there a "significant other" with whom she lives? Is there a support system for her emotional/financial needs?

- Is she nutritionally deprived?

- Her occupation and that of her mate, particularly if it is other than skilled or professional. If she is working, does she stand at work or do heavy lifting? Is she exposed to harmful substances? Does she have the opportunity to sit, to raise her legs, to eat a regular lunch and take breaks for snacks? Is there a provision for maternity leave?

- Is she emotionally stressed (showing fears, anger, hostility)?

- How much or how little education does she have?

- Was this pregnancy planned?

- How do the man and woman feel about the pregnancy?

- To what extent will this pregnancy and the infant alter the couple's plans for their career/employment, education, and life-style?

- Do they plan to take childbirth and parenting education classes?

Family Violence/Battering

Battering during pregnancy has multiple effects on both the mother and child, among them the risks of spontaneous abortion, alcohol or drug abuse, and a low-birthweight infant (Ladewig, London & Olds, 1990; Hilton, 1986). Approximately 50% of all battered women report having been abused during pregnancy. Esposito (1993) reports approximately 37% of pregnant women are abused, irregardless of class, race, or education level. She further reports, in one hospital emergency department, 21% of pregnant women had been battered and these women had two times as many miscarriages as non-battered women. Identification is the nurse's first step toward helping the battered woman, followed by support to help her increase her decision-making abilities and decrease the potential for further abuse Providing a safe environment for the woman and her baby may call for referrals to community resources such as emergency shelters, the police, and legal or counseling services. Chronic psychosomatic symptoms and nonspecific or vague complaints may indicate abuse. Old scars on the head, chest, arms, abdomen, or genitalia must be assessed, and bruising or evidence of pain must be evaluated. There may be a decrease in eye contact, silence when the partner is present, or a history of nervousness, insomnia, or drug or alcohol abuse.

The nurse should assess the woman for battering away from the partner and any other children. It is important to maintain eye contact and explain that battery screening is a routine procedure. If battery or violence is suspected, the nurse should describe the cycle of violence and encourage the woman to describe her situation. Nurses are often the first professionals to whom women acknowledge their problems. Once diagnosed, the patient must be asked if she feels safe at home and provided with options. Of great importance is education concerning the signs of escalating physical danger, including the partner's access to or use of weapons, an extension of his assaults to other family members, forced sexual encounters, and accusations of infidelity. Nurses can provide the battered woman with dignity and protection by treating battering as a health issue, by using a private, nonjudgmental approach, and by recognizing that denial may be part of the coping mechanism.

Discussion of case findings among staff is to be discouraged, and nurses must examine their own feelings and prejudices concerning battering.

Substance Abuse

Drug and alcohol abuse is commonplace in our society, and with its increased prevalence among young people, drug abuse in pregnancy has become a frequent occurrence (ACOG, 1986). Many abused drugs have well-documented effects on the fetus, and in many cases the drug-abusing woman is prone to complications during pregnancy due to her life-style. Her nutritional deficiencies can lead to anemia, fetal growth retardation, and preeclampsia. STDs and other infectious diseases may occur. IV drug users risk endocarditis, hepatitis, and AIDS. Many of these women may also have an uncooperative attitude toward medical care. Advice may be ignored and nutritional supplements disregarded. The nurse may enhance cooperation by using a tactful, nonthreatening approach.

The initial prenatal visit should include questions concerning the use of any drug, including tobacco, caffeine, prescribed medication, over-the-counter (OTC) medications, as well as illicit substances. The presence of needle marks or evidence of poor nutrition should prompt direct questioning about the use of specific drugs. Commonly used illicit substances include amphetamines, barbiturates, hallucinogens, cocaine/crack, heroin, and other narcotics (Ladewig, London & Olds, 1990). Antepartum care of the pregnant addict must include medical, socioeconomic, and legal considerations; ideally it calls for a team approach with the inclusion of social services. Urine screening should be done regularly to identify the type and amount of substance being used. The nursing assessment should focus on the woman's general health status with special attention paid to skin abscesses and infections. The nurse must anticipate noncompliance, coupled with neglect of the baby.

Ideally, drug abusers should give up their habit before conception; however, the nurse must assume that this will not happen and therefore reinforce factors that will improve perinatal outcome—prenatal visits and good nutrition. Delivery should be arranged in a facility with access to support for the management of neonatal complications, since the chief victim of the mother's addiction is the neonate.

Alcoholism also is high among women between ages 20 and 40 and can cause malnutrition, bone marrow suppression, increased infection, and liver disease in the mother. The effects of fetal alcohol syndrome (FAS) are both physical and mental (refer to Fetal Alcohol Syndrome, page 201). Since no absolutely safe intake level has been identified, the woman should avoid alcohol completely during the weeks of organogenesis, and ideally throughout pregnancy. Assessment for alcohol intake should be an important part of the medical history, with questions asked in a direct but non-judgmental manner. If heavy consumption is involved, an immediate referral should be made to an alcoholic treatment program. The program's counselor must be made aware of the pregnancy before drug therapy (some of which may be teratogenic) is instituted.

Smoking doubles the risk of spontaneous abortion or stillbirth. Infants of smoking mothers have a lower birth weight than infants of nonsmokers, and studies show that intrauterine growth decreases with the number of cigarettes smoked (Ladewig, London & Olds, 1990). Smoking may also cause pre-term delivery, congenital anomalies and developmental problems in the child. Nurses should strongly advocate smoking cessation with their patients, stressing the need to protect the unborn child.

OTC medications: Very few pharmacologic agents given to the mother, including those given by mouth, do not affect the fetus. If the medication, whether a prescription or OTC drug, is given during the first trimester (at the time of organogenesis), it may be teratogenic (causing fetal malformations). Often OTC medications are used by the woman to treat the discomforts of pregnancy. Knowledge of their adverse effects is limited, and fetal harm is unlikely unless they are taken over long periods of time or the recommended dose is exceeded. Nevertheless, periodic questioning about the patient's use of OTC drugs is necessary, since many patients do not consider them medications. Women should check with their physician/midwife before taking any medication.

Environmental Hazards

With increased numbers of women working, their exposure to chemical and environmental pollutants bas risen. Those in their childbearing years are at particular risk (Ladewig, London & Olds, 1990; NAACOG, 1985). Women working in the microelectronic industry are exposed to lead, arsenic, radiation, and glycol ethers and risk spontaneous abortion and babies with birth defects. Women who work with heavy metals such as lead or mercury (or those whose mates do) risk spontaneous abortion, stillbirths, and premature delivery, and their offspring risk impaired growth and neurological damage. Mercury has been found in the placentas of pregnant dental workers and nurses. Other women working in operating rooms with anesthetic gasses risk low fertility, spontaneous abortions and low-birthweight babies. Nurses who administer antineoplastic drugs evidence increased spontaneous abortions and fetal anomalies. Wives of workers exposed to vinyl chloride and chloroprene (used in manufacturing rubber products) have increased spontaneous abortions, and stillbirths. PCBs, used in the manufacture of plastics and electrical products, have caused low-birthweight babies with cola-colored skin, premature tooth eruption, and eye defects, while women exposed to pesticides risk spontaneous abortion, still or premature birth, and some degree of mental retardation in their children.

Psychosocial Factors

The changes and stresses of pregnancy may result in crises, producing disequilibrium until a means of coping is found. If, upon assessment, the nurse determines that the woman is not adapting to changes and not accomplishing the tasks of pregnancy, additional support and guidance is indicated and a referral to counseling may be in order (Ladewig, London & Olds, 1990; Pohodich, Ramer & Sasmor, 1981). While obtaining data for the psychosocial assessment, the following possible risk factors must be considered:

- **Marital status:** Single parenthood; bereavement; lack of emotional support; marriage required due to pregnancy; age disparity; illness in family; economic problems; lack of emotional support

- **Family history:** Illness and its stresses; fear of hereditary problem; broken home; bereavement; isolation; fear of complications; effect of perceptions of parental role; negative or unrealistic attitude toward childrearing; difficulty assessing role as parent

- **Current pregnancy:** Conflicts over career, education, employment, finances; hostility toward self, husband, or fetus; confusion; fear; denial; rejection, guilt; isolation; lack of family and peer group support; financial problems

- **Status of mother:** Anger; depression; attempted abortion; denial; disgust; resentment; physical discomforts causing negative attitude toward pregnancy; problems with attachment to infant; unrealistic expectations; difficulty adjusting to emotional, physical, sexual, and psychological changes; problems coping with responsibility; difficulty in assuming responsibility for parental role due to lack of skills and knowledge

- **Age of mother:** A maternal age of under 16 or over 35.

Cultural Factors

The woman's actions during pregnancy are much determined by her cultural beliefs. Thus, any nursing plan must reflect the nurse's awareness of the woman's needs, personal preferences, cultural focus, and beliefs (Ladewig, London & Olds, 1990; Johnston, 1980). When a conflict exists between established protocol and the practices of the patient, rather than imposing her own values on the patient, the nurse should try to be understanding and attempt to determine the following:

- Are these customs or practices harmless? If they have no obvious effect on health, they are best ignored. A good example is the ritual disposal of the placenta and cord practiced in some groups, which has no untoward medical effect and may put the patient at ease, since her conditioned behavior is not interfered with or denied.

- Are these practices harmful? Certain dietary or exercise regimes may have detrimental effects on the mother and/or baby and should be modified, perhaps with the assistance of someone from within the patient's cultural group.

Those practices over which there is uncertainty should be left unopposed pending investigation. Some examples of this include the use of herbs and folk remedies, the swaddling of infants, and the abdominal binding of mothers.

MEDICAL MANAGEMENT OF THE NORMAL PREGNANCY

Prenatal Visits

Schedule of visits and the physical exam

The nursing objectives in the first prenatal visit include determining the factors in the patient's, partner's, and family's history that may affect the prenatal course, the outcome of the pregnancy, and the patient's and baby's long-term health; assessment of the patient's past and present health; informing both the patient and her partner about her pregnancy and her prenatal needs; and the establishment of patient/healthcare provider rapport (Neeson, 1987).

Calculation of the EDD (estimated delivery date) is made at this time, and a health history is collected. This should include demographic data, menstrual history, assessment of risk factors, medical history of the patient and her family, a review of systems, and any past pregnancies (Raff & Freisner, 1989). At the first prenatal visit a general physical examination is performed that includes palpation of the thyroid, auscultation of maternal heart rate, inspection and palpation of breasts and abdomen, measurement of fundal height, and auscultation of fetal heart rate. An obstetrical exam includes an evaluation of the pelvis for shape, size, external and internal measurements, a vaginal exam to determine pregnancy (Goodell's sign and Chadwick's sign), and a Pap smear.

Subsequent visits in an uncomplicated pregnancy are done every four weeks from the first to the 28th week of gestation; every two weeks from the 28th to the 36th week; then every week until delivery (Ladewig, London & Olds, 1990). At each visit the nurse must determine the status of the pregnancy between visits, perform a nutritional assessment; and do a physical exam, including blood pressure and weight (Neeson, 1987).

A random urine toxicology test may also be desirable at the first prenatal visit for high-risk women. The nurse should, however, verify that there is a written physician's order or written protocol or policy governing the collection of specimens for drug screening. The patient's informed consent for the test should be obtained (May & Mahlmeister, 1994).

Lab tests to be done at the initial visit include CBC *(see appendix lab values)*, Rh and blood typing; antibody screening; rubella titer; VDRL; urinalysis and/or urine culture; Pap and GC screening; hemoglobin electrophoresis (sickle cell screening in blacks); hepatitis screening; purified protein derivative (PPD) testing; chlamydia culture; and wet mount of vaginal secretions as indicated (Neeson, 1987).

At each prenatal visit, a urine dipstick test for glucose, proteins, and ketones is done. CBC or hemoglobin testing may be done each trimester to assess anemia. In the Rh negative, unsensitized patient, antibody screening is repeated at the 28th week. A cervical smear for GC may be done again in the third trimester. A vaginal secretion wet mount is repeated if signs of vaginal infection are present.

Problem Identification

The nurse must impress upon the patient and family the necessity of immediately reporting to her health care provider any danger signs that occur. These include the following (Neeson, 1987; Ladewig, London & Olds, 1990; Raff& Freisner, 1989):

- Abdominal pain, cramping, or bleeding; which may herald premature labor or abruptio placentae.

- Loss of vaginal fluid, which may indicate premature rupture of the membranes.

- Fever of over 101°F (38.3°C) indicating infection.

- Absence of fetal movement, which may be caused by maternal medication, obesity, or fetal death.

- Emotional stress.

- Severe headache, edema of extremities, sudden weight gain, visual changes, dizziness, muscular irritability, convulsions, epigastric pain. Any of these may indicate preeclampsia or eclampsia.

- Dysuria, a sign of urinary tract infection.

- Oliguria, possibly indicating renal impairment or decreased fluid intake.

Fetal Surveillance

Many caregivers are now encouraging the mother to monitor her fetus's activity and keep fetal movement records and/or a fetal diary (Ladewig, London & Olds, 1990). This serves a dual purpose: assurance that no problem exists and, should overt activity occur, a documented record is available for additional evaluation. Beyond the mother's monitoring, the caregiver monitors fetal well-being by several other means. Most diagnostic tests are done on an outpatient basis, so the nurse will have limited interaction with the patient during these procedures. However, support and counseling should be given before any procedure, along with information concerning the test, its purpose, benefits, risks, and alternatives. This is of paramount importance, for it can help allay the patient's fears about possible unfavorable test results. Common diagnostic tests include the following:

Biophysical profile

Biophysical profiles (BPP) assess five variables: fetal breathing movements, body movements, muscle tone, amniotic fluid volume, and fetal heart rate reactivity. The reactivity is evaluated via a non-stress test while the remaining four variables are assessed via abdominal ultrasound. Each of the five components are scored 2 points (normal) or 0 (abnormal). A score of 8–10 is considered normal; a score of 6 is considered equivocal (test

should be repeated within 12–24 hrs); and a score of 4 or less is abnormal. The five components are given 2 points if the following criteria are met:

1. Reactive NST.

2. One or more episodes of rhythmic fetal breathing movements of 30 seconds or more within a 30 minute period.

3. Three or more discrete body or limb movements within 30 minutes.

4. One or more episodes of extension of a fetal extremity with return to flexion.

5. Presence of a single pocket of amniotic fluid exceeding 2 cm in two perpendicular planes.

Biochemical Assessment

Triple screen

It is recommended that all women have a triple screen blood test performed between 15–19 weeks gestation. This test evaluates the amount of maternal serum alpha-feto-protein (MSAFP), human chorionic gonadotropin (hCG) and estriol (μE3). Research has indicated abnormal levels of one or more of these indicators may be associated with an increased risk of developmental and/or genetic disorders. For example, if the MSAFP is elevated while the hCG and μE3 are normal, there is an increased risk for the infant to have an open neural tube defect (NTD), fetal demise, ventral wall defects (i.e. omphaloceles), skin abnormalities, trisomy 13 and 18, oligohydramnios and placental tumors. If all three values are low, there is increased risk of trisomy 18 without a ventral wall defect. Elevated MSAFP and hCG levels in the presence of a normal μE3, is associated with placental problems which can lead to oligohydramnios and IUGR. Decreased levels of MSAFP and μE3, in combination with elevated hCG levels, is associated with trisomy 21. Items which can cause false positives include incorrect gestational dating and multiple gestation.

Group B strep

Group B strep (GBS) is the leading cause of perinatal bacterial infections in the United States. Approximately 15–40% of pregnant women are asymptomatic carriers of GBS. Risk factors which have been identified for selection of patients most likely to benefit from intrapartum antibiotic chemoprophylaxis include maternal colonization with GBS PLUS:

- Pre-term labor or

- Pre-term, premature rupture of membranes, or

- Prolonged rupture of membranes (>18 hours) or

- Sibling affected by symptomatic GBS infection, or

- Maternal fever during labor.

Treatment of choice for symptomatic GBS infection of mother or baby is penicillin or ampicillin. Mothers who are allergic to these medications may receive Erythromycin or Clindamycin instead. Selective intrapartum chemoprophylaxis can prevent GBS early-onset neonatal disease and reduce maternal puerperal morbidity. There does not appear to be an effect on late-onset neonatal disease.

Amniocentesis and genetic studies

Amniocentesis is the process of removing amniotic fluid from the amniotic sac through a needle inserted in the abdominal wall in conjunction with ultrasound. It is usually done after the 14th week of pregnancy, and is used to detect genetic defects in the fetus due to chromosomal abnormalities (such as Down's syndrome), enzyme deficiencies (such as Tay-Sachs disease), inborn errors of metabolism (such as cystic fibrosis), neural tube defects, and sex-linked defects (such as hemophilia). Fetal well-being is determined by AFP testing, the color of the amniotic fluid, and bilirubin determination.

Amniocentesis can also be used in estimating fetal maturity, in determining Rh problems, testing for phosphatidyl glycerol, and in taking the L/S (lecithin/sphingomyelin) ratio, which measures surfactant levels in the fetal lung. It can also be used therapeutically to relieve hydramnios, to give an intrauterine transfusion, and to perform a therapeutic abortion in the second trimester. Its risks are hemorrhage, hematoma, premature labor, amniotic fluid leak, syncope, infection, and fetal puncture (Ladewig, London & Olds, 1990; Raff & Freisner, 1989).

Electronic Assessment (Antenatal Testing)

1. Ultrasonography is a scanning procedure using sound waves to display two-dimensional images of an area. It is painless and does not expose the patient to radiation. It can detect pregnancy as early as the fifth or sixth week of gestation, identify multiple pregnancy, and be used to measure the fetal head or femur, thus helping to determine fetal age and growth status. It can also help detect abnormalities, identify amniotic fluid pockets, locate the placenta, observe fetal heart beat and respiration, grade the placenta, and determine fetal position, presentation, or death.

2. Fetoscopy is an experimental technique in which a fetoscope is introduced into the abdominal cavity through the abdomen. Performed at the 17th week by ultrasound, it is used for direct visualization of the fetus and fetal blood and for fetal skin sampling.

3. Chorionic villus sampling, done by ultrasound, tests for chromosomal and biochemical disorders, but cannot detect neural tube abnormalities. A sample of chorionic villi from the placenta is aspirated through a catheter. Performed in the first trimester, the test provides for the option of terminating an abnormal

pregnancy but carries with it the risk of septic shock.

4. Percutaneous umbilical blood sampling is a new technique wherein a needle is inserted into the umbilical cord using ultrasound to view the fetus, allowing fetal blood sampling for assessment of blood counts, liver function, blood gases and acid/base balance.

5. Magnetic resonance imaging (MRI) provides a detailed and precise image of the entire fetus in one scan. Done during the second or third trimester, it is used to obtain confirmation of fetal abnormalities that may have been suggested by ultrasound. It is also done for purposes of pelvimetry and for assessing placental localization and size (Neeson, 1987; Ladewig, London & Olds, 1990).

Fetal Movement Counting

Healthy fetuses are very active and may have up to 30 to 32 movements in one hour. When fetuses become stressed, however, their activity and movements decrease. Decreased fetal movements may also occur during fetal sleep, which may last as long as 60 minutes. Keeping a daily record of fetal movements during a specified period of time is very important in monitoring the well-being of the fetus and to potentially reduce the incidence of antepartum fetal death, especially in women who are already experiencing complications during the pregnancy. Counting fetal movements is usually begun around the 28th gestational week. Patients should be carefully instructed how to follow the protocol and when to notify their health care provider.

A method of counting fetal movements recommended by Moore and Piaquadio (1989) is as follows:

1. The patient should begin counting when the fetus is most active. For most fetuses this is the evening.

2. It is easiest to count kicks or movements when she is lying on her side and quiet.

3. Record the time on the sheet when counting started.

4. Continue counting until 10 separate fetal movements are felt. A movement can be a kick, roll, turn, or flip.

5. If 60 minutes pass with less than 10 movements, start over with a new count. If 10 movements are not felt before the end of the second hour, the patient is to come immediately to the hospital.

6. The patient should also come to the hospital for further evaluation if she does not feel the baby move all day, and if it is taking longer and longer each evening to get to the 10th movement.

7. The patient should bring the record to each prenatal visit for review by the health care provider.

Non-stress testing: Non-stress testing is performed with the use of an electronic fetal monitor. It evaluates the baseline variability and acceleration of the fetal heart rate in relation to fetal movement and can determine the presence or absence of intrauterine hypoxia. A reactive non-stress test indicates fetal well-being. It is quick to perform, easy to interpret, inexpensive, without risks, and can be done in an office or clinic setting. However, a suitable tracing cannot always be obtained, and the patient may find it uncomfortable to lie still for the 20 minutes required for testing (refer to chapter 7).

Vibroacoustic stimulation uses vibration and sound to induce fetal reactivity during a non-stress test. The nurse applies an artificial larynx or fetal acoustic stimulator over the fetus' head for 1–5 seconds.

Contraction stress testing (CST) is performed to evaluate the oxygen/carbon dioxide exchange of the placenta and identify the fetus at risk for asphyxia (Ladewig, London & Olds, 1990). During contractions, intrauterine pressure increases and blood flow to the placenta is reduced, thereby decreasing oxygen transport to the fetus (Raff & Freisner, 1989). A healthy fetus can tolerate this reduction. A CST is indicated when there is risk of placental insufficiency or fetal compromise; it is contraindicated where there is a risk of premature delivery, in third trimester bleeding, and in women with previous Cesarean deliveries. Contractions may occur spontaneously or they may be induced by intravenous administration of oxytocin (Pitocin) or by nipple stimulation, since the body produces oxytocin in response to stimulation of the breast or nipples. An electronic fetal monitor is used throughout to provide information regarding the fetal heart rate and uterine contractions. CSTs are usually begun at 32–34 weeks and repeated weekly until intervention is necessary or the woman delivers. A negative CST implies adequate placental support, while a positive CST may indicate fetal compromise. However, false positives are common, and when a positive CST occurs, further investigation is indicated.

Clinical Assessments

Fundal height may be used as a measure of uterine size, but is accurate only within about four weeks and cannot be used late in pregnancy. Using a centimeter tape measure, the abdominal distance is measured from the top of the symphysis pubis to the top of the fundus (McDonald's method). The fundal height generally equals the gestational age until the third trimester (for example, 20 cm equals 20 weeks gestation). This measurement will vary in extremely tall or short women. The absence of increased fundal height may indicate intrauterine growth retardation, while a sudden increase may indicate multiple pregnancy or hydramnios (Ladewig, London & Olds, 1990).

Leopold's maneuvers (see *figure 3-3*) are a systemic method of evaluating the maternal abdomen, but may be difficult to perform on the obese woman or the woman with excessive amniotic fluid. The patient must first empty her bladder, then lie on her back with her feet on the bed and her knees bent (Ladewig, London & Olds, 1990).

The four Leopold maneuvers provide a clinical assessment tool to determine the following information on fetal presentation and position (Martin, 1990):

1. Is the lie longitudinal or transverse?

2. What presents at or in the pelvic inlet?

3. Where is the back?

4. Where are the small parts?

5. What is in the uterine fundus?

6. On which side is the cephalic prominence?

7. Has engagement taken place?

8. How high in the abdomen is the uterine fundus?

1st maneuver: Facing the woman, palpate the upper abdomen with both hands. Note the shape, consistency, and mobility of the palpated part. The fetal head is firm, hard, and round, and moves independently of the trunk. The buttocks are softer and move with the trunk.

2nd maneuver: Move the hands toward the pelvis and palpate the abdomen with gentle, deep pressure. The fetal back feels smooth and the arms, legs, and feet feel knobby and bumpy.

3rd maneuver: With one hand above the symphysis note whether the palpated part feels like the head or the buttocks and whether the presenting part is engaged.

4th maneuver: Face the woman's feet. With both hands on the lower abdomen, move fingers gently down the sides of the uterus toward the pubis. Note the cephalic prominence or brow.

FIGURE 3-3
Leopold Maneuvers

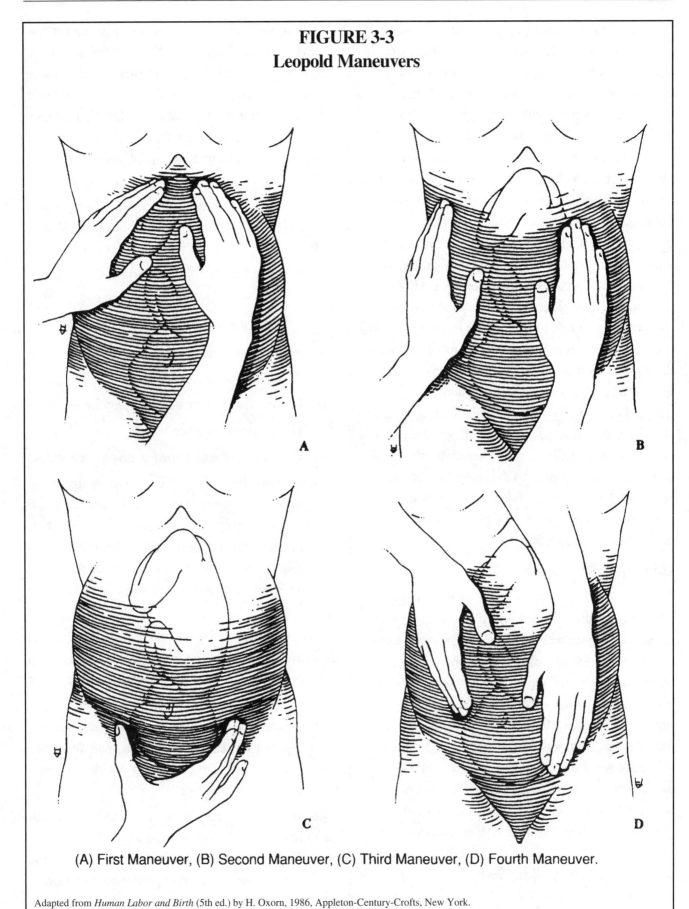

(A) First Maneuver, (B) Second Maneuver, (C) Third Maneuver, (D) Fourth Maneuver.

Adapted from *Human Labor and Birth* (5th ed.) by H. Oxorn, 1986, Appleton-Century-Crofts, New York.

Possible Complications During Pregnancy

Gestational diabetes mellitus (GDM)

Gestational diabetes mellitus (GDM) is abnormal carbohydrate metabolism first diagnosed during pregnancy. It is recommended all pregnant women have a 1-hour (50 gram) glucose test between 26–28 weeks gestation. If the results are greater than 135mg/dl, a 3-hour (100 gm) glucose tolerance test can be performed for further diagnosis. If two or more of the following results are exceeded, the diagnosis of GDM is made: fasting, 105mg/dl; one hour, 190mg/dl; two hour, 165mg/dl; and three hour, 145mg/dl. GDM affects approximately 2–3% of all pregnant women and is due to the insulin-antagonistic effects of human placental lactogen (hPL), cortisol, and progesterone. Women who develop GDM have a 30–40% incidence of developing diabetes mellitus in the future. Management GDM includes careful monitoring of diet, exercise, insulin administration and patient education. Oral hypoglycemic agents are contraindicated during pregnancy because of teratogenic effects upon the fetus. Women are taught how to self-monitor their blood glucose levels. They are usually monitored four times/day; fasting blood sugar (FBS) and 2 hours post prandial. Target glucose levels for the FBS is generally <100mg and post prandial <120mg. Maternal complications of GDM include increased incidence of pre-eclampsia, possible birth trauma due to fetal size, increased chance of post partum hemorrhage, polyhydramnios and urinary tract infections. Newborn complications include hyperinsulinemia, respiratory distress syndrome, prematurity, macrosomia, and intrauterine fetal demise.

Hyperemesis gravidarum

A condition in which there is persistent, severe vomiting, early in pregnancy, which lead to weight loss, fluid and electrolyte imbalance, dehydration and metabolic imbalance. If untreated, it can be fatal. Though the exact cause is unknown, it has been associated with hormone levels (esp. human chorionic gonadotropin hCG), trophoblastic activity and psychological factors. Uteroplacental circulation is decreased following dehydration and delivery of nutrients to the fetus is affected, possibly leading to intrauterine grown retardation (IUGR). If the patient cannot be managed at home with antiemetics, high-carbohydrate meals and rest, hospitalization may be required. Treatment then includes intravenous hydration, electrolyte replacement and the continued use of antiemetics such as promethazine or hydroxyzine. Patients are maintained NPO and fluids and solids are reintroduced slowly. A "dry" diet consists of a patient first eating dry, plain crackers followed by a fluid 1 hr later. Once she can tolerates that diet, she is slowing advanced to a liquid, soft and house diet.

Premature rupture of membranes

Premature rupture of membranes (PROM) is defined as the rupture of the amniotic membranes one or more hours prior to the onset of true labor. PROM occurs in approximately 10% of term pregnancies due to unknown causes. Some predisposing factors of PROM include malpresentation, weakened areas within the chorion and amnion, and an incompetent cervical os. Following PROM, prevention of infection is of prime importance since the ruptured membranes provide a portal of entry for microorganisms. PROM can be diagnosed either via nitrazine paper which turns blue (alkaline) when in contact with amniotic fluid or the fern test where a swab of vaginal fluid is applied to a microscope slide. Once it dries, amniotic fluid assumes a fern-like appearance under a microscope. Nursing interventions include frequent monitoring of amount/color/odor of fluid leaking from the vagina, monitoring of uterine contractions, and frequent changing of bed pads and provision of perineal care.

EXAM QUESTIONS

CHAPTER 3
Questions 11–13

11. Leg cramps can be relieved by

    a. increasing calcium intake.

    b. rubbing calves to stop cramp.

    c. wearing an ace wrap.

    d. having regular exercise and calf stretching.

12. A practical method for assessing fetal well being during pregnancy is

    a. measuring fundal height.

    b. performing Leopold maneuvers.

    c. performing serial ultrasounds.

    d. monitoring daily fetal movements.

13. A warning sign of a complication developing during pregnancy is

    a. weight gain of 1lb. a week in the second or third trimester.

    b. sudden increase in facial or hand/feet edema.

    c. Braxton Hicks contractions.

    d. nausea and vomiting during the first trimester.

CHAPTER 4

CHILDBIRTH EDUCATION AND FAMILY PREPARATION

CHAPTER OBJECTIVE

After studying this chapter, the reader will be able to recognize the purpose of childbirth preparation and identify major methods and philosophies for providing effective prenatal educational support.

LEARNING OBJECTIVES

After reading this chapter, the student will be able to

1. Recognize the goal of childbirth education and preparation.

2. Differentiate between various philosophical approaches to childbirth education.

3. Identity the role of the "coach" or support person.

4. Specify the responsibilities of the childbirth educator in providing effective prenatal and new-parenting education.

INTRODUCTION

Childbirth education in the United States began in the early 1900s with the American Red Cross and the Maternity Center Association of New York, whose goal was to meet public health needs and improve the health of women and children (ICEA, 1986). Subsequently, other childbirth education classes were developed for the purpose of meeting women's pain-reduction needs during labor and delivery. Early contributors, such as Dick-Read and Lamaze, formed the basis of today's childbirth education class, which, in addition to pain management, is designed to help women cope with childbirth through active participation and increased decision-making (AHA & AAP, 1990). Now, with lower infant and maternal mortality rates, the focus of childbirth education has shifted. The public health aspect is no longer the major factor; instead, childbirth education now emphasizes making childbirth a more rewarding experience for the mother, her mate, and her entire family.

THE PURPOSE OF CHILDBIRTH EDUCATION

According to the American Childbirth Association, today's ideal program should focus on wellness, health promotion, risk reduction, self-involvement, informed consent, birth as a unique experience, and the use of non-medical and self-care techniques for the normal pregnancy, labor, and birth (ICEA, 1986). Childbirth education, in its broadest definition, should include preparation for pregnancy, labor, birth, and parenting, and should address breastfeeding, sexuality, changes in the couple's relationship, and family planning.

GOALS OF EDUCATIONAL PROGRAMS

Antepartal education programs vary in content, leadership techniques, and teaching methods (Ladewig, London & Olds, 1990). A class's content is usually directed by its goals. Before making a referral to a program, the nurse should first assess the couple's needs for information, for self-care measures, and for assistance in coping. Acting as a parent advocate, the nurse should then provide information and refer the couple to programs that show respect for the couple's dignity and rights and promote the health and safety of both the mother and fetus. The ideal childbirth education program should help the couple to cooperate through the "problem" of labor in a manner satisfactory to both. It should provide them with coping skills and the impetus to practice what they have learned, and it should encourage mutual participation (AHA & AAP, 1990). Their feelings concerning labor and parenthood should be brought out and discussed; and, since the class's atmosphere should be one of total acceptance, they should feel free to bring out any negative feelings that exist and receive help in resolving them. As the couple works toward assuming an active and independent role in the childbirth experience, they will learn to become more flexible, and their potential for working together in future situations will be enhanced. Therefore, the objectives of childbirth education should include the following:

- Providing a supportive milieu
- Reducing anxiety
- Providing factual information
- Providing practical tools for labor
- Maintaining a focus on current concerns (Ladewig, London & Olds, 1990).

METHODS AND PHILOSOPHIES

Psychoprophylaxis (Lamaze method) (see *table 4-1*). Using Pavlov's stimulus-response theory to decondition women in labor, Dr. Fernand Lamaze developed a method of "painless childbirth" that became popular in the 1960s and is now one of the most frequently used methods of childbirth education (Raff & Freisner, 1989). Lamaze classes consist of two components:

- Education to dispel fears, coupled with training to achieve relaxation of body musculature.
- Conditioning for labor, achieved through the development of consciously controlled activity that displaces the pain sensations of contractions in the brain. Relaxation is achieved by means of breathing techniques for each stage of labor and by massage and counter-pressure. Positioning is used as a means to assist in increasing maternal comfort, and exercises to strengthen pelvic musculature are taught (Ladewig, London & Olds, 1990).

Modified Lamaze

Childbirth educators have enhanced the Lamaze method by adding information on prenatal nutrition, infant feeding, cesarean birth and variations from the usual labor, discussions concerning sexuality, and parenting and coping skills for the postpartum period (see *table 4-1*.) Many educators have modified Lamaze's original exercises, particularly in changing the pace of breathing (Jiminez, 1980). The original Lamaze theory specified the presence of a female monitor, now a father-husband coach is encouraged, along with a medical attendant. Whereas exercise was originally seen as necessary to build the body for an athletic event, it is now used to enhance comfort in pregnancy and birth. But perhaps the most important modification involves a change in philosophy concerning the goals of expectant parents. The original Lamaze theory virtually demanded that in order to have a successful childbirth experience, the delivery was to be painless and without anesthetic. In many cases, the parturient who was unable to fulfill this goal was left with a feeling of inadequacy. Today, childbirth educators encourage the couple to set their own goals, supplying them with the tools for accepting these goals while providing reassurance and information about other options for those who cannot achieve a pain-free and anesthetic-free delivery (Ladewig, London & Olds, 1990).

Bradley

This method of partner-coached, natural, and pain-free childbirth developed by Dr. Robert Bradley involves exercises used to accomplish relaxation and slow, controlled, primarily abdominal breathing. It is based on the behavior of lower animals in labor, and adapted for humans. The patient's mate and her physician are essential for support. The technique of abdominal breathing is taught, and the spiritual, mystical nature of birth is stressed. Psychic harmony and mental relaxation are achieved by means of disassociation from the present—an imitation of sleep, in a dark and quiet room, with the eyes closed (Ladewig, London & Olds, 1990).

Dick-Read

This psychophysical approach is based on Dr. Grantly Dick-Read's movement toward "natural childbirth," a term he coined, and on his theory that fear causes tension, which in turn causes pain. Dick-Read believed the fear-tension-pain syndrome could be alleviated by education and proper use of the body. His method consists of education about pregnancy and childbirth, with the goal of dispelling fears and misapprehensions, coupled with exercises aimed at strengthening and increasing the flexibility of the muscles used in labor. It includes muscle-relaxing techniques and abdominal breathing in harmony with contractions. Initially a medical attendant was stressed, but now

the father/husband/coach is welcomed. The Dick-Read method also stresses psychic harmony, a positive mental attitude, passive relaxation, and withdrawal into oneself.

Harris

This approach has the advantage of being easy to learn, and can be taught in labor to couples who have not attended childbirth education classes. Based on the dual philosophy that childbirth is intended to be a bonding experience, and that labor, which may be painful, must be coped with, the Harris theory stresses physiological control, mental relaxation, slow breathing, and touch-relaxation. If taught in a prenatal setting, exercise is stressed for achieving comfort during pregnancy and birth. The husband/coach serves as the focal point (Ladewig, London & Olds, 1990).

Kitzinger

This psychophysical approach developed by Sheila Kitzinger, concentrates on the psychosexual aspects of birth and a close relationship with the mate, using sensory memory to help the parturient to understand and work with her body in preparation for birth. The father/husband is highly significant. Prenatal exercise is stressed, as is emotional preparation, conscious active relaxation, the use of touch, rhythmic coordination of breathing with contractions, and detailed pushing technique (Ladewig, London & Olds, 1990).

Hypnosis

Hypnosis, in obstetrics, is also called the hypno-reflexogenous method. It is a combination of hypnosis and conditioned reflexes. Although it does not teach specific techniques of producing anesthesia or analgesia, these are thought to be by-products of the method (Jiminez, 1980).

TABLE 4-1
Content Outline for Lamaze Prepared Childbirth Classes

A. **Theory of the Lamaze Method**

B. **Anatomy and Physiology as They Relate to:**
- Pregnancy
- Labor and birth
- The postpartum period (the mother)
- The newborn

C. **Emotional Responses of Expectant Parents to:**
- Pregnancy experience
- Childbirth experience
- Early parenting experience (include role changes)

D. **Physical Conditioning for Childbirth**
- Prenatal exercises
- Posture/body mechanics
- Guidelines for exercises

E. **Stages and Phases of Labor**
- Overview
- First stage
  Latent phase
  Active phase
  Transition phase
- Second stage
- Third stage
- Woman's physical responses
- Woman's emotional responses
- Coach's role

F. **Nonpharmacological Analgesia**
- Progressive relaxation
- Touch relaxation
- Imagery
- Focusing techniques
- Effleurage
- Massage
- Comfort measures (back rub. positioning, and the like)
- Support (role of the coach, birthing agency staff and physician or midwife)

G. **Pharmacological Analgesia and Anesthesia**
- Types used (describe and explain)
- Route and when administered
- Effects on expectant mother and baby

H. **Breathing Techniques**
- Respiratory theory and principles
- Respiratory techniques
  Slow paced
  Modified paced
  Patterned paced
- Second stage expulsion
  Physiologic techniques
  Modified Valsalva technique

I. **Birthing Process**
- Vaginal birth
- Cesarean birth
  Indications
  Procedures
  Use of prepared childbirth techniques
  Coach's role
- Precipitous birth

J. **Variations in Labor and Birth**
- Back labor
- Amniotomy
- Fetal monitoring: External/Internal
- Induction and augmentation
- Forceps and vacuum extraction
- Episiotomy (use of perineal massage)

K. **Birthing Agency Procedures**
- Admission
- Labor and birth
- Postpartum care (mother and baby)
- Parent-infant interaction

L. **Provision for Other Content**
- Nutrition
- Infant feeding (breast or bottle)
- Signs of premature labor (prevention of prematurity)
- Grieving and loss in unexpected outcomes
- Postpartum "blues"
- Family planning (contraception)

M. **Consumer Advocacy (integrated throughout classes)**
- Is a balanced viewpoint (positive and negative aspects) of procedures presented regarding:
  Pregnancy?
  Childbirth?
  Parenting?
- Are family-centered options presented?
- Are alternatives to "standard" or "routine" practices that are inconsistent with the philosophy of family-centered maternity care and a physiologic approach to child-birth explored?
- Is the development of effective communication skills promoted between:
  Pregnant woman and her labor partner?
  Pregnant woman and her obstetrical care provider?
- Are realistic expectations and birth plans promoted?
- Are information and guidelines provided so that expectant parents can make informed decisions?

Source: Guidelines for Developing a Teaching Plan, ASPO/Lamaze Teacher Certification Program for Childbirth Educators. Washington D.C.: American Society for Psychoprophylaxis in Obstetrics, 1987.

TEACHING CONTENT

Childbirth preparation classes are designed to help the couple make informed decisions during the childbearing year and should contain information regarding changes in the woman and the development of the fetus. They are best conducted in chronological sequence, with both parents taught breathing and relaxation techniques, infant care, and coping strategies.

The First-Trimester Class

Suggestions for the content of the first-trimester class include the following: early gestational changes; self-care during pregnancy; fetal development and environmental dangers for the fetus; sexuality in pregnancy; birth settings and types of care providers; nutrition, rest, and exercise suggestions; relief measures for common discomforts of pregnancy; psychological changes in pregnancy; information for getting pregnancy off to a good start (Ladewig, London & Olds, 1990). This class should also highlight factors that place the woman at risk for pre-term labor and discuss its signs and symptoms. The pros and cons of breastfeeding and bottlefeeding should be covered, since many women make their decisions regarding feeding before the third trimester.

Second- and Third-Trimester Classes

Later classes should focus on preparation for labor, birth, and early parenthood, stressing (and allowing practice time for) body conditioning, relaxation, breathing techniques, and other measures that promote comfort and participation during the birth experience. Birth choices should be outlined: does the woman want an episiotomy, medications, fetal monitoring? Postpartum self-care should be taught, as well as early adjustment to parenthood and infant care including feeding, family nutrition, child health and safety, growth and development, infant stimulation, and family development. Of particular importance is a discussion of the car seat: how to choose it, how it works, how vital it is to the baby's safety. In most states, a car seat is required as early as the infant's trip home from the birthing center.

Refresher Courses

In many areas, birth preparation refresher courses are now given for experienced parents who have previously taken a course in prepared childbirth and who want to update their skills and knowledge. These classes review the process of labor and delivery as well as methods of promoting comfort and participation during childbirth. They most often include a segment on sibling adjustment.

Adolescent Parenting Classes

The adolescent has special learning needs during pregnancy and is best suited to a teen pregnancy and parenting program. These offer help and support to the young woman, teaching her about bodily changes and preparation for the baby and often making referrals to community resources that can help her following the baby's birth. The emphasis is on the adolescent's particular nutritional requirements, baby care activities, combining motherhood with schooling, and the exploration of feelings during pregnancy and early parenthood. Studies have shown that the following are the pregnant teenager's primary concerns: how to be a good parent; how to care for the new baby; health dangers to the baby; how to recognize when the baby is sick; how to protect the baby from accidents; how to make the baby feel happy and loved; healthy foods to eat during pregnancy. These areas should be covered in prenatal classes, and, ideally, some provisions should be made for ongoing educational support after the birth of the baby.

Prenatal Breastfeeding Classes

In recent years, the number of programs offering information on breastfeeding has increased. Often the father is included in these classes, since his support and encouragement is vital. Many hospitals, health clinics, and birthing centers now have lactation consultants who offer comprehensive educational programs on breastfeeding. These feature individual or group instruction and generally cover the advantages and disadvantages of breastfeeding, counseling on breastfeeding techniques and management methods of breast preparation, and adjusting the routine to allow for demand feeding. Consideration is given to the pregnant woman who has special needs. For example, the mother who wishes to return to work while breastfeeding will be taught methods of expressing and storing her milk for later use. La Leche League International is an organization of nursing mothers that encourages and assists women who wish to breastfeed, and that provides literature, advice, and support. Chapters are located in most major cities.

Grandparenting Classes

The birthing process and infant care have changed drastically since the time that most expectant grandparents had their own babies. For this reason, many centers now offer "grandparenting classes," which are often attended by the pregnant couple as well as their parents. Many offer slide presentations or a birth film in addition to a discussion of current beliefs and practices in childbearing. Ideally, the class will also provide tips on being a supportive grandparent, since grandparents are a vital source of support for new parents. For those who want to participate in the labor and birth experience, information is provided on the techniques of coaching.

Cesarean Birth Preparation Class

With cesarean birth constituting one out of five deliveries, preparation for the possibility should be included in every childbirth education class. To help the couple avoid the feelings of anger, loss, and grief that can occur with cesarean birth, it should be approached as a normal event, with the instructor stressing the similarities between it and vaginal birth. Information should be provided that

will help a couple make personal choices and participate in the experience. The curriculum should cover the details of a cesarean delivery and describe what the mother and father will feel as well as what they can do. Every couple should be encouraged to speak with their physician or nurse-midwife concerning their needs and desires in the event a Cesarean is indicated, and also to learn what approach will be taken. Their choices include participation in selecting an anesthetic and the option of the father/coach being present during the cesarean birth.

For the couple who know ahead of time that cesarean birth is planned (for instance, the handicapped woman or the woman with pelvic insufficiency), many centers and local groups provide more detailed cesarean preparation classes. These classes are also given to couples anticipating a repeat cesarean birth and are particularly beneficial for those who have had negative experiences. They are afforded the opportunity to discuss the factors that contributed to their negative feelings, identify what changes they would like made, and review interventions that will make the subsequent experience more acceptable. Those who have had positive experiences require reassurance that the upcoming cesarean will again meet their needs, and any fears or anxieties (particularly the anticipation of pain) should be discussed, with reassurance given. The instructor should stress that for the woman whose first cesarean was preceded by a long or strenuous labor, there will be much less fatigue the second time around.

Vaginal Birth After Cesarean (VBAC) Class

In the past, the theory was "once a cesarean, always a cesarean," and indeed there was a time when a woman who had undergone a cesarean birth was advised never to become pregnant again. All of that has changed with increased knowledge and technology, and many women who have had cesarean births can now anticipate vaginal deliveries. However, their needs are substantially different, and thus special VBAC classes have been developed in which couples are encouraged to ask questions, share experiences, and form bonds with each other. The instructor supplies details of attempting a trial of labor and identifying decisions regarding the birth experience. Often two birth plans are given, one for vaginal and one for cesarean birth. This appears to help couples take more control of the birth experience and increase the positive aspects of the experience. Following the initial session, classes are often divided according to the couples' needs, with those who have had recent coached childbirth experience needing only a refresher course, and others being referred to regular classes.

Sibling Preparation Class

Becoming a sibling in early childhood can be a stressful experience, affecting the child's cognitive, social, and emotional development (Ladewig, London & Olds, 1990; Honig, 1986). To ease the transition, programs have been created to prepare children for the birth of a sibling to help them develop positive feelings toward their new sibling, and to encourage collaboration in the experiences of pregnancy, birth, and siblinghood. The ideal program promotes the child's cognitive and emotional growth and helps establish a foundation for bonding. With the increased emphasis on family-centered childbirth, children are now being included in the birthing process, often visiting during labor, being present at the birth, and visiting during the postpartum period. Proponents claim this fosters family unity and closeness, that it is a learning experience for the child, and that it helps eliminate feelings of jealousy and rivalry (Ladewig, London & Olds, 1990; Honig, 1986).

Sibling preparation classes usually include a tour of the maternity ward, a view of the newborn nursery, and a visit to a birthing room. Following the tour, children are taught (using books, audiovisual materials, models, discussions, classes, and play experience) how babies are born, what babies are like, and what happens to parents and newborns in the hospital. Their feelings about a new baby are elicited. Parents are also given teaching resources and advised to involve the child in the pregnancy, including listening to the fetal heartbeat. Classes may vary according to age groups.

Whether a sibling should be present at birth is the parents' decision. Those siblings who will be present must be made familiar with what to expect during labor and delivery, including the mother's sounds, the sight of blood, the equipment, and how the baby will look at birth.

Prenatal Exercise Class

A well-conditioned body will perform better and more reliably under the stress of labor than a body in poor physical condition (De Santo & Hassad, 1983). However, because of the body's changes during pregnancy, the pregnant woman must learn how to exercise safely and effectively, to condition her body with minimum risk to herself and the fetus (Raff & Freisner, 1989). Thus, a number of prenatal exercise classes have evolved that take into consideration the pregnant woman's increased heart rate, the softening of her connective tissues, and her postural imbalance (Ladewig, London & Olds, 1990). These classes should be taught by teachers with current knowledge of and experience with the unique needs of pregnant women. The American College of Obstetricians and Gynecologists (ACOG) has published specific guidelines for exercise during pregnancy; these should be incorporated into the class curriculum. In addition, an exercise prescription from the woman's physician is encouraged. The goal of these exercises is to strengthen muscle tone in preparation for delivery and promote faster restoration of muscle tone after delivery. The criteria for the exercises are as follows:

- They must be free of sudden, exaggerated movements that could stress the joints or ligaments.

- They must be performed in a way that motion can be controlled.

- The pelvis must be stabilized.

- They must not increase the lordotic curve of the spine.

- They must not cause excessive compression of the uterus.

- They should be enjoyable.

Among the exercises taught are the pelvic tilt *(see chapter 3)*, abdominal exercises (tightening abdominal muscles in synchronization with respiration, partial sit-ups), inner-thigh exercises (done cross-legged in tailor position), and Kegel's exercises to strengthen the perineal muscles.

Groups with Special Needs

Preparation for pregnancy and parenting classes can also be tailored to other groups of women and families with special needs. Individual or small group classes can be extremely valuable to women at high risk for developing or who have developed complications during their pregnancy, such as pre-term labor, pregnancy-induced hypertension, or bleeding disorders. They may require home care and be on limited activity or bedrest at home or in the hospital. High-risk women generally want more detailed information on warning signs and anticipated interventions that they may encounter. Information on the care of high-risk infants should also be discussed.

HIV-positive women, lesbian women who are pregnant, single women who are pregnant, and couples who have conceived after infertility treatment all have unique learning needs that must be addressed individually or in separate group classes. New parenting classes can also be adapted for adopting couples (May & Mahimeister, 1994).

Effectiveness of Prenatal Education

Prenatal education serves many purposes on many different levels. Although prepared childbirth does not preclude the use of medication when necessary, it allows for a decreased use of analgesics and anesthetics during labor, thereby lowering the probability of drug-related side effects to mother and baby (Raff & Freisner, 1989). It also intensifies the mother-father-child relationship by allowing for full participation in the birth process. It reduces fear, anxiety, and pain by providing knowledge and understanding, helping to make the experience of parenthood one of joy. In sharing experiences with other couples, lateral supports are strengthened, reducing the couple's feelings of isolation. The understanding gained concerning changes in the woman's body during pregnancy, labor, and the postpartum period provides a feeling of preparedness and calm. Added to this are the benefits of increased circulation and respiratory exchange, a reduced perception of contractions as painful, and increased confidence in the couple's ability to cope with the discomforts of labor.

As counselor, teacher, professional, and friend, the childbirth educator helps parents evaluate their feelings. Since pregnancy and birth are "normal crises of life," the educator helps parents gain internal as well as external resources for handling crisis situations, which aids them in achieving a satisfactory and healthy adjustment. In the open and permissive classroom atmosphere, the educator encourages parents to examine their feelings and discuss how and why they react the way they do to situations. Through discussions and role-playing, the responsibility of learning to adjust is placed on the parents, and the educator guides them through the process of exploring their reactions and trying new ones. And with the proper guidance, it becomes easier to choose appropriate responses in labor and cope with the stresses of the postpartum period.

TABLE 4-2
Coaching Help Sheet

ENCOURAGEMENT/MOTIVATION ROUTINE
Assist the laboring woman when discouraged about her labor progress by reminding her of the:
1. Normalcy of her labor pattern and her discouragement.
2. Progress she has made.
3. Techniques—reinforcing the learned behaviors of relaxation, paced breathing, and other coping strategies.
4. Need to take each contraction separately, one at a time, rather than focusing on the entire remaining labor.

Give her:
Attention—lots of it.
Support—both verbal and physical.
Confidence—remain calm and controlled and communicate to her that she can cope effectively.

PANIC ROUTINE
Assist the laboring woman to cope more effectively during labor.
1. Recognize the signs of panic—inability to use breathing patterns or other coping strategies, and the expression of need for help, or desire to give up.
2. Use eye-to-eye contact. Without words, this says, "I'm here and I can help."
3. Hold her firmly and send message, "I can help you and I know what to do."
4. Engage her total attention: Bring your face within 10 inches of her face. Use your hand to turn her face towards yours. Breathe with her using a loud, throaty sound starting where she is and then changing to a paced breathing pattern to lead her back into the use of appropriate controlled breathing. Move your face to reinforce the breathing pattern.

CONFLICT ROUTINE FOR THE COACH
When the labor coach must make a difficult decision during the labor process:
1. **Relax:** Take 2 or 3 deep breaths and release your muscles.
2. **Realize:** Realize what is happening. Think to yourself, "I'm getting upset. I've got to stay calm." Catch the conflict by preparing for it, confronting it early, and coping with feelings of being overwhelmed.
3. **Focus:** Get your mind off the problem and on to the alternatives.
4. **Avoid:** Don't get hooked into "tunnel thinking" (focusing on only one solution).
5. **Explore:** Look at the consequence of each alternative.
6. **Decide:** Make the best decision you can with the information you have.
7. **Forget it:** The decision is past and you did your best.

Adapted from Campbel, A., and Worthington, E. Teaching expectant fathers how to be better labor coaches. *MCN: the American Journal of Maternal-Child Nursing* 7:28, 1982.

The Role of "Coach" or Support Person

Providing a supportive milieu is one of the most important functions of childbirth preparation programs. The childbirth coach, an integral member of the support team, goes to class with the expectant mother, asks questions regarding issues of concern, and uses the discipline of repetitive practice with the expectant mother to begin the process of conditioning (Ladewig, London & Olds, 1990). The coach's role is to help the mother use the techniques she has learned *(see table 4-2)*. During labor, the coach comforts and supports the woman with caretaking activities such as soothing conversation, touching, staying close by, giving back rubs, applying cool cloths to the face and forehead, and maintaining eye contact. Using verbal clues the couple has practiced together, the coach reinforces learned responses while encouraging and working with the laboring mother to achieve a satisfying birth experience. The coach is particularly important in helping the woman time contractions, identifying the beginning of each one and breathing through it with her or encouraging and supporting her as she breathes.

The Role of the Childbirth Educator

The childbirth educator has three responsibilities: assessment of parents, intervention, and fulfillment of their educational needs (Raff & Freisner, 1989).

Assessment includes determining the accuracy and completeness of the parents' information regarding parenting, determining their misconceptions (if any) about the maternity cycle, determining their ability to understand information and instructions, assessing their motivation to learn, and becoming familiar with any personal or cultural values that may influence their acceptance of information and their compliance with instructions.

Intervention may include parents' classes, dispensing of literature appropriate to their level of understanding and educational level, and individual counseling and teaching. Teaching effectiveness is enhanced by choosing the time of optimum readiness for motivation to learn (for example, not teaching labor and delivery during the first trimester); limiting the amount of new information given at one time; summarizing and writing down points; providing a feedback mechanism to assess learning, such as asking clients to repeat information, asking if they understand material, and verifying their understanding by nonverbal clues; and providing an atmosphere where questions can be asked freely.

Educational needs may include anatomical and physiological changes in pregnancy, the labor and delivery process, signs of labor, nutrition, signs of complications in pregnancy, the rationale for early and regular prenatal care, safety precautions, hospital admission and daily routine procedures, hospital policies affecting mother-child interaction, the rights of health care consumers, planning and purchasing the layette and other items, preparation for natural childbirth, exercises, hygiene, fetal development, general health care, and newborn care.

EXAM QUESTIONS

CHAPTER 4
Questions 14–16

14. A goal of most childbirth education programs is to

    a. eliminate the need for medications during labor.

    b. guarantee a normal, vaginal delivery.

    c. reduce the incidence of cesarean delivery.

    d. provide factual information in a supportive environment.

15. Most of the childbirth education philosophies include content on

    a. fear-tension-pain syndrome.

    b. psychosexual component.

    c. hypnoreflexogenous method.

    d. relaxation and breathing methods.

16. The term given to the person who supports the laboring woman with caretaking activities, and who practices conditioned techniques for relaxation and breathing is a

    a. childbirth educator.

    b. "coach" or support person.

    c. physician.

    d. patient advocate.

CHAPTER 5

THE INTRAPARTUM PERIOD

CHAPTER OBJECTIVE

After studying this chapter, the reader will be able to differentiate normal labor stages and patterns and select appropriate nursing interventions to support the laboring patient and family.

LEARNING OBJECTIVES

After reading this chapter, the student will be able to

1. Identify the four forces of labor and select variables in these forces that affect the progress of labor.

2. Choose appropriate nursing interventions in caring for women experiencing pre-term labor.

3. Recognize standards of care for supporting patients during each stage of labor.

4. Identify potential maternal complications that may occur during labor and select their specific effects on the fetus.

INTRODUCTION

Labor is a process that involves a series of integrated uterine contractions occurring over a period of time, leading to the development of expulsive forces adequate to propel the fetus through the birth canal against the resistance of soft tissue, muscle, and the bony structure of the pelvis (Martin, 1990). It depends on both the expulsive forces of the muscles of the uterus and the compliance of the cervix.

LABOR FORCES

Theories of Causation

Although much research has been done on the topic, the exact mechanisms that initiate labor are not known (Raff & Freisner, 1989; Ladewig, London & Olds, 1990). For some reason, at the appropriate time for both the uterus and the fetus, labor starts. In all probability, labor is caused by an interaction of factors in the maternal, placental and fetal systems—hormones, the aging of the placenta, and uterine distention. Some of the theories regarding the initiation of labor include the following:

- **The hormonal theory,** which suggests that hormones may interact. Progesterone exerts a relaxing effect on the uterus, and when there is a balance between progesterone and other hormones—oxytocin, prostaglandins, estrogen, and fetal cortisol—no contractions occur. Oxytocin is known to stimulate contractions, but while it alone will not initiate labor, the preponderance of oxytocin along with an increase in prostaglandins and estrogen (which stimulate smooth muscle contractions), may cause labor to start. In addition, as the fetus approaches term, it produces an increased amount of cortisol, which is thought to inhibit progesterone production while stimulating the precursors to prostaglandins.

- **The uterine distention theory** suggests that a full organ tends to contract and empty itself when stretched, but due to the relaxing effect of progesterone, the uterus does not contract, even though stretched. As the production of progesterone decreases, irritability of the small muscles of the uterus may increase, which in turn may stimulate the production of prostaglandins.

- **The aging of the placenta theory** suggests that as the placenta ages, its function decreases, thus causing a decrease in uterine blood flow, which in turn causes increased uterine activity (Martin, 1990).

- **The fetal-maternal communication theory** was postulated by Hippocrates in 400 B.C. Current research indicates that, in a manner as yet unidentified, the fetus may play a major role in the initiation of labor by sending out chemically-mediated signals that bring about a retreat from pregnancy maintenance (Martin, 1990).

Cervical ripening—softening, thinning, and dilatation of from 1 cm to 3 cm—thought to be promoted by hormones, is essential to labor. When ripened, the cervix will respond to the forces of uterine contractions, leading to gradual dilatation (Martin, 1990).

Research continues, aimed toward identifying of the physiological events that initiate labor. The most recent theories suggest that intermediate chemicals and mechanisms, which operate between the already known biophysical processes, play a part in labor, but at this time many questions remain to be answered about this complex human event.

The Four Forces

Four forces, commonly called the "Four P's" are of critical importance in labor and delivery. They are passage, passenger, power, and psyche. The passage involves the size of the pelvis, its shape, the ability of the cervix to dilate, and the vagina's ability to stretch. In a normal pregnancy, the pelvic anatomy (passage) must be adequate for the fetus. The fetus (passenger) must be in an advantageous position, and the contractions of the uterus (power) must be rhythmic, coordinated, and efficient. The maternal efforts (psyche) must be adequate to accomplish delivery of the fetus (Neeson, 1987; Ladewig, London & Olds, 1990).

Powers

As the passenger moves through the passage, the powers involve the frequency, duration, and intensity of the contractions of the uterus (Neeson, 1987; Ladewig, London & Olds, 1990). They also involve the effectiveness of abdominal pressures from pushing during the second stage of labor. Primary and secondary powers work in concert, accomplishing the expulsion of the fetus, the fetal membranes, and the placenta from the uterus. The primary power is the contraction of the uterine muscles, which causes the changes in the first stage of labor—the effacement and dilatation of the cervix. The secondary power is the use of the abdominal muscles in pushing during the second stage of labor. This pushing adds to the primary power following full dilatation of the cervix.

Uterine contractions

The purposes of uterine contractions are the effacement and dilatation of the cervix, the facilitation of the descent and rotation of the fetus, the separation and expulsion of the placenta following birth, and the maintenance of hemostasis after expulsion (Neeson, 1987; Ladewig, London & Olds, 1990; Martin, 1990). Uterine contractions are rhythmic and intermittent; between each one is a period of relaxation. The relaxation serves two purposes, providing a respite for the mother and the uterine muscles and permitting restoration of utero-placental circulation.

Contractions have three phases:

- The *increment* or *building-up,* which is usually the longest part of the contraction;

- The *acme* or *peak,* which is the shortest but most intense part;

- The *decrement* or *letting-up,* a rapid diminishing of the contraction.

In describing labor contractions, the terms *frequency, regularity, duration,* and *intensity* are used.

- **Frequency** is the time between the beginning of one contraction and the beginning of the next. Contractions may start at 10 to 15 minutes apart, progressing to intervals as close as 2 to 3 minutes apart in later labor.

- **Regularity** refers to the rhythmic pattern of contractions that occurs as labor becomes well established.

- **Duration** is measured from the contraction's increment to its decrement. In early labor, the duration is usually about 30 seconds, but in later labor, a range of 45 to 90 seconds is normal.

- **Intensity** is the strength of the contraction during the acme. It may be established sujectively by palpation (judging the amount of indentability of the uterine wall at the acme) by indirect or external tocodynamometer, or may be measured directly by the use of an intrauterine pressure catheter. Intensity, which increases as labor intensifies, is assessed subjectively as mild, moderate, or strong. In normal labor, the intensity or amplitude of the contraction varies from 30 to 55 mm Hg intrauterine pressure, with a frequency of 2 to 5 contractions every 10 minutes. In prolonged labor, the intensity may be less than 25 mm Hg, with a frequency of less than 2 per 10 minutes. No labor is occurring if the intensity is less than 15 mm Hg.

The Passage

The passage is determined by the maternal pelvic anatomy—the bony pelvis and the muscles of the pelvic floor and perineum (*see figure 5-1*). The true pelvis, which forms the bony canal through which the baby travels, is composed of three planes: the inlet, the pelvic cavity or mid-pelvis, and the outlet. In an adequate pelvis, the pubic arch should be wide and rounded at 90 degrees or more, and the ischial spines should be blunt. A flat or convex sacrum will increase the pelvic capacity. With the exception of some relaxation of the pelvic joints, due to hormonal influences, the pelvis cannot expand. The relationship of fetal head size to the pelvis is a very important factor in labor, as is the ability of the fetal head to change its shape (mold) to fit through the pelvis (Neeson, 1987; Ladewig, London & Olds, 1990; Martin, 1990).

There are four classic types of pelves, differentiated by their shapes, diameters, and angles:

1. The *gynecoid,* or typical female pelvis, found in 50% of women, is adequate for labor and birth.

2. The *android,* or typical male pelvis, characterized by narrow dimensions, is found in 20% of women. It often causes slow descent of the fetal head, a stoppage of labor, and the necessity of forceps delivery.

3. The *anthropoid,* or apelike pelvis, is found in 25 to 40% of women. It is narrowed from side to side and widened from front to back. Its diameters are generally adequate for labor and birth.

4. The *platypelloid* pelvis, characterized by front to back narrowing and side-to-side widening, is found in 3 to 5% of women. Its diameters usually are not adequate for vaginal birth, and this

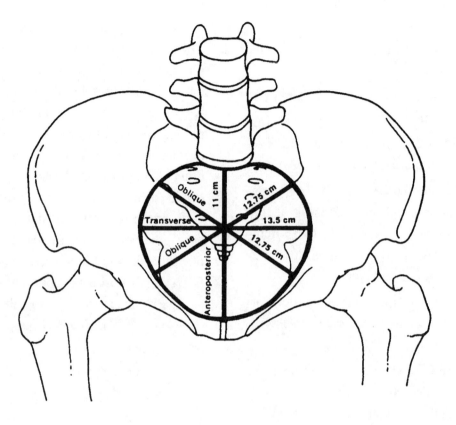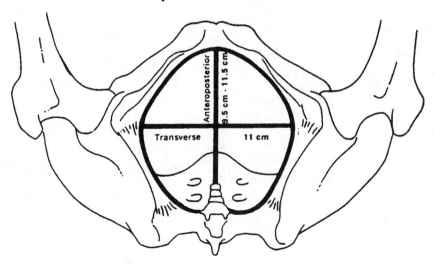

FIGURE 5-1
The Normal Female Pelvis

pelvic inlet

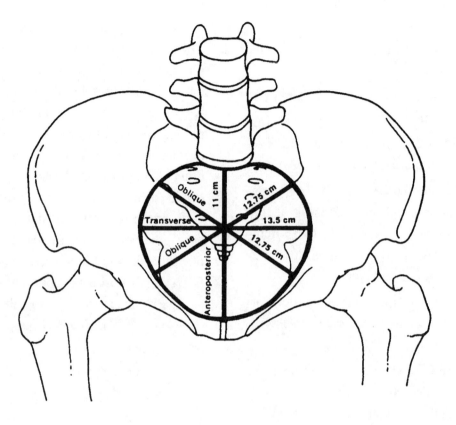

pelvic outlet

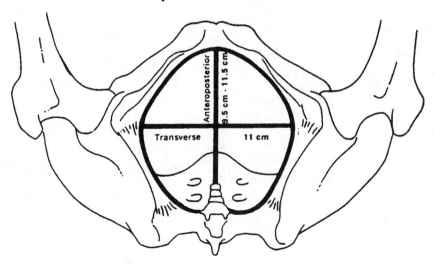

Source: Ross Labs, © 1980

type of pelvis frequently causes a delay in the descent of the fetus.

Women may have a combination of characteristics from these classic types of pelvises.

Measurements of the pelvis can be done by pelvic examination, usually at the time of the first prenatal visit and again toward the end of the pregnancy or during labor.

The cervix: effacement and dilatation

As the myometrium (uterine musculature) contracts, the uterus divides into two segments. This process is known as the physiological retraction ring, during which the upper (contractile) segment thickens, shortens, becomes more powerful, and with each contraction exerts a longitudinal traction on the cervix. The lower portion of the uterus, which includes the cervix, becomes thinner, softer, and more relaxed, allowing the baby to be pushed out at birth. As the fundal segment contracts, the downward pressure is transmitted to the cervix, causing effacement, a thinning and dilatation of the cervix. Partial or complete effacement often precedes labor in a primapara. In the multipara, the cervix may be effaced as much as 50% before labor. Effacement is evaluated in percentages during labor, from 0%, indicating no effacement, to 100%, meaning complete effacement (Neeson, 1987; Ladewig, London & Olds, 1990; Martin, 1990).

Cervical dilatation is the opening or enlargement of the external cervical os, from a few mm during pregnancy to as much as 10 cm at complete dilatation. It results from the hydrostatic pressure of the amniotic sac and from the elongation of the uterus that occurs with each contraction (Ladewig, London & Olds, 1990). As the fetal body straightens out, its upper portion presses against the fundus of the uterus, and its presenting part is thrust toward the lower uterine segment and the cervix (fetal axis pressure). As the cervix is drawn up over the baby into the uterine side walls, it becomes

transformed from a long, thick structure to one that is as thin as tissue paper, thus allowing for the baby's descent. When the cervix is totally dilated, it can no longer be palpated. The round ligament then pulls the fundus forward, thus aligning the fetus with the bony pelvis.

The Passenger

Fetal head landmarks

In labor and birth, the head is generally the presenting, most important, largest, and least compressible part of the fetus (Neeson, 1987). It is composed both of fixed and flexible bony parts, which can make childbirth either easier or more difficult (Ladewig, London & Olds, 1990). Once the head has been delivered, the birth of the rest of the body is usually accomplished without difficulty (Martin, 1990). The fetal head is composed of three major divisions: the face, the base of the skull (or cranium), and the vault of the cranium (or roof) (Ladewig, London & Olds, 1990). The bones of both the cranial base and the face are fused and fixed. At the cranial base are two temporal bones, each having a sphenoid and ethmoid bone. The vault is composed of two frontal bones, two parietal bones, and the occipital bone, none of which are fused, thus allowing this part of the head to adjust in shape as the passenger travels through the narrow portions of the pelvis. The cranial bones have the ability to "mold" or overlap under the pressure of labor, generally without damage to the underlying tissue. This molding can be felt during vaginal examination (Neeson, 1987; Martin, 1990).

Identifying landmarks of the fetal skull will assist you in performing vaginal examinations to determine the progression of the mother's labor and the position of the fetal skull. Suture and fontanel landmarks are used in describing the fetal head. The sutures are membranous spaces between the cranial bones. The fontanels are spaces covered by membranes, located at the intersections of the cranial sutures (Ladewig, London & Olds, 1990).

The important sutures of the cranial vault are, the saggital suture, the coronal suture, and the lambdoidal suture (Martin, 1990). The two clinically useful landmarks formed by the sutures are:

- The diamond-shaped anterior fontanel (or bregma), measuring 2 cm to 3 cm, which permits growth of the brain by remaining unossified for up to 18 months following birth; and

- The posterior fontanel, which is smaller, triangular-shaped, and marks the meeting point of the saggital and lambdoidal sutures. If not already closed at birth, it closes within the first three months of life.

Other important landmarks of the fetal skull are the sinciput (brow), the vertex (the area between the anterior and posterior fontanels), the occiput (the area beneath the posterior fontanel where the occipital bone is located), and the mentum (fetal chin) (Martin, 1990).

Fetal attitude

Fetal attitude is the relation of the fetal parts to each other. The normal fetal attitude is one of moderate flexion of the head, with the arms flexed onto the chest and the legs flexed onto the abdomen (Neeson, 1987; Ladewig, London & Olds, 1990; Martin, 1990). Changes in fetal attitude, particularly in the head's position, cause the fetus to present larger diameters of its head to the pelvis. These changes often contribute to difficult labor.

In the attitude of extension, with the head bent back and the chest and abdomen slightly curved, the fetal face is the leading part as it travels through the pelvis. This attitude causes fetal trauma and often prevents vaginal delivery, since a larger diameter of the fetal head is presenting than in the normal attitude of flexion.

The military attitude occurs when the fetal position is not one of flexion nor extension. Partial extension occurs when there is a moderate extension of the head.

The cephalic prominence is that part of the fetal head felt by placing both hands on the sides of the uterus and feeling down toward the pelvis (Martin, 1990). In normal flexion, the cephalic prominence is felt on the opposite side of the fetal back. In hyperextension, the cephalic prominence is felt on the same side as the fetal back.

Fetal lie

Fetal lie is the relationship of the long (cephalocaudal) axis of the fetus to the long (cephalocaudal) axis of the mother (Raff & Freisner, 1989). The fetus can assume either a longitudinal or transverse lie. A longitudinal lie, which occurs in 99.5% of all pregnancies, occurs when the cephalocaudal axis of the fetus is parallel to the mother's spine (Neeson, 1987). A transverse lie, found in .5% of pregnancies, occurs when the cephalocaudal axis of the fetus is at right angles to the mother's spine (Ladewig, London & Olds, 1990). Only a longitudinal lie is normal. A longitudinal lie can be either cephalic or breech. When the head is leading, it is called a cephalic lie (Martin, 1990). If the buttocks come first, it is called a breech lie. A transverse lie often occurs in grandmultiparity (women having five or more pregnancies), in women with a small or contracted pelvis, or in placenta previa. Vaginal delivery is not possible with a transverse lie.

Fetal presentation

Fetal presentation is determined by the fetal lie and by the body part that enters the pelvic passageway first (see figure 5-2). This portion of the fetus is called the presenting part (Ladewig, London & Olds, 1990). The most common presentation, cephalic (or vertex), occurs in 95% of labors. Breech presentations occur in about 4% of labors. Shoulder presentations, which occur infrequently, result from a transverse lie (Martin, 1990).

In a cephalic presentation, the head is the presenting part. Cephalic presentations are further classified according to the degree of flexion or extension (attitude) of the fetal head (Ladewig, London & Olds, 1990; Martin, 1990):

- The most common type of cephalic presentation is the vertex, in which the head is completely flexed on the chest, the chin in contact with the thorax, and the occiput presenting.

- In a face presentation, the neck may be sharply extended so that the occiput and back come in contact. The face is the presenting part.

- In the sinciputal (or military) presentation, the head is moderately flexed in a position intermediate between a vertex and face presentation, with the large fontanel presenting.

- In the brow presentation, the fetal head is partially extended so that the brow becomes the presenting part.

The type of presentation will largely determine the course of labor. Cephalic presentations pose the least risk to mother and baby, since the presenting part has the smallest diameter. A brow presentation poses a greater degree of risk to mother and baby, since the largest diameter of the head is the presenting part. However, as labor progresses in a delivery with a sinciputal or brow presentation, there is often a conversion to a vertex presentation by flexion, or to a face presentation through extension. Delivery with a brow presentation can result in severe perineal laceration to the woman, and in excessive molding of the baby's head. In some cases of persistent brow presentation, a Cesarean delivery is indicated. A face presentation also increases the risk of perineal laceration, and often causes bruising and swelling of the baby's face, with its head appearing elongated and flat. However, these conditions will gradually disappear, with no resulting permanent damage.

Breech presentations are classified in several ways, according to the attitude of the fetus' hips and knees (Pillitteri, 1995) *(see figure 5-2)*. In all variations of breech presentations, the sacrum is the landmark to be noted. The classifications are as follows:

- *Complete breech,* in which the feet and legs are flexed on thighs, thighs are flexed on abdomen. The buttocks and feet present to the maternal pelvis.

- *Frank breech,* in which the fetal hips and thighs are flexed, and the legs and knees are extended over the anterior surfaces of the body. The buttocks present to the maternal pelvis.

- *Foot or footling breech* (also called *incomplete breech)* is designated when one or both feet present. The fetal hips and legs are extended in this presentation.

- *Incomplete foot or knee presentation,* in which one leg may retain position for full or frank breech, while the other foot or knee may present.

- A *kneeling breech,* in which one or both knees are the presenting part.

A shoulder presentation occurs when the fetus has assumed a transverse lie (Martin, 1990). The scapula, trunk, or arm can be the presenting part. Generally, the fetus is in an attitude of complete flexion, with one shoulder lower and the back facing the mother's back or abdominal wall. In this case, a Cesarean delivery is usually indicated.

Compound presentations, in which a fetal extremity presents along with the presenting part, are rare. The most common type of compound presentation is a hand alongside the presenting head. This presentation generally causes no problems, since the hand either remains in the same position or else slides upward into the uterus as the head advances. If the arm does not rise, fundal pressure may be used to push it upward. Some compound presentations are complicated by prolapse of the umbilical cord, and in this situation immediate obstetrical manipulation or Cesarean delivery is indicated.

FIGURE 5-2 *(1 of 2)*
Categories of Presentation

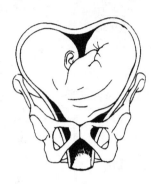

Shoulder Presentation

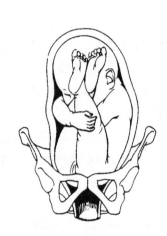

Frank Breech

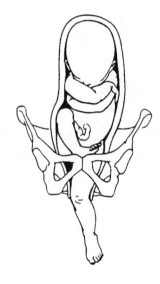

Incomplete Breech

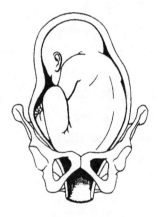

Left Sacral Anterior

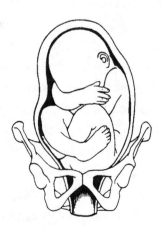

Left Sacral Posterior

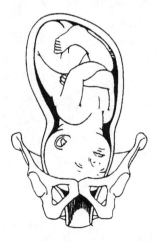

Brow Presentation

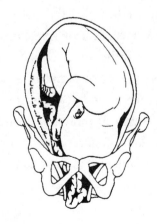

Prolapse of Cord

FIGURE 5-2 *(2 of 2)*
Categories of Presentation

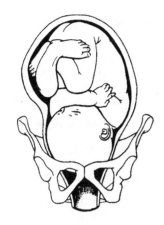
Left Occipital Posterior

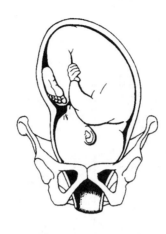
Left Occipital Transverse

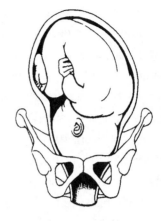
Left Occipital Anterior

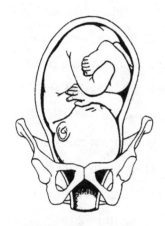
Right Occipital Posterior

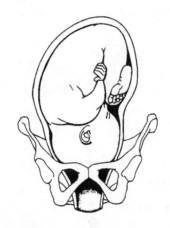
Right Occipital Transverse

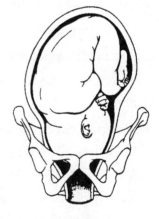
Right Occipital Anterior

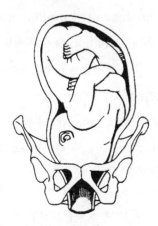
Left Mentum Anterior

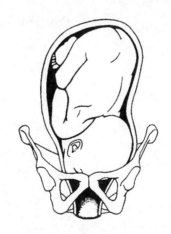
Right Mentum Posterior

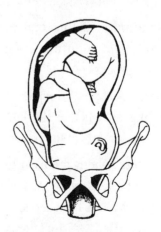
Right Mentum Anterior

Fetal position

In addition to the lie and presentation of the fetus, its position must also be established. To determine position, a point (or landmark) of the fetus' presenting part is described in relation to the mother's right or left side and to her front or back. The landmark of the fetus' presenting part is stated in relation to four imaginary quadrants of the pelvis: left anterior, right anterior, left posterior, and right posterior (Neeson, 1987; Ladewig, London & Olds, 1990; Martin, 1990). These quadrants describe whether the presenting part is directed toward the front, back, left, or right of the passage. Fixed points on the fetus are designated as:

- Occiput, in a vertex presentation.
- Frontum (or forehead), in a brow presentation.
- Mentum, in a face presentation.
- Sacrum, in a breech presentation.
- Acromion process of the scapula, in a shoulder presentation.

If the landmark is directed toward the center of the side of the pelvis, the fetal position is designated as transverse rather than anterior or posterior.

In describing fetal position, three notations are used:

1. Right (R) or left (L) side of the maternal pelvis.
2. The landmark of the fetal presenting part: Occiput (O); mentum (M); sacrum (S); acromion process (A).
3. Anterior (A), posterior (P), transverse (T), depending on whether the landmark is in the front, back, or side of the pelvis.

These abbreviations are used by the healthcare team to describe fetal position. For example, when the occiput faces to the front and left of the pelvis, the abbreviation used is LOA (for left-occiput-anterior).

"Dorsal," referring to the fetus' back, denotes a transverse lie (Ladewig, London & Olds, 1990). In this situation, RADA would indicate that the scapula's acromion process faces the mother's back and that the fetus' back is anterior.

Positions in the vertex presentation are

ROA	Right-occiput-anterior
ROT	Right-occiput-transverse
ROP	Right-occiput-posterior
LOA	Left-occiput-anterior
LOT	Left-occiput-transverse
LOP	Left-occiput-posterior

Positions in the face presentation are

RMA	Right-mentum-anterior
RMT	Right-mentum-transverse
RMP	Right-mentum-posterior
LMA	Left-mentum-anterior
LMT	Left-mentum-transverse
LMP	Left-mentum-posterior

Positions in breech presentation are

RSA	Right-sacrum-anterior
RST	Right-sacrum-transverse
RSP	Right-sacrum-posterior
LSA	Left-sacrum-anterior
LST	Left-sacrum-transverse
LSP	Left-sacrum-posterior

Positions in the shoulder presentation are

RADA	Right-acromion-dorsal-anterior
RADP	Right-acromion-dorsal-posterior
LADA	Left-acromion-dorsal-anterior
LADP	Left-acromion-dorsal-posterior

Fetal position exerts a vast influence on labor and birth. The most common position is occiput-anterior, and in this position labor generally proceeds normally. A posterior position, which increases pressure on the mother's sacral nerves, causes backache and pelvic pressure in labor, and may cause excessive bearing down and pushing earlier than normal. In the last trimester, the fetus' position and presentation can be provisionally determined by routine abdominal inspection and palpation. However, changes in position may occur before engagement (the time when the widest segment of the presenting part has passed through the pelvic inlet).

Other methods of determining presentation and position are vaginal examination, ultrasonography, magnetic resonance imaging (MRI), and X-ray examination. However, since frequent X-rays and those done in early pregnancy can harm the fetus, X-rays are taken only when there is no other means of determining fetal position.

Fetal station

Fetal station refers to the relationship of the fetus' presenting part to an imaginary line drawn between the ischial spines, the blunted prominences that are about halfway between the mother's pelvic inlet and pelvic outlet (*see figure 5-3*) (Ladewig, London & Olds, 1990; Martin, 1990). In a normal pelvis, the ischial spines mark the narrowest diameter through which the fetus must pass. As a landmark, the ischial spines are designated as "zero station," thus, when the presenting part of the fetus is at the level of the ischial spines, it is said to be at zero station. (This is called engagement.) The long axis of the birth canal above and below the ischial spines is divided into thirds. If the presenting part is higher than the spines, a negative number is assigned, noting centimeters above zero station. Thus, if the presenting part is at the level of the pelvic inlet, it is said to be at -3 station. If it has descended two-thirds the distance past the inlet, it is at -1 station. A similar division is assigned to the distances between the ischial spines and the pelvic outlet. If the presenting part is one-third to two-thirds the distance between the spines and the outlet, it is at +1 or +2 station. When it descends into the bony outlet, it is at +3 station, and when it is at the outlet, it is at +4 station.

In normal labor, the presenting part moves from negative stations to the mid-pelvis at 0 station, then into the positive stations. Failure of the presenting part to descend under the influence of strong contractions may be due to a disproportion between the maternal pelvis and the presenting part or to a short and/or entangled umbilical cord. Descent can be determined by vaginal examination.

The Psyche

The psychosocial adaptation of a woman to her labor and delivery is of utmost importance (Neeson, 1987; Ladewig, London & Olds, 1990). For the woman facing her first labor, and even for the multipara, each labor is a new experience, bringing many attendant fears and doubts—fear of physical injury, doubt about meeting her and her family's expectations of her as a parent, worry about life style disruption, and concerns about ongoing relationships and self-image. The woman's perception is influenced by her self-confidence, her manner of coping with uncertainty and stress, her attitudes and expectations about labor and birth, her expectations about her family and healthcare providers, and her response to pain, anxiety, and other alterations of functioning. Certain psychosocial factors may predict progress in labor. Those women who have prepared for labor by attending childbirth education classes, by reading, or by networking, seem to cope better with the rigors of labor. Fantasizing about labor also seems to prepare the woman to cope. Other factors associated with a positive birth experience include the woman's motivation for pregnancy, her sense of competence or mastery, a positive relationship with her mate, maintaining control during labor, support from her mate or other person during labor, and not being left alone in labor. Researchers have also found that the manner in which the woman views the birth experience after delivery may significantly influence her mothering behavior.

SIGNS AND SYMPTOMS OF LABOR

In primiparas as well as in multiparas, the premonitory signs of labor are as follows (Raff & Freisner, 1989; Ladewig, London & Olds, 1990):

- **Lightening (or engagement),** at which time the fetal head begins to settle into the pelvic inlet *(see figure 5-3)*. As the fetus descends, the uterus moves downward, and as the fundus ceases to press on the diaphragm, the woman is able to breathe more easily. Lightening generally occurs ten days to two weeks before labor in a primagravida, but may not happen until true labor begins in a multigravida. As the downward pressure of the presenting part increases, the woman may evidence pain or cramps in her legs due to pressure within the obdurator foramen in the pelvis, increased vaginal secretion due to congestion of the vaginal mucous membranes, urinary frequency, or increased venous stasis leading to edema.

- **Ripening of the cervix**

  A few days before the onset of labor, the cervix will soften (or ripen), and will commence to efface and dilate slightly. Ripening is a biochemical mechanism due to changes in the cervix's connective tissue.

- **Bloody show**

  During pregnancy, a mucous plug accumulates cervical secretions and seals off the uterine cavity as a protective device. As softening and effacement occur, and as small cervical capillaries rupture, the mucous plug often is expelled. Blood will mix with the mucous, resulting in pink-tinged secretions.

- **Rupture of the membranes (ROM)**

  In about 12% of women, the amniotic sac

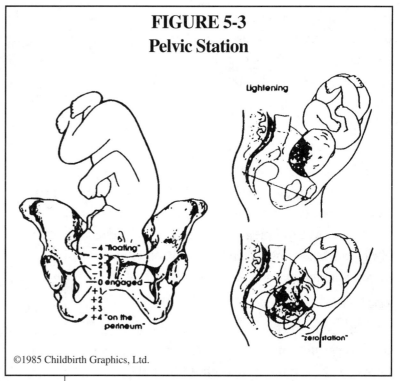

FIGURE 5-3
Pelvic Station

©1985 Childbirth Graphics, Ltd.

(membranes) rupture prior to labor's onset, causing either a gush or a leakage of amniotic fluid. However, in the majority of cases, ROM will occur during the actual labor process. When rupture occurs before the onset of labor, 80% of women will go into spontaneous labor within 24 hours. If ROM occurs when the pregnancy is near term and if labor does not ensue within 12 to 24 hours, it may be necessary to induce labor. If the membranes rupture before engagement, in addition to the risk of umbilical cord prolapse, the woman runs the risk of infection due to the open pathway to her uterus. Patients must be taught to notify their healthcare providers immediately following ROM, and told to proceed immediately to the hospital or birthing center. In addition, the patient must be taught to check the source of leakage to distinguish between slight leakage and urinary incontinence, which may be associated with urgency, coughing, or sneezing.

- A sudden burst of energy may occur a day or two before labor, often referred to as the "nesting instinct." Nurses should advise patients not to overexert or tire themselves excessively when this occurs, in order to conserve their strength for labor.

- Early contractions, experienced as low back pain, may occur due to sacroiliac pressure as the relax in hormone exerts its influence on the pelvic joints.

- Abdominal cramps

- Diarrhea, indigestion, nausea, or vomiting

- Weight loss of 1 to 3 pounds, caused by fluid loss and hormonal changes

False Labor

False labor is characterized by Braxton-Hicks contractions which are irregular and do not increase in intensity, duration, or frequency, and are usually confined to the lower abdomen, groin, or back. Contractions may cease with walking or a change of position, and will generally stop with the use of relaxation techniques. There is no change of fetal position, no further descent of the head, and the cervix will not further soften or efface (Neeson, 1987; Raff & Freisner, 1989; Ladewig, London & Olds, 1990).

True Labor

In true labor, contractions occur at slow, regular intervals. The interval between the contractions progressively shortens, while the intensity increases. True labor contractions are generally felt in the back and radiate to the abdomen, and are not stopped by the use of relaxation techniques. There will be an increase in cervical dilatation and effacement, and a further descent of the fetus' presenting part will be noted.

Because false labor is common and cannot be distinguished from true labor except by vaginal examination, the patient must be advised to contact her healthcare provider and to come in for an assessment of her labor. The patient should also be taught the characteristics of true labor and labor's premonitory signs.

THE FOUR STAGES OF LABOR

The four stages of labor have clear lines of demarcation. The first stage starts with the beginning of true contractions and terminates with full dilatation and effacement of the cervix. The second stage starts at full dilatation and ends when the delivery of the baby has been completed. The third stage begins following the infant's birth and ends with the delivery of the placenta. The fourth stage follows delivery of the placenta and continues until the uterus is fully contracted and bleeding is controlled at the placental site (Raff & Freisner, 1989; Ladewig, London & Olds, 1990; Martin, 1990).

The First Stage

The first stage of labor is divided into three phases: the latent (early) phase; the active phase; and the transition phase (see *figure 5-4*).

The latent phase begins with the first true contraction, as the cervix starts to dilate and to efface. In the primigravida, the latent phase generally lasts from 6 to 18 hours, but should not exceed 20 hours. In multiparas, the range is from 2 to 10 hours, with the average about 5.3 hours and the top limit 14 hours. Uterine contractions become established, increasing in frequency, duration, and intensity. They may start mildly, occurring at 20 to 30 minute intervals, with short duration and mild intensity, then become moderate, lasting from 30 to 40 seconds, and occurring every 5 to 7 minutes. During this phase the woman is usually able to cope with the discomfort, although she may evidence anxiety and/or elation.

During the active phase, contractions occur approximately every 2 to 3 minutes, generally last about 60 seconds, with stronger intensity. The cervix dilates from about 3 to 4 cm to 8 cm, and fetal descent progresses. The woman's anxiety

FIGURE 5-4
Phases of the First Stage of Labor

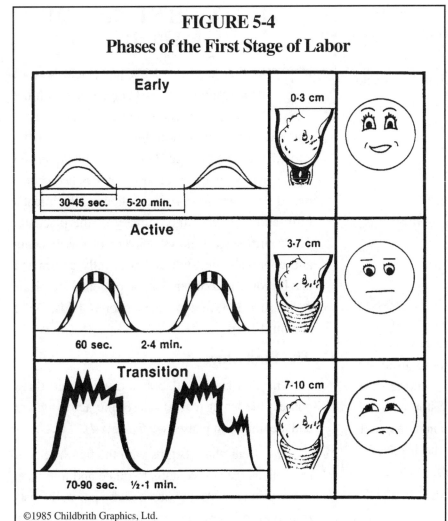

©1985 Childbrith Graphics, Ltd.

increases, and she may have a decreased ability to cope.

The transition phase ends the first stage of labor, with contractions coming every one and one half to two minutes, lasting from 60 to 90 seconds, with increased intensity. The woman may become significantly anxious, restless, and experience fear of abandonment. She should be assured that she will not be left alone. She may also become withdrawn, may doubt her ability to cope, or become apprehensive and irritable. She may be restless, bewildered, and have difficulty understanding directions. Other characteristics of the transition phase are hyperventilation, profuse perspiration, nausea, vomiting, and violent shaking. Rectal pressure increases as dilatation approaches 10 cm, and the woman will have an uncontrollable desire to bear down. Bloody show and rupture of the membranes may occur.

The Second Stage

The second stage of labor starts at full dilatation of the cervix (10 cm) and lasts until the baby is born. Contractions continue at one and one-half to two minutes, lasting from 60 to 90 seconds, and are of very strong intensity. This stage usually lasts from 30 minutes to 3 hours in a primigravida, and from 5 to 30 minutes in a multigravida. The bearing-down reflex appears spontaneously, bloody show increases, and pressure on the rectum causes the woman to have the desire to defecate. As the fetal head descends, the perineum bulges, flattens, and moves anteriorly, and the labia begin to part.

"Crowning" occurs when the fetal head becomes visible on the perineal floor between contractions. "Caput" (the baby's head) becomes visible, and birth is imminent. At this point, the childbirth-prepared woman may feel relief, coupled with a sense of control, while the unprepared woman may evidence fear, fight contractions, and reject the attempts of others to persuade her to push.

The Third Stage

This stage occurs following the birth of the baby until placental separation, and usually lasts from 5 to 10 minutes. The uterus contracts, causing the placenta to separate, resulting in a gush of bleeding. The uterus becomes globular as the membranes peel off the uterine wall, and the umbilical cord and the placenta descend into the vagina. Bearing down by the mother aids expulsion.

The Fourth Stage

From 1 to 4 hours following delivery, the mother recovers from any anesthesia that she has been given, and her vital signs, bleeding, and fundal muscle tone stabilize. The uterus remains contracted, nausea and vomiting cease, and the woman may become thirsty, hungry, or chilled. This stage is critical because of the danger of hemorrhage.

LABOR PATTERNS

Friedman Curve

Evaluation of the intensity, frequency, and duration of contractions does not fully document the progress of labor. However, it is possible to further document progress by an objective means, using a graph that evaluates three factors: uterine activity, cervical dilatation, and fetal descent. The graph, which resulted from studies done by Dr. Emanuel Friedman, an obstetrician, shows that cervical dilatation and fetal descent occur within time frames that can be plotted. Use of the graph has helped establish normal time limits for different phases of labor in the nullipara and the multipara (Ladewig, London & Olds, 1990; Martin, 1990).

The Friedman curve requires special graph paper as well as special skill in determining cervical dilatation and fetal descent. The numbers at the bottom of the graph indicate hours of labor. Vertically, at the left, dilatation is measured in centimeters. Vertically, at the right, fetal station is indicated, also in centimeters. By plotting cervical dilatation and fetal descent, a basic pattern emerges. An "S" curve represents dilatation, and an inverse "S" curve indicates descent. Evaluating the progress of labor by means of the Friedman curve helps the healthcare team identify normal and abnormal labor patterns.

By using the graph, Dr. Friedman identified some of the patterns that emerge in normal labor:

- Most nulliparas achieve exactly 2 cm of dilatation during the 4th hour of labor. At 10 hours, 3 cm of dilatation has occurred. After this, dilatation progresses rapidly, and the nullipara achieves full dilatation after 14 hours of labor.

- The multiparous woman reaches full dilatation after an average of eight hours of labor.

- The rate of cervical dilatation during the active phase is 1.2 cm or more per hour in nulliparas, and 1.5 cm or more per hour in multiparas.

- The length of the first stage of labor ranges from 13.3 hours to 28.5 hours for the nullipara, and from 7.5 hours to 20 hours for the multipara.

- Fetal descent in the nullipara occurs at about 1 cm per hour in the active phase; in the multipara, it occurs at about 2 cm per hour or faster in the active phase.

VARIABLES AFFECTING LABOR

In most instances, labor and birth are accomplished with few problems. However, when complications do arise, they develop quickly and present risks both to mother and baby. Healthcare providers must identify the problem and swiftly intervene to reduce or limit detrimental effects (Neeson, 1987). Some of the variables are discussed below:

Dystocia is defined as an abnormal or difficult labor due to mechanical factors produced by the fetus or the maternal pelvis, or due to inadequate uterine or other muscular activity (Ladewig, London & Olds, 1990). To successfully complete the gestational period, the four forces (passage, passenger, powers, and psyche) must function harmoniously. Disruptions in any of these four components may affect the others and cause dystocia (Neeson, 1987). It may result from malpresentation or malposition, such as a large, less compressible head delivering last in breech position, and may cause the fetus muscle damage, or cause it to aspirate amniotic fluid or meconium (Ladewig, London & Olds, 1990). Shoulder dystocia occurs when the fetal head is born but the shoulders are too broad to deliver between the symphysis and the sacrum. This condition is often found in large neonates with high birth weight, such as those born of diabetic or prediabetic mothers. Dystocia can also be caused by a tight pelvic outlet.

Dysfunctional labor is caused by complications of the powers, and involves problems with the frequency, duration, and intensity of contractions and/or the resting tone of the uterus between contractions (Ladewig, London & Olds, 1990). The deviations in dysfunctional labor are hypertonic labor, hypotonic labor, prolonged labor, and precipitate labor (Martin, 1990). Dysfunctional labor can occur either in a prolonged phase or an active phase, as slow progress (protraction) or failure of progress (arresting).

Hypotonic labor, formerly called secondary uterine dysfunction, occurs during the active phase, causing ineffectual contractions and a lack of progression of labor (Ladewig, London & Olds, 1990). It is characterized by irregularly occurring contractions (less than two to three contractions within a 10-minute period) of short duration, which do not cause the mother much discomfort. Causes may include overstretching of the uterus by a multiple pregnancy, a large fetus, hydramnios, grandmultiparity, bladder or bowel distention, weak abdominal muscles, emotional factors, cervical rigidity, too early use of analgesia, fatigue, pelvic disproportion, and fetal malposition. Hypotonic labor exposes the fetus to the dangers of anoxia, brain injury, and sepsis, and puts the mother at risk for exhaustion, dehydra-

tion, infection, hemorrhage, and mental strain (Raff & Freisner, 1989).

Hypertonic labor, formerly called primary uterine inertia, is one in which ineffectual uterine contractions of poor quality occur in the latent phase, before acute cervical dilatation begins and when the myometrium's resting tone increases (Ladewig, London & Olds, 1990). Contractions may become more frequent and painful, but are weak, ineffectual, and uncoordinated, and do not dilate or efface the cervix. Causes of hypertonic labor include muscle weakness, nerve defects, overdistention of the uterus due to multiple births or hydramnios, and emotional factors. It causes fetal distress, since contractions and increased resting tone interfere with the uteroplacental exchanges. Prolonged pressure on the fetal head may also result in cephalhematoma, caput succedaneum (swelling or edema of the fetal scalp), and excessive molding. The mother risks discomfort from lack of oxygen to the uterine muscle cells, and also risks fatigue, dehydration, infection, and stress (Raff & Freisner, 1989).

Prolonged labor lasts over 24 hours without spontaneous delivery. Generally the first stage is prolonged with the latent or active phase longer than normal. Prolonged labor is more common in nulliparas, and its principal causes are myometrial dysfunction, cephalopelvic disproportion, malpresentations, malpositions, and cervical dystocia. It can also be influenced by the overuse of analgesics, anesthetics, and sedatives during the latent phase of labor. It poses the risk of fetal distress, infection, and cord prolapse after ROM, if the presenting part is not well engaged. Maternal implications include exhaustion, intrauterine infection, and bleeding due to inadequate uterine contractions in the third stage and the postpartum period (Neeson, 1987; Ladewig, London & Olds, 1990; Martin, 1990).

Precipitate labor is when labor lasts for less than 3 hours before spontaneous delivery. It occurs when there is a low resistance of the soft parts of the maternal tissue, permitting easy and fast passage of the fetus through the passageway; in multiparity; in women who have had previous precipitate labors; when the fetus is small and in the vertex position; and when contractions are strong (Raff & Freisner, 1989; Ladewig, London & Olds, 1990; Martin, 1990).

Precipitate labor and precipitate delivery are not the same. A precipitate delivery is unexpected, sudden, and frequently unattended. In a precipitate labor, maternal problems are rare when the tissues are pliable and the cervix is effaced and dilated. The mother risks complications when the cervix is long and firm, when contractions are sufficiently vigorous to cause uterine rupture, when maternal tissues are firm and resistant to stretching, causing lacerations of the cervix, vagina, and perineum. Other risks include uterine rupture, amniotic fluid embolism, postpartal hemorrhage due to undetected lacerations and/or inadequate post-delivery contractions, and loss of the ability to cope. The fetus risks distress, hypoxia from decreased uteroplacental circulation caused by intense contractions of the uterus, and trauma to the head (Raff & Freisner, 1989; Ladewig, London & Olds, 1990; Martin, 1990).

Nursing Care in the Unexpected Delivery

Labor may sometimes progress so quickly that the nurse must assist with the actual precipitate birth. This may happen if the woman has had a history of rapid labors, if she is having a precipitate labor, if she must travel a distance in active labor, or if the baby is very small. However, an emergency delivery can be well planned and can provide a safe and satisfying experience for the woman (Neeson, 1987; Ladewig, London & Olds, 1990; Martin, 1990). The signs of an impending delivery have been discussed earlier in this chapter (see "The second stage of labor," page 74). In this event, the nurse must support and reassure both the mother and her support person, and must alleviate the mother's fear of abandonment by staying with her. Other important objectives for nurses attending an unexpected birth include preventing maternal trauma, infection (i.e., by using Standard Precautions), and neonatal hypothermia; establishing effective neonatal respiratory effort; and, minimizing maternal blood loss (May & Mahlmeister, 1994). Each work environment should have specific policies, procedures, and training to address these objectives.

Auxiliary personnel can contact the physician or nurse-midwife and retrieve the "precip pack," a sterile emergency birth pack that should be kept ready at all times. A typical pack will contain the following: 4 by 4 gauze sponges, 2 absorbent towels, a soft bulb syringe, a small drape, 2 clamps (Kelly or Rochester), a cord clamp or umbilical tape, scissors, gloves, a baby blanket, and a suction catheter.

While reassuring the mother and encouraging her to take a comfortable position, the nurse scrubs (time permitting), puts on sterile gloves, and places a sterile barrier on the woman's hips. The nurse instructs the woman to "feather blow" to control her expulsion efforts and explains that skin cleansing is being done. She then soaks the sterile swabs in antiseptic solution and scrubs the pubis, thighs, and perineal and rectal areas thoroughly—again, only if time permits. The nurse may "iron the perineum" to prevent laceration by placing an index finger inside the lower portion of the vagina and a thumb on the perineum. It is of utmost importance *not* to hold back delivery of the head by pushing against it or by crossing the woman's thighs.

When the head crowns, the woman must be instructed to pant, thus decreasing the pushing urge. If the amniotic sac is intact, the nurse uses the pads of the thumb, index, or middle fingers, or the cupped palm of the hand, to maintain flexion of the head and provide control, while she tears the sac to prevent the infant from aspirating amniotic fluid with its first breath. The nurse then allows the baby to be born between contractions.

As the woman pants, the nurse inserts one or two fingers along the back of the fetal head to check the umbilical cord. If it is wound around the neck (nuchal cord), the nurse bends her fingers and gently pulls it over the baby's head, checking that it is not wound around more than one time. If it cannot be slipped over the head, the cord must be clamped in two places, then cut between the clamps and unwound.

After the birth of the head, the nurse suctions the baby's mouth, throat, and nasal passages. Then, with one hand on either side of the head, she applies gentle downward traction until the anterior shoulder passes under the symphysis pubis. Gentle upward traction will help the delivery of the posterior shoulder. Instructing the woman to push gently, the nurse then supports the newborn as it emerges. The baby will be slippery, so it must be held carefully at the level of the uterus as it is again suctioned, then dried off.

Once the nurse determines that its respirations are adequate, the baby is placed on the mother's abdomen with its head slightly lower than its body, to aid drainage of fluid or mucus. Its weight will stimulate its mother's uterine contractions, which will aid in placental separation. The umbilical cord must *not* be pulled. Watching for signs of placental separation (a gush of dark blood, lengthening of the cord, or a change in the shape of the uterus to globular), the nurse instructs the mother to push and delivers the placenta, determining whether it is intact. The fundus is then massaged gently to stimulate contractions and reduce bleeding, and the baby may be put to its mother's breast.

Now the umbilical cord is cut by placing two sterile clamps about 1 to 3 inches from the newborn's abdomen and cutting between them with sterile scissors. A sterile cord clamp can be placed between the clamp on the newborn's abdomen and the actual abdomen, but it must not be placed snugly against the abdomen. Next, the area under the mother's buttocks is cleansed, and the perineum is inspected for lacerations. If bleeding has resulted from lacerations, a clean perineal pad is placed against the perineum and the woman's thighs.

Immediate care of the mother includes assessment of the firmness and position of the uterus, noting the color and amount of lochia, observing and recording her vital signs every 15 minutes, assessing the status of her bladder, and providing warmth and rest. In the event the newborn has respiratory distress, it must be transferred immediately to the nursery. No baby should be sent to the nursery without proper identification affixed.

Record-keeping must include the following: fetal presentation and position at birth; presence of cord around neck or shoulder; date and time of birth; Apgar scores at 1 and 5 minutes after birth; the newborn's sex; time of placental delivery; method of placental expulsion; appearance of cord; appearance and intactness of placenta; any lacerations to maternal tissue; any medication given to the mother or baby according to agency protocol; presence of birth injuries or abnormalities in the baby; estimation of maternal blood loss; anything unusual about the birth; first stooling or voiding by the baby; vital signs of both mother and baby; the nurse's name.

Untoward Situations

If meconium staining is present in the amniotic fluid, as soon as the head is delivered, and before the shoulders deliver, the oropharynx and nasopharynx must be suctioned out.

If shoulder dystocia occurs, do not use fundal pressure. Have the mother flex her knees as if in the knee-chest position, and have another staff member place both palms above the pubic bone to apply reasonable suprapubic pressure.

If excessive postpartum bleeding occurs, massage the top of the uterus, administer oxygen if needed, increase the rate of administration of intravenous fluids, and take and record blood pressure and pulse.

If there is laceration of the cervix or vagina, place the woman in a Trendelenburg position and increase the rate of administration of intravenous fluid.

When hematoma of the perineum or vagina occurs, send for a physician, increase intravenous fluid to greater than 125 ml/hour, take and record blood pressure and pulse, and chart the amount, color, and type of blood loss.

When the emergency delivery is a breech, avoid excessive handling of the delivering breech and prevent stress on the cord by gently pulling a loop free. After the breech, apply a warm towel to the baby, as if in a harness, and lift the body with the towel to deliver the shoulders. Lower the body after the shoulders deliver. Use suprapubic pressure to keep the head flexed. Once the baby's hairline is visible, use the towel to raise its body, and deliver the chin, mouth, nose, forehead, and top of the head. Cleanse the airway as soon as you see the mouth and nose.

If the nurse finds that she is assisting a woman giving birth unexpectedly, and they are not in a hospital or birthing center, the objectives previously discussed are still appropriate and attempts must be made to attain them as best as the situation and available equipment allow. The delivering woman should be coached to prevent expulsive pushing efforts and assisted into a Sims' or lateral position. The nurse should avoid touching the vagina during the birth process, but should support the perineum with a clean cloth or paper as the baby's bead begins to crown. After delivery, the

newborn should be held in a head-down position, cleared of mucus in the mouth, and then stimulated if necessary to initiate effective breathing. The baby should then be dried and wrapped in clean soft cloth if possible and put to the mother's breast to help promote uterine contractions. Placing the baby skin to skin on the mother, then wrapping them together will provide the most warmth. As soon as the baby is delivered, the nurse needs to observe for signs of placental separation as discussed previously. If transportation to a health care facility is imminent or anticipated within the next two hours, and the placenta has delivered, the cord can be tied off but left intact. The placenta should be wrapped in paper, plastic, or cloth and kept near the baby; the cord should not be pulled or subjected to traction. Finally, the nurse must stay with the mother and baby until help arrives. As soon as possible, a report regarding the birth should be made to the patient's health care provider (May & Mahlmeister, 1994).

Abnormal Presentations and Positions

Fetal presentations and positions have been discussed earlier in this chapter. A malpresentation can result in the failure of the presenting part to engage in the pelvic inlet, in turn causing uterine inertia or arrest of labor. A transverse lie and breech, face, brow and compound presentations are considered abnormal and can lead to dystocia. Also, a persistent occiput posterior, which can lead to uterine inertia, is abnormal (Ladewig, London & Olds, 1990; Martin, 1990).

The most common cause of malpresentation is a contracted or very small pelvis. Other causes leading to an unfavorable position for labor and descent are lax abdominal muscles, fibroid tumors blocking the passageway, uterine malformations, and placental size or location abnormalities. Fetal factors leading to malpresentation include breech presentation or transverse lie, abnormal fetal attitude, multiple pregnancy, fetal abnormality, and hydramnios.

Malpresentation prolongs the labor process, due to inefficient, weak, and irregular contractions. This causes slow and incomplete cervical dilatation, failure of the presenting part to descend, and increases the need for an operative delivery as well as the risk of uterine rupture. For the mother exhaustion often occurs, along with a greater risk of lacerations, heavy bleeding, infections, and decreased peristalsis of the bladder and bowels. The fetus will excessively mold, its presenting part will become edematous, and it runs a high risk of anoxia, brain damage, or intrauterine death. In this situation, there is a high incidence of either Cesarean or forceps delivery, and a high risk of prolapsed cord. Delay of over 30 minutes in delivering the baby increases the risk of fetal mortality fourfold.

The nurse is often the first person to recognize a malpresentation (Martin, 1990). Early diagnosis by abdominal and vaginal examinations, and careful, continuous monitoring during descent can improve the prognosis for a safe delivery. It is essential to inspect the perineum, listen to fetal heart tones, and conduct a vaginal examination in all patients who have a breech presentation or any presentation that does not fit the pelvis well. A vaginal examination must be performed when the presenting part is high, when the membranes rupture with a high presenting part, and when a woman presents with a malpresentation. If malpresentation is expected, the nurse must alert the primary caregiver immediately, must not leave the patient alone, and must closely monitor her status, her labor progress, and her baby.

INDUCTION AND AUGMENTATION OF LABOR

According to the American College of Obstetricians and Gynecologists (ACOG), induction of labor is the deliberate initiation of uterine contractions before their spontaneous onset. Induction may be elective or medically indicated because of the presence of a maternal or fetal problem. Elective induction is the initiation of labor for the convenience of an individual at term pregnancy who is free of medical indications. Its advisability is questionable because of risks to the mother and the possibility of delivering a pre-term infant (Ladewig, London & Olds, 1990).

Medically indicated induction is considered when the following conditions exist: diabetes mellitus; renal disease; severe pregnancy-induced hypertension (PIH); abruptio placenta; premature ROM; post-term pregnancy; fetal hemolytic disease; and intrauterine fetal death.

Any contraindications to spontaneous labor and vaginal delivery are also contraindications to induction. Maternal contraindications include client refusal, previous uterine incision, cephalopelvic disproportion, active herpes virus 2, centrally-located placenta previa, overdistention of the uterus. Fetal contraindications include severe fetal distress or a positive contraction stress test, a pre-term fetus, and a breech or transverse presentation. Before induction, fetal maturity must be assessed.

Candidates (Bishop's Score)

Vaginal examinations assist in determining whether cervical changes favorable to induction have occurred. Bishop's score, a prelabor scoring system, has been devised to assist in predicting if an induction will be successful. The score assesses five components: cervical dilatation, effacement, consistency, position, and fetal station. Each component is given a score of 0 to 3. The higher the score, the more likely labor will ensue. A favorable cervix is the most important criterion for a successful induction (Ladewig, London & Olds, 1990).

Induction Methods

Stripping of amniotic membranes is a less common method of induction that is performed during a vaginal exam. The amniotic membranes are manually separated (or "stripped") from the lower uterine segment near the uterus. Before the procedure is done, presence of placenta pervia or abnormal fetal presentation or lie should be ruled out. There remains risks of premature rupture of membranes and infection (May & Mahlmeister, 1994). Stripping of a membranes, in addition, can pose a serious problem by exposing the endocervical veins to amniotic fluid after rupture of the amniotic sac. The patient would then be at increased risk of possible amniotic fluid embolus (Whitley, 1985).

Amniotomy, artificial ROM by a physician, is the most common and most successful procedure. Always done during a sterile vaginal examination, once the presenting part is engaged, in order to avoid a prolapsed cord, an amnihook or other rupturing device is introduced into the vagina and a small tear is made in the amniotic membrane. Fetal presentation, position, and station are first assessed to ascertain engagement, and the fetal heart rate is assessed both before and after the procedure. Labor generally ensues within 12 hours of rupture.

This procedure permits examination of the amniotic fluid for blood or meconium stains and allows for placement of intrauterine monitoring devices when indicated. Once amniotomy is done, delivery must occur in spite of any findings that arise to delay birth. In addition, amniotomy may not be effective, and a Cesarean delivery may have to be done.

The risks of amniotomy are: maternal uterine infection as well as fetal infection, increased incidence of early deceleration of labor, prolapsing or compression of the umbilical cord; and an increase in compression and molding of the fetal head. The advantages of amniotomy are that contractions are similar to spontaneous labor, there is usually no risk of hypertonia or uterine rupture; the woman does not require as close surveillance as with an oxytocin infusion; and fetal monitoring is facilitated, since amniotomy does not interfere with fetal scalp blood sampling, fetal electrode application, or intrauterine catheter placement (ACOG, 1995).

Oxytocin infusion is the administration of oxytocin, a synthetic hormone that initiates uterine contractions. It may also be used to augment or enhance ineffective contractions. When hypotonic dysfunctional labor occurs, the same principles for oxytocin administration are used, but lower doses are given. During administration, the goal is to achieve contractions of good intensity, lasting from 40 to 50 seconds and occurring every two to three minutes, with the uterus relaxing between contractions. Oxytocin should be initiated only by a physician with privileges to perform Cesarean delivery, and while it is being administered, an electronic fetal monitor should record the fetal heart rate and contractions. The risks of oxytocin administration include hyperstimulation of the uterus, fetal distress due to decreased placental perfusion, rapid labor and delivery with the danger of laceration of the perineum or cervix, uterine rupture, and water intoxication when large doses are given in an electrolyte-free solution (NAACOG, 1988). Detailed policies and procedures for administering oxytocin infusion should be available in each institution and reviewed by the nurse before initiating the treatment. General guidelines are also available for reference from AWHONN.

Prostaglandin induction. In order to help the cervix dilate, soften and efface, the physician may utilize either Laminaria or prostaglandin E2 (PGE2). Laminaria is composed of sterile, dried and compressed seaweed which, when inserted into the cervical os, absorbs moisture and swells to 3 to 5 times its original size. Within several hours, Laminaria lead to cervical changes. In 1992, the U.S. Food and Drug Administration approved a prostaglandin E2 gel preparation for cervical ripening in women at or near term who have a medical or obstetric indication for inducing labor. It is available in a 2.5 ml syringe which contains 0.5 mg of dinoprostone (Prepidil, a form of prostaglandin E2). The intracervical route causes little uterine activity and enhanced efficacy in the very unripe cervix. A prostaglandin vaginal insert (Cervidil, 10 mg of dinaprostone) was also approved by the FDA and is commercially available. While in the supine position, the medication is inserted into the vagina or cervix. After 30 to 120 minutes of bedrest during which time her vital signs, fetal heart rate and contraction pattern are assessed, the woman may be discharged with instructions to return to the hospital in the morning at which time oxytocin (Pitocin) may be started intravenously. A second dose may be given if there are insufficient cervical changes within 6 to 12 hours. A potential complication of prostaglandin gel is hyperstimulation during which there are tetonic contractions which do not allow for uterine relaxation between contractions. If this occurs, a tocolytic such as Terbutaline is administered to help relax the uterine muscles. Maternal systemic effects often associated with prostaglandin E2, (fever, vomiting, and diarrhea) are negliable due to the low dose (ACOG, 1995).

Augmentation of Labor

When labor has begun but it is dysfunctional or it has stopped altogether, labor can be effectively stimulated or augmented with several methods. Amniotomy and oxytocin infusion can be used for augmentation as well as for induction of labor.

Ambulation is another method to help augment labor. Walking helps stimulate mild or ineffective uterine contractions by increasing the downward pressure from the presenting part against the cervix. This may lead to a more efficient contraction pattern (Martin, 1990).

Nursing Role

The nurse who assumes the responsibility of managing an induction of labor should have additional educational preparation, including a knowledge of the physiology of normal labor, potential labor complications, intravenous therapy, electronic fetal monitoring, techniques of induction, risks and benefits of the procedure, and pharmacodynamics. The nurse's database must include a comprehensive history, laboratory results, and physical and obstetrical findings. The patient will have special needs related to her condition, but she will also have the same nursing needs as the woman in spontaneous labor. The nurse must assess the educational focus for the patient, then determine nursing priorities, providing assistance, support, and intervention when necessary. She must assess the woman's support system, her relationship with the support person, her degree of anxiety, her response to labor, and her ability to cope. Continual accurate observation is essential.

In amniotomy, the nurse explains the procedure to the woman, assesses fetal presentation, position, and station, then places the woman in a semi-reclining position and drapes her. The fetal heart rate, assessed before and immediately after the procedure, is compared. If there are changes, the nurse must check for cord prolapse. Amniotic fluid must be inspected for amount, color, odor, and presence of meconium or blood. Following the procedure, the perineal area is cleansed and dried, with underpads changed frequently for comfort. Temperature is monitored every 2 hours and vaginal examinations are kept to a minimum, with strict sterile technique observed.

During an oxytocin infusion, the nurse must make constant and accurate assessments. Baseline data (temperature, pulse, respirations, blood pressure, and fetal heart rate) are obtained prior to infusion. In many institutions a fetal monitor is applied 15 minutes before infusion. Before each time the infusion rate is stepped up, the nurse must assess blood pressure and pulse, and the rate and reactivity of fetal heart rate tracings. During infusion, continual assessments must be made of the following: contraction status, including frequency, intensity, duration, and resting tone between contractions; and urinary output, to identify retention, fluid deficit, or water intoxication. Vaginal examinations are performed to evaluate cervical dilatation, effacement, and station. Client teaching should include the purpose and procedure for the induction, an explanation of nursing care to be provided, assessments, comfort measures, and a review of breathing techniques for labor.

PRE-TERM LABOR

Pre-term labor is the onset of rhythmical uterine contractions that produce cervical change, effacement, and/or dilation after fetal viability is established but before fetal maturity is achieved. It usually occurs between the 26th and 37th week of gestation, and should be treated as an obstetrical emergency (NAACOG, 1984). It is the most common complication of the third trimester, and occurs in approximately 10% of pregnancies. The greatest problem posed by pre-term labor is the delivery of a low birth weight baby. Nearly two-thirds of infant deaths during the neonatal period are associated with low birth weight (Raff & Freisner, 1989).

Pre-term labor can be caused by fetal, maternal, or placental factors. Premature ROM is the causative factor in 30% of cases. In others, causation is unknown, but among the many theories are the following: cervical incompetency; uterine anomalies; polyhydramnios; multiple births, which increase uterine distention and contractilty; fetal anomaly; abruptio placenta or placenta previa; fetal death; previous pre-term delivery or late abortion; maternal systemic disease; hormonal changes; personal life style factors (smoking, drinking, use of drugs, fatigue, overwork, poor nutrition); traumatic cervical manipulation or aggressive sexual intercourse; and DES exposure.

Screening

Pre-term labor is diagnosed when ultrasound confirms evidence of pre-term gestational age and/or fetal weight of 500 to 2499 grams, and the presence of labor-like uterine activity associated with progressive cervical effacement and dilation. Frequently, the diagnosis is made on contraction frequency alone—in most instances, contractions lasting 30 seconds, occurring every 10 minutes, and recurring for 30 to 60 minutes. Once diagnosed, a decision must be made by the physician whether or not to attempt inhibition.

Indications for inhibition are gestational age of 26 to 36 weeks, intact membranes, absence of fetal and maternal contraindications, adequate fetal weight, uterine irritability with progressive cervical effacement and/or dilation, fetal lung immaturity, and urinary tract infection.

Nursing Interventions

Dealing with the woman in pre-term labor requires specific nursing care. The identification of pre-term labor and the assessment of the patient must be done systematically. Candidates for inhibition must be recognized and treated in order for inhibition therapy to be successful. All pregnant women must be screened to identify those at risk, and a prevention and follow-up program must be instituted (NAACOG, 1988; Raff & Freisner, 1989).

Once a woman at risk for pre-term labor has been identified, the nurse must work to help the patient reduce stress-related biochemical changes through counseling, development of support systems, avoidance of stressful situations, and the use of relaxation techniques. The patient must be taught to recognize the signs of pre-term labor, however subtle, and must also be taught how to palpate and time her uterine contractions. She must be advised to be alert for contractions that occur regularly every 10 minutes or less, with or without a low, dull backache, constant or intermittent menstrual-like cramps in the lower abdomen, intermittent pelvic pressure, abdominal cramping with or without diarrhea, and any change or increase in vaginal discharge, especially if it is mucous, watery, or tinged with blood. If contractions occur, she must lie down on her side immediately for at least an hour; if they continue, she must notify her physician or nurse-midwife immediately. Her daily rest periods should be increased to lessen pressure on the uterus and increase blood flow to the fetus. Lying one hour three times a day in left lateral position is recommended.

The patient must be advised to report any signs of urinary infection immediately; maintain a balanced diet with no dieting or fasting; avoid stimulation of the nipples in preparation for breastfeeding; either abstain from sexual intercourse or ensure sexual relations are as gentle as possible; and decrease strenuous activities. Those women at high risk may have to wear an ambulatory tocodynamometer to record uterine contractions; they should also have weekly follow-up monitoring of cervical change. During monitoring, extreme care must be taken not to irritate or traumatize the uterus.

In the hospital or birthing center, care of the woman in pre-term labor is more intense. Again, left lateral position is advisable. In addition, the nurse must do the following: take a thorough history and investigate possible causes of infection; monitor the fetal heart rate and uterine activity electronically; assess the hydration level; strictly monitor intake and output; weigh daily; monitor vital signs hourly until stable, with blood pressure and fetal heart rate baseline; observe for changes after treatment is initiated; check baseline laboratory studies (CBC, blood glucose, electrolytes); assess baseline breath and bowel sounds; and monitor reflexes to determine central nervous system status. Catheterized urinalysis with culture may be ordered to rule out urinary tract infection, and EKG may be ordered before the administration of inhibitory medication.

In-Hospital Management

There are three categories of care for women in pre-term labor. Nursing care in all categories includes the evaluation of stress and anxiety levels and using nursing measures to alleviate these when necessary (NAACOG, 1988; Raff & Freisner, 1989).

Category 1 describes the woman whose contractions cease with bedrest and cause no cervical changes. This woman is placed on bedrest in left-lateral position and monitored with an external monitor. A gentle baseline cervical examination is performed, and if no changes exist the woman is sent home, careful follow-up care is planned, and moderate bedrest is advised.

Category 2 describes the woman whose contractions do not cease with bedrest but cause no cervical changes. The patient is placed on bedrest, a gentle baseline cervical examination is performed, uterine activity is carefully monitored, and the cervix is rechecked. If no changes have occurred, she is sent home on moderate bedrest and careful follow-up care is instituted.

Category 3 describes the woman with persistent uterine activity and cervical change. She is also put on bedrest, a baseline cervical examination is performed every 12 hours, she is placed on continuous electronic monitoring, and drug therapy is instituted.

Those women who present with uterine contractions, cervical effacement of over 80%, and dilation of more than 3 cm are generally treated for short-term prevention of labor, consisting of bedrest and drug therapy. Usually they are subsequently transferred to a tertiary care center where the premature infant can receive appropriate care.

Tocolytic Therapy

Tocolytic drugs are used as a means of managing pre-term labor by quieting or inhibiting smooth muscle activity; the myometrium of the uterus is made up of smooth muscle. Tocolytic drugs in use today generally fall into four categories: (1) beta-adrenergic stimulants, such as ritodrine, and terbutaline sulfate, (2) smooth muscle relaxants, such as magnesium sulfate; (3) calcium channel blockers, such as nifedipine; and, (4) prostaglandin synthetase inhibitors like indomethacin. Of note, ritodrine is the only drug currently approved by the FDA for labor inhibition; the others, are used on an experimental basis throughout the country (Martin, 1990; May & Mahlmeister, 1994).

Tocolytic therapy is usually contraindicated, especially with the use of beta-adrenergic drugs, when the following conditions exist: fetal death confirmed by ultrasound; fetal anomaly incompatible with life; fetal distress; antepartum hemorrhage; severe preeclampsia/eclampsia; cervical dilatation of over 3–4 cm; maternal cardiac or renal pathology; pulmonary hypertension; hyperthyroidism; gestational age under 20 weeks; ruptured fetal membranes; chorioamnionitis; or the mother is already taking betamimetic therapy (Martin, 1990;

NAACOG, 1988; Raff & Freisner, 1989). The benefits of labor suppression should be weighed carefully with regard to the risks to the patient and fetus for developing life-threatening cardiopulmonary complications that may occur with certain tocolytic drugs. Each situation should be assessed thoroughly and nurses must be knowledgeable of the actions and alert to the side effects of each tocolytic agent selected.

Nursing Implications in Tocolytic Therapy

Ritodrine, and terbutaline sulfate can each be administered orally, and intravenously; terbutaline sulfate can also be given subcutaneously. Terbutaline sulfate has been used subcutaneously by continuous pump infusion for long-term suppression of labor. By receiving a low dose, and continuous infusion, with intermittent boluses, the woman can benefit from home management of pre-term labor (Bobak & Jensen, 1993). Nursing care involves thorough patient education on the signs and symptoms of labor, how to palpate uterine contractions, when to call the health care provider, and (if applicable) how to operate the infusion pump. Frequently, uterine activity monitoring using a tocodynamometer with a recording unit and transmitter can be implemented for home use. Assessments and personal support are provided by a home care nurse in collaboration with the patient's physician.

Indomethacin, and nifedipine can each be administered orally; nifedipine can initially be given rectally for a more rapid absorption. Magnesium sulfate is only administered intravenously. The nurse should consult with the institution's policies for tocolytic drug dosages, and routes, and should carefully verify the physician's orders for specific tocolytic therapy.

The side effects of tocolytic agents depend upon their category and specific action, but they have significant implications for nursing care in terms of assessment and prompt intervention.

Ritodrine and terbutaline sulfate are beta-adrenergic stimulants that inhibit smooth muscle (e.g., uterine) contractibility. These drugs cause a degree of hypotension, an increase in the maternal heart rate and pulse pressure, and may decrease serum potassium levels, leading to potential arrhythmia. Maternal side effects from either of these drugs may be life-threatening and may include increased pulse rate, palpitations, headache, dyspnea, chest tightness, tremors, anxiety, tachypnea, shortness of breath, and cough. The fetus may also suffer tachycardia, cardiac dysrhythmia, and/or decreased pH. The neonate may have a disturbed glucose level and suffer from irritability, tremors, hypotension, and ileus. Patent ductus arteriosis and sepsis may be masked. The most serious maternal complication is pulmonary edema. Implications for nursing care include preparing the patient for potential side effects, careful monitoring of vital signs every 15 minutes, careful monitoring of contractions and fetal heart rate; strict bedrest in correct position; strict intake, output, and weigh daily; being extremely alert for overhydration, pulmonary edema, and respiratory distress syndrome. Antiembolism stockings are usually applied on the lower extremities. The antidote (Inderal) should be readily available.

Magnesium sulfate inhibits smooth muscle contractibility by decreasing the amount of acetylcholine at the neuromuscular junction. It has been used for over 50 years without causing gross harm to mother or baby. Some of its maternal side effects may be drowsiness, impaired sensorium, slurred speech, heavy eyelids, flushing, slower reflexes, decreased gastrointestinal tract action, and decreased respiration. If toxic levels are reached, maternal respiratory depression and arrest and decreased urinary output can occur. In the fetus and neonate it can cause central nervous system depression, evidenced as lethargy, reduced muscle tone, reduced sucking reflex, reduced respirations, and increased serum magnesium levels. However, these conditions are usually transient.

Nursing care must include careful monitoring of the woman, including her reflexes, respiratory rate, and urinary output. Concurrent use of narcotics must be avoided, and the diet must be planned to avoid ileus. Resuscitation equipment must be readily available, as well as the antidote (10% IV calcium gluconate).

Nifedipine is a calcium channel blocker that inhibits the transport of calcium across the cell membrane so that the uterine muscle relaxes. Maternal side effects that may occur include flushing, headache, hypotension, tachycardia, syncope, nausea, diarrhea, fever, or dyspnea. Careful monitoring and documentation of the patient's cardiopulmonary status, and fetal well-being are crucial.

Indomethacin, on the other hand, suppresses labor by inhibiting prostaglandin synthesis, thereby inhibiting uterine muscle contractions. Maternal side effects from this agent may include nausea, heartburn, GI ulceration, or decreased renal function. Indomethacin is not administered after 32 weeks gestation since it can cause closure of the fetal ductus arteriosus, oligohydramnios, or pulmonary hypertension in the newborn (May & Mahlmeister, 1994).

Home Care

For the woman at risk for pre-term labor, there are several self-care measures the nurse can recommend (Ladewig, London & Olds, 1990). These include:

- Resting two to three times daily on the left side.

- Drinking two to three quarts of water or fruit juice daily, avoiding caffeine drinks.

- Emptying the bladder at least every two hours when awake.

- Avoiding lifting heavy objects (have children climb onto mother's lap).

- Avoiding prenatal breast preparation .

- Avoiding overexertion.

- Curtailing or eliminating sexual activity.

- Focusing on pleasurable activities to compensate for limitation of activities.

- Focusing on one day or one week at a time.

- Getting dressed and resting on a couch, rather than remaining in bed when on bedrest.

MATERNAL WELL-BEING

Standards of Care

The well-being of the woman in labor is the primary concern of the nurse (Ladewig, London & Olds, 1990). The major needs of the woman are met by assessing her labor progress, keeping vaginal examinations to a minimum, providing her the opportunity to empty her bladder at least every two hours, giving support and encouraging her support person, providing proper positioning, providing comfort measures, using pain-control measures, and ensuring hydration (Martin, 1990).

Admission Procedures

Upon the patient's admission, the nurse should identify herself and secure proper patient identification. Vital signs (temperature, pulse, respirations, blood pressure, and FHR) are taken, and a history and physical examination are done. The history should include the following: obstetrical status (primigravida, multipara, estimated date of confinement); symptoms of patient in this labor (show, ROM, character and duration of contractions); allergies; current or recent illness in mother or her family; time of last meal; plans for breast- or bottlefeeding; when she last slept and whether she is fatigued; presence of discomfort; physical prob-

lems or disabilities; blood incompatibilities; and lab results (Raff & Freisner, 1989; Martin, 1990).

The physical examination includes the woman's general and obstetrical status. The obstetrical examination will determine the stage and progress of her labor. The woman's knowledge of and attitudes toward labor and delivery must be determined, including her desires regarding the management of her labor and delivery, her preparation for childbirth, and her fears and concerns. Her family relationships must be assessed, which include her marital status, her wishes regarding the presence of a family member or friend during labor and delivery, and the arrangements or concerns she has regarding her children at home. Nursing intervention is based on the rationale that fear and anxiety increase muscular tension, leading to an increased perception of pain.

The patient must receive orientation to the hospital, an explanation of the institution's routines, and an introduction to its staff. She must be given information about the status of her labor, what to expect as labor progresses, and mechanisms to reduce pain. Medications are given as ordered and as desired by the patient. A patient record must be established, provisions made for draping and for screens to ensure her privacy, and any deviations from the norm in her general or obstetrical status must be reported.

Patient Teaching

Having determined the woman's knowledge base, the nurse then assesses the factors affecting her communication and anxiety levels. Then, having also assessed the labor process, the nurse can determine the amount of time available for teaching. If the woman is in early labor and needs additional information, teaching should be directed toward the essentials of nursing care during labor.

After reviewing with the patient the aspects of the admission procedure, the nurse presents aspects of ongoing physical care, such as when to anticipate assessment of her vital signs, fetal heart rate, and contractions. If electronic fetal monitoring is to be used, it should be shown to her; then she must receive orientation on how it works and the information it will provide. Its sights and sounds should be explained, as well as what "normal" data will look like and what characteristics are being watched for. The patient must be advised that assessments will increase as labor progresses, in spite of the fact that during this transition phase her strongest desire will probably be to be left alone. The nurse must provide information regarding the assessments, making it clear that they will be done to keep the mother and baby safe. It is of great importance to stress the support the woman will receive during labor. The patient should be able to verbalize the assessments that will be made during labor, and also discuss with the nurse the support and comfort measures that will be available to her.

Using a cervical dilatation chart for illustration, the nurse then explains the vaginal examination and what information it provides *(see appendix)*. Then, comfort and breathing techniques are reviewed, and after ascertaining which ones the woman believes will be effective, the nurse should have her demonstrate them. At this time, the nurse and patient should also review and discuss positioning, backrub, effleurage, touch, distraction techniques, and ambulation. If time permits, a tour of the birthing area is advisable (Ladewig, London & Olds, 1990).

Labor Support

Kind and sensitive support during labor provides the laboring woman with many advantages (Martin, 1990). It enables her to cope better, relax more readily, cooperate with treatment, more positively recall the labor and birthing experience, and adjust more easily to parenthood. A family member or friend should be encouraged to stay with her and support her, but this support person will also need help. The nurse must remember to show support

persons how to help the laboring woman, not forgetting to praise them for their efforts (Ladewig, London & Olds, 1990).

It is of utmost importance that the woman in active labor not be left alone. Support also includes comfort measures—prompt changing of soiled and damp linen; providing mouth care (ice chips, mouth lubrication, or mouth rinses); massaging the abdomen, back, or legs as the patient desires; providing good ventilation in the room; and adjusting the labor room's environment to the mother's wishes (lights, quiet, privacy). The nurse and support person should encourage frequent changes of position, and should assist in ambulation during early labor.

There are various positions a laboring woman can use to alleviate discomfort and aid labor progress. Some positions are more effective to some women than to others.

The nurse should be familiar with positions such as the ones listed below and offer guidance to the patient as to the benefit of each position (Michels, 1992):

- **Standing:** spinal flexion lowers the lumbar curve to provide the fetus with a straighter path through the birth canal.

- **Upright:** the uterus falls forward and away from the maternal spine and pelvic vessels. When the uterus is supported by the anterior abdominal wall, most of the weight is directed toward the pelvic inlet.

- **Multiple positions:** present a variety of angles between the fetal head and the pelvic inlet to provide increased chances to help deflexed, transverse, or OPs to find the right fit.

- **Squat:** the weight of the body exerts a passive stretch on the muscles attached to the ischial tuberosities to help separate them; Widening of the intertuberous diameter aids rotation and descent.

- **Seated:** maternal weight placed on the ischial tuberosities encourages their separation which aids fetal rotation and descent.

- **Lithotomy:** maternal weight is placed largely on the sacrum and coccyx which restricts the posterior movement of the sacrum and decreases the pelvic outlet dimensions.

- **Walking:** alternate weight bearing on each leg shifts pressures and changes the shape of the pelvis to encourage fetal rotation and descent.

- **Flexion of maternal spines:** (e.g., Pelvic rock and hands/knees) redirects the downward force transmined by the fetal spine-flexing head and makes rotation more likely.

As labor progresses to the active phase, the woman must be encouraged to maintain breathing patterns and should be given a quiet environment to reduce external stimuli. She now needs reassurance, encouragement and support, and both she and her support person must be kept informed of her progress. She will get some relief from backrubs, sacral pressure, a cool cloth on her forehead, help with position changes, support with pillows, effleurage, and mouth care. She must be reminded to void every two hours. During the transition phase, she must be encouraged to rest between contractions. If she sleeps between contractions, she must be awakened at the start of a contraction in order to begin her breathing pattern. She will need support, encouragement, and praise at this time. She and her support person must be kept informed of progress. However, during transition, she may not wish to be touched, so make provisions for privacy if necessary.

During the second stage, assist the woman in pushing, encouraging her to assume a position of comfort. Provide praise, encouragement, and information about her progress. Ice chips may be given to relieve dryness of the mouth. If the woman desires privacy, respect her wishes.

Assessment and Documentation of Labor Progress

If a normal baseline fetal heart pattern has been obtained upon admission of a woman in early labor, the FHR evaluation may be carried out less often than every 15 minutes, but should nevertheless be done at least hourly (Martin, 1990). At the inception of active labor, evaluation intervals of 15 to 30 minutes are appropriate. Vital signs and other assessments should be monitored according to the schedule shown below.

The FHR is taken for 30 seconds immediately after a contraction. When the cervix is dilated 8 to 10 cm, FHR should be taken after every contraction when the mother is pushing. If the membranes have ruptured, temperature should be taken every 2 hours. An increase in pulse rate may precede an elevation in temperature.

Identifying Complications

Hemorrhage

The most common cause of intrapartal hemorrhage is abruptio placentae, a major emergency in both labor and delivery that calls for immediate, effective intervention *(see figure 5-5)*. It is defined as separation of the placenta from the site of implantation in the uterine wall before delivery of the infant. Its cause is unknown, but there are theories attributing it to decreased blood flow to the placenta through the sinuses during the last trimester. Other suggestions for causation include excessive intrauterine pressure caused by hydramnios or multiple pregnancy, uterine trauma, maternal hypertension, violent labor, cigarette smoking, alcohol ingestion, cocaine use, increased maternal age and parity, trauma, and sudden changes in intrauterine pressure (Raff & Freisner, 1989; Ludewig, London & Olds, 1990).

Hemorrhage is subdivided into three types:

1. **Central,** in which the placenta separates centrally and the blood is trapped between the pla-

FIGURE 5-5
Abnormalities of the Placenta

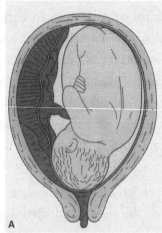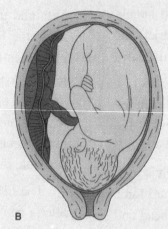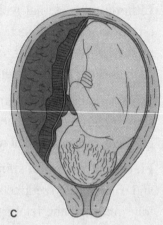

ABRUPTIO PLACENTAE **A** Marginal abruption with external hemorrhage. **B** Central abruption with concealed hemorrhage. **C** Complete separation.

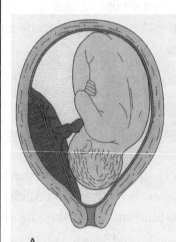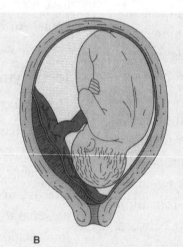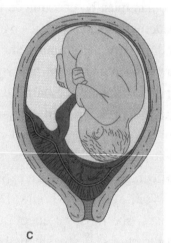

PLACENTA PREVIA **A** Low placental implantation. **B** Partial placenta previa. **C** Total placenta previa.

Source: *Maternal Newborn Nursing Care,* 4th ed., Ladewig, P.W., London, M.L. & Olds, S.B., 1998, Addison-Wesley, Longman, Inc. New York, NY

centa and the uterine wall. This leads to concealed bleeding, and the abdomen will be rigid, with acute pain in the area. Blood pressure is decreased *(see figure 5-5).*

2. **Marginal,** in which blood passes between the fetal membranes and the uterine wall and dark, red blood escapes vaginally. The abdomen is not rigid, there is tenderness over the uterus, and blood pressure is decreased *(see figure 5-5).*

3. **Complete,** in which massive vaginal bleeding is seen in the presence of total separation. The

abdomen is rigid, with acute pain, and the patient is in profound shock. In severe cases of central abruptio placentae, blood invades the musculature of the uterus and, if it continues, the uterus turns blue. After delivery, the uterus contracts poorly, frequently necessitating hysterectomy. In addition, central abruptio placentae can cause fibrinogen levels to drop in minutes to the point at which blood will no longer coagulate. Maternal mortality is approximately 6%, depending on the severity of bleeding, coagulation defects, and the time elapsed between separation and birth. Moderate to severe hemorrhage results in hemorrhagic shock, which can be fatal if not reversed *(see figure 5-5).*

Postpartally, the mother is at risk for hemorrhage and renal failure, vascular spasm, intravascular clotting, or a combination of all three. Fetal mortality ranges between 15% and 100%, depending on the fetus' level of maturity. The most serious complications come from pre-term labor, anemia, and hypoxia. If unchecked, hypoxia will lead to brain damage or death. Treatment consists of close monitoring of the blood and cardiovascular status of the mother, giving transfusions as needed, and developing a plan for delivery, either by Cesarean or by induction of labor. Nursing care consists of electronic monitoring of contractions and resting tone. Abdominal girth measurements may have to be taken hourly. Another method of evaluating uterine size (which increases as bleeding persists) is by placing a mark at the top of the fundus, and evaluating the distance between the fundus and the symphysis pubis hourly.

The nurse must observe, record, and report blood loss, and must evaluate the decrease in blood volume by monitoring respirations, pulse, and blood pressure. Urine output must also be monitored, and the skin inspected for pallor, coolness, and clamminess. Blood loss can also be evaluated by counting and weighing pads used. Postpartally, the uterus must be massaged and evaluated every 15 minutes for one hour, every 30 minutes for one hour, and every 60 minutes for two to four hours. The woman must be kept informed of her status, provided with accurate information, given answers to her questions, and permitted to participate in decision making if possible. A trusting nurse-patient relationship is paramount in this situation.

Hypertension

Hypertension disorders in pregnancy have four classifications (Neeson, 1987; Raff & Freisner, 1989; Ladewig, London & Olds, 1990):

- Pregnancy-induced hypertension (PIH), which includes preeclampsia and eclampsia

- Chronic hypertension preceding pregnancy

- Chronic hypertension with superimposed pregnancy-induced hypertension, which includes superimposed preeclampsia and superimposed eclampsia

- Transient hypertension

Hypertension is defined as a sustained blood pressure increased to levels of 140mm Hg systolic or 90mm Hg diastolic. Although earlier reports suggested that an increase in blood pressure of ≥30mm Hg systolic or ≥15mm Hg diastolic from second-trimester values was also of diagnostic value, this concept is no longer considered valid. Results from one study found that 73% of primigravid patients with normotensive pregnancies demonstrated an increase in diastolic blood pressure of more than 15mm Hg at some stage during pregnancy, while 57% of these patients demonstrated an increase in diastolic pressure of more than 20mm Hg during pregnancy (ACOG, 1996).

PIH is the most common hypertensive disorder of pregnancy, most often seen in the last 10 weeks of gestation, during labor, or within 48 hours of delivery. It is defined by blood pressure of 140/90 during the second half of pregnancy in a previously normotensive woman. Nursing assessment for women at risk for PIH includes screening of the patient at each visit for elevated blood pressure, proteinuria, weight gain, and edema. Protein and excessive salt intake must be assessed, and the patient must be encouraged to drink 8 to 10 glasses of no-sodium, no-sugar fluids daily.

preeclampsia is a progressive disease requiring medical intervention. It is characterized by hypertension with proteinuria and/or edema. Eclampsia is defined as a convulsion, and is the leading cause of maternal death in the United States. PIH, however, rarely progresses to eclampsia, due to today's available treatment and early diagnosis. Those at particular risk for PIH are older primigravidas, teenagers of lower socioeconomic status, women with a family history of of PIH, those with a large placental mass due to multiple gestation, women with chronic hypertension and/or renal disease, and diabetics.

The cause of PIH is unknown, despite many existing theories. It affects all the major systems of the body. Central nervous system changes include hyperreflexia, headaches, and cerebral edema. In severe cases, the woman is at risk for renal failure, abruptio placentae, disseminated intravascular coagulation, ruptured liver, pulmonary edema, and pulmonary embolism.

HELLP is an acronym for hemolysis, elevated liver function tests, and low platelet count, a syndrome viewed as a variant of PIH. Fetal and neonatal risks include low birth weight, prematurity, and mortality. The neonate may also be oversedated due to medication given the mother, or may have hypermagnesemia due to its mother's management with large doses of magnesium sulfate.

Medical management's goals are prompt diagnosis; prevention of convulsion, hematologic, renal, and hepatic diseases; and birth of an uncompromised newborn as close to term as possible. In mild preeclampsia, this is accomplished by a high-protein diet with adequate calories, frequent rest periods in the lateral position, and careful monitoring of prescribed medication. Fetal well-being is closely monitored by means of fetal movement record, nonstress testing, ultrasonography, contraction stress testing, and amniocentesis.

Nursing assessment for women at risk for PIH includes screening of the patient at each visit for elevated blood pressure, proteinuria, weight gain,

and edema. Protein and excessive salt intake must be assessed, and the patient must be encouraged to drink 8 to 10 glasses of no-sodium, no-sugar fluids daily.

In the event of fetal distress, induction is done, even if the fetus is immature. Severe preeclampsia requires hospitalization, with complete bedrest, a high-protein, moderate sodium diet, anticonvulsants (generally magnesium sulfate), fluid and electrolyte replacement, sedatives, and antihypertensives.

In the event of eclampsia, immediate treatment is given. Magnesium sulfate is administered intravenously to control convulsions, the lungs are auscultated for pulmonary edema, and the woman is observed for circulatory and renal failure and signs of cerebral hemorrhage. Signs of magnesium sulfate toxicity include respiratory rate (<12/min) hyporeflexia, oliguria, reduced consciousness and elevated magnesium sulfate serum levels (>7mg/100mg). The antidote to magnesium sulfate is 10% IV calcium gluconate (1 gram over 2 minutes).

Following stabilization, induction of labor is considered if the fetus is mature. The woman and her partner must be given a careful explanation of her status, the status of the fetus, the treatment, and plans for further treatment and delivery. Cesarean delivery may be necessary even with an immature fetus. Oxytocin and magnesium sulfate may be used simultaneously. Demerol, a pudendal block, or an epidural block may be used for delivery, with birth accomplished in a semi-sitting position. A pediatrician or neonatal nurse practitioner should be available to care for the newborn at birth. Generally, the woman improves after delivery, but seizures can occur up to 48 hours postpartum.

In the event of hospitalization, the following must be assessed: blood pressure, temperature, pulse, respirations, and fetal heart rate (every 2–4 hours); urinary output, urine protein, and urine specific gravity; edema; weight; pulmonary edema (by auscultation and observation for coughing); deep tendon reflexes; signs of placental separation; headaches; visual disturbances; epigastric pain; level of consciousness; emotional response; and the effects of any medications. In addition, laboratory blood tests are done daily *(see table 5-1)*. A high-protein diet is ordered. Ultrasound may be prescribed to assess placental function, and antihypertensive drugs will be administered intravenously.

Women at risk for convulsions require special nursing care. They should be placed in a darkened room to reduce central nervous system stimuli and provided with seizure precautions. Urinary output is measured hourly with a Foley catheter. Blood pressure and pulse are recorded every 15 minutes until the patient is stabilized, then every 30 to 60 minutes. Deep tendon reflexes are tested every 2–4 hours for hyperreflexia or clonus. The fetal monitor is observed for signs of fetal distress or spontaneous onset of labor, and magnesium sulfate intra-venous infusion and other medications are given as ordered. The normal loading dose of magnesium sulfate is 4 grams over 20 minutes followed by 2–3 gm/hr via a controlled infusion pump. If pulmonary edema occurs, the patient is transferred to the intensive care unit.

Throughout, the woman with PIH requires constant support and teaching in order to deal with her many concerns—the fear of losing her fetus, her relationship with her mate and children, her finances, and boredom. The nurse can offer explanations, information, and referrals to community agencies. She must also teach the family which symptoms are significant and the purpose of medical therapy.

During labor, the patient must have all the care necessary for normal labor, as well as the special care needed for managing PIH. Both the woman and her support person must be kept informed of progress and the plan for care, and their wishes concerning the birth experience should be respected whenever possible.

TABLE 5-1
Commonly Ordered Tests to Evaluate preeclampsia

TEST	ABNORMAL RESULTS
Uric acid	>10 mg/dl
Creatinine	>2 mg/dl
Blood urea nitrogen	>10 mg/dl
Liver enzymes AST LDH	 >50 U/L >350 IU/L
Proteinuria (24 hr)	≥5 gm
Magnesium sulfate levels	8–10 mg/100ml - patellar reflex disappears 10–12 mg/100ml - respiratory depression ≥15 mg/100ml - cardiac conduction defects
Platelets	<100,000/mm^3

Sources: Gilbert & Harmon (1993) and Pillitteri (1995)

Postpartally, vaginal bleeding must be assessed, and the woman must be observed for signs of shock. Pulse and blood pressure are monitored every 4 hours for 48 hours, hematocrit is checked daily, urinary intake and output are measured, and the woman is assessed for further signs of PIH. Postpartal depression may be relieved by frequent maternal-infant contact and by visits from family members.

The woman should be cared for by the same nurses throughout her hospital stay, and should be provided with family planning information before discharge.

Infection

Maternal infection, whether contracted before or during pregnancy, poses severe risks both to the mother and her baby. Premature delivery or spontaneous abortion may result, and the risk of morbidity to mother and baby increases. Since the mother may not present any signs or symptoms of infection, it is essential that diagnosis and treatment be made promptly (Neeson, 1987; Ladewig, London & Olds, 1990).

The acronym TORCH stands for a group of infectious diseases that pose great risk of developmental anomalies to the embryo or fetus, particularly if exposure occurs during the first 12 weeks of gestation. These are toxoplasmosis, rubella, cytomegalovirus, herpesvirus type 2, and other infections.

Toxoplasmosis, caused by a protozoan, can be acquired when the pregnant woman eats raw or insufficiently cooked meats or when she comes into contact with infected cats. It may be asymptomatic and therefore not diagnosed properly, or the woman may develop myalgia, malaise, rash, splenomegaly, or enlarged cervical lymph notes. Diagnosis is made by serologic testing, and treatment consists of sulfadiazine and pyrimethamine. If diagnosed before 20 weeks gestation, therapeutic abor-tion is considered. Fetal effects include spontaneous abortion, stillbirth, intrauterine growth retardation, and congenital infection. In neonates, jaundice, hepatosplenomegaly or encephalitis may result. Those who survive risk microcephaly, cerebral calcification, chorioretinitis, and mental retardation. Nursing intervention consists of instructing the patient about the source of the disease and counseling her to thoroughly cook meats and avoid contact with cat feces. She should also be advised to wear gloves when gardening and to avoid areas where cats congregate.

Rubella, or German measles, is transmitted by nasopharyngeal droplet. Its effects are not severe for the mother, but it poses great risk to the fetus and neonate. Prevention is the best therapy, and experts recommend that all women of childbearing age be tested for immunity, then immunized if they are susceptible and not pregnant. Symptoms include swollen lymph nodes preceding a rash that begins on the face and spreads to the neck, chest, abdomen, and extremities. Joint pain is common in adults. If a woman develops rubella during the first trimester, therapeutic abortion is suggested, and nursing support and understanding are vital to the couple. They must be informed of the fetal effects of rubella, which include stillbirth, spontaneous abortion, and gross abnormalities such as microcephaly, heart defects, cataracts, and deafness. Infants born with congenital rubella syndrome are infectious and must be isolated. The expanded rubella syndrome may affect children years after the infection. Defects include insulin-dependent diabetes mellitus, sudden hearing loss, glaucoma, and slow, progressive encephalitis (Neeson, 1987; Ladewig, London & Olds, 1990).

Cytomegalovirus is transmitted through contact with body fluids and causes both congenital and acquired infections called CID (cytomegalic inclusion disease). In pregnancy, the virus is transmitted across the placenta to the fetus. It can also be transmitted by the cervical route during birth. Antibodies from prior exposure are found in 50-60% of pregnant women, and, although asymptomatic, the virus tends to become activated during pregnancy. Fetal effects range from subclinical to severe, and include hyperbilirubinemia, hepatosplenomegaly, pneumonitis, and encephalitis. Of those with encephalitis, 5% will die and 85% will have central nervous system abnormalities. Newborn infants should be isolated, since the virus is shed in saliva and urine. There is no known treatment or immunization (Neeson, 1987; Ladewig, London & Olds, 1990).

Herpes virus type 2 is transmitted by sexual contact, by contact with cervical mucus, or transplacentally. Found mostly in young adults, the primary infection exhibits painful vesicles on the labia, vagina, or cervix, accompanied by fever, malaise, headache, and anorexia. In recurrent infection, there are localized painful lesions whose presence in the genital tract can profoundly affect the fetus, causing abortion in early pregnancy, pre-term labor in later pregnancy, a 60% risk of mortality, and severe neurologic sequelae in 50% of those infants who survive. The infant is asymptomatic at birth, but within 2 to 12 days may develop fever, jaundice, seizures, and poor feeding. One-half of infected infants develop vesicular skin lesions.

There is no definitive treatment available. Diagnosis is made by culturing lesions periodically, and if a positive culture is found within 72 hours before delivery, Cesarean section is indicated. The newborn is isolated and observed for signs of infection. Treatment of the mother is directed toward relieving vulvar pain, with sitz baths and blow-drying of the vulva. Bedrest may help, and wearing cotton panties is advisable. The drug acyclovir reduces the infectious period, but its effects on pregnancy are unknown. The virus is not found in breast milk, so breastfeeding is acceptable, with a strong warning to the mother to wash her hands thoroughly before handling the baby.

Client education during pregnancy is of great importance, focusing on the effects of herpes on the fetus, the possibility of Cesarean delivery, and the possible association of herpes with cervical cancer. A yearly Pap smear must be emphasized. Since no cure exists, the patient must be given realistic information about dealing with herpes both physically and emotionally. Counseling may be advisable to deal with the anger, shame, and depression that often accompany this condition (Neeson, 1987; Ladewig, London & Olds, 1990).

Among the other infectious processes that put pregnancy at risk are urinary tract infections, vaginal infections, and sexually transmitted diseases.

Women with urinary tract infections may develop cystitis or pyelonephritis in the third trimester if not treated. Oral sulfonamides taken in the last weeks of gestation may lead to neonatal hyperbilirubinemia and kernicterus. When urinary tract infections remain untreated, and pyelonephritis results, there is an increased risk of premature delivery and intrauterine growth retardation.

Vaginal infections pose additional problems. The woman with an untreated monilial or yeast infection can deliver an infant infected with thrush. The treatment for bacterial vaginitis, metronidazole, has potential teratogenic effects, as has clotrimazole, the treatment for trichomoniasis.

HIV/AIDS

An increasing number of females are HIV+ and AIDS is now the third leading cause of death for females between 25 and 44. (Bland, 1995) The woman who tests HIV+ may exhibit any of the following symptoms: fatigue, anemia, weight loss, lymphadenopathy, diarrhea, fever, neurologic dysfunction, immunodeficiency and evidence of purplish or reddish brown lesions called Kaposi's sarcoma. Women constitute 14% of reported AIDS cases and there are approximately 80,000 HIV+ women of childbearing age in the U.S. The Centers for Disease Control estimates 7,000 of these women give birth each year. Based on a perinatal transmission rate of 15 to 30%, an estimated 1,000 to 2,000 infants are estimated to be HIV infected (Taylor, 1996). These infants will fail to thrive, have enlarged livers and spleens, interstitial pneumonia, recurrent infections, immunodeficiency, Epstein-Barr virus and neurologic abnormalities. The infant's facial characteristics may include microcephaly, a prominent forehead, large spaces between the eyes, a flat nasal bridge and a mild obliquity of the eyes (Ladewig, London & Olds, 1990). Since routine screening of blood and blood products have essentially eliminated this route of transmission in children, virtually all new infections in infants and children are transmitted perinatally. HIV is transmitted from mother to infant during pregnancy, labor and delivery or postpartum by breastfeeding. Approximately 65 to 70% are infected at or around the time of delivery, with the remainder during pregnancy. Though HIV+ women are advised not to breastfeed, about 1% of perinatal transmission is via this route in the United States. *The AIDS Clinical Trials Group Protocol 076*, published in 1994, showed a two-thirds reduction (from 25% to 8%) in the rate of perinatal transmission of HIV by asymptomatic infected women whose CD_4 cell count was greater than 200, had never taken zidovudine (AZT) before and were between 14 and 34 weeks gestation. The women were treated with AZT orally during pregnancy and intravenously during labor, and their infants received oral AZT for 6 weeks after birth (Taylor, 1996). These result have lead to the recommendation that all pregnant women who are HIV+ be offered AZT.

In the past, HIV testing was recommended only for those women who fell into high risk categories such as prostitutes, intravenous drug users, and women whose current or previous partners were HIV+ or bisexual. Current recommendations encourage health care providers to offer HIV testing to all pregnant women so that, if positive, early intervention with antiretroviral therapy can begin. Women must receive extensive pre and post counseling. If women opt to use AZT, informed consent must be obtained since physicians are not 100% certain of potential short and long term effects of AZT upon the fetus/infant.

Sexually transmitted diseases have enormous implications on pregnancy (Neeson, 1987; Ladewig, London & Olds, 1990). Chlamydial infection is treatable with tetracycline, which is not given to pregnant women because it can discolor fetal teeth. Instead, treatment with erythromycin is given. Infants born to woman with untreated chlamydial infection may be born prematurely, suffer fetal death, or develop newborn conjunctivitis or chlamydial pneumonia. Syphilis can be transmitted to the fetus via the placenta, and, if untreated with penicillin, can cause second trimester abortion, stillbirth at term, or a congenitally infected infant. Pregnant women (and their partners) are treated for gonorrhea with penicillin or spectinomycin. Untreated women with a gonorrheal infection present at birth may deliver a baby with ophthalmia neonatorum.

Fetal Distress/Cord Prolapse

Although this topic will be discussed in more detail in a later chapter on fetal heart rate monitoring, cord prolapse is briefly mentioned here because it poses such a great risk to the newborn. A prolapsed cord results when the umbilical cord precedes the presenting part, placing pressure on the cord as it is trapped between the mother's pelvis and the presenting part (Neeson, 1987; Ladewig, London & Olds, 1990; Martin, 1990). This situation may lead to a Cesarean delivery or to the death of the baby. It occurs in about 1 of 200 pregnancies, resulting from abnormal fetal position, multiple gestation, premature ROM, fetopelvic disproportion, a low-lying placenta, or an abnormally large umbilical cord. Compression of the cord causes decreased blood flow to the fetus, leading to fetal distress. If labor is occurring, the cord is further compressed with each contraction, and if not relieved, the fetus will die. The fetal survival rate, if delivered within an hour of prolapse, is 70% to 75%. If delivery is delayed by over one hour, more than 50% of infants will die. Umbilical cord prolapse also can lead to prematurity, birth trauma, meconium aspiration, and hypoxia.

Prevention of prolapse is the preferred approach, but when prolapse occurs, relieving compression is vital. Bedrest is essential for laboring women with a history of ROM until engagement occurs with no prolapse. When membranes rupture spontaneously, or when amniotomy is performed, the FHR must be auscultated for a full minute, again at the end of a contraction, and after a few contractions. If fetal brachycardia is detected, the woman must be examined to rule out cord prolapse. If the cord prolapses, and if electronic monitor tracings show severe, moderate, or prolonged variable decelerations with baseline bradycardia, vaginal examination is indicated. If the cord's loop is discovered, the gloved fingers should be left in the vagina and attempts made to lift the fetal head off the cord until a physician arrives. This will save the baby's life.

Oxygen should be administered, and the FHR monitored to determine whether cord compression has been adequately relieved. Gravity can also be employed to relieve compression. The bed should be adjusted to Trendelenburg position and the woman placed in Sims' position while she is transported to the operating or delivery room. The cord may be occult prolapsed, with a loop extending into the vagina or lying alongside the presenting part. It may also be pulsating, and if the pulsations are weak, it will be difficult to determine whether the fetus is alive.

A new method to relieve cord compression from a prolapsed cord involves inserting a Foley catheter into the bladder and rapidly infusing 1000 cc of sterile saline. This technique helps to elevate the presenting part away from the cord (May & Mahimeister, 1994).

The nurse should advise all pregnant women to contact their caregivers when membranes rupture, and go to the clinic, birthing center, or office immediately. A sterile vaginal examination will determine whether the danger of cord prolapse exists. If engagement has taken place, the risk of prolapse is minimal and ambulation is permitted. If the presenting part is not well engaged, bedrest is recommended.

Since cord prolapse is often associated with fetal death, some caregivers insist on bedrest after ROM, regardless of engagement status. When in labor, any alteration in the FHR or any indication of meconium in the amniotic fluid indicates the need to assess for cord prolapse. Vaginal delivery is possible with cord prolapse when the cervix is fully dilated and when pelvic measurements are adequate. Otherwise, Cesarean birth is necessary.

EXAM QUESTIONS

CHAPTER 5

Questions 17–26

17. Upon physical exam, the physician notes the patient's pelvic type is gynecoid. What are the implications of this finding?

    a. The patient most likely will need a cesarean delivery.

    b. This type of pelvis is seen in only 5 to 10% of women.

    c. This is a typical female pelvis.

    d. The use of forceps is likely.

18. The *primary power* is the contraction of the uterine muscles which causes

    a. dilation and effacement of the cervix.

    b. expulsion of the fetus.

    c. expansion of the pelvic diameter.

    d. changes in the fetal attitude.

19. The term for a breech presentation in which the fetal hips and thighs are flexed and the buttocks presents toward the maternal pelvis is

    a. Frank breech

    b. Complete breech

    c. Footling breech

    d. Kneeling breech

20. The fetal position that would result in the most backache and pelvic pressure for a laboring woman is

    a. acromion-dorsal-posterior

    b. occiput posterior

    c. right sacrum transverse

    d. occiput anterior

21. Frequency of contractions is best described by which of the following statements?

    a. The time from the start of a contraction to the end of that contraction.

    b. The time between the beginning of one contraction and the beginning of the next contraction.

    c. The time from the start of a contraction to the end of the next contraction.

    d. The time between the end of one contraction and the beginning of the next contraction.

22. Which of the following drugs can be used as an antidote to terbutaline sulfate?

    a. Inderal

    b. Nefedipine

    c. Indomenthacin

    d. Yutopar

23. The nursing intervention that is crucial in caring for the pre-term labor patient on magnesium sulfate is

    a. monitoring the patient's respiratory rate

    b. padding the side rails

    c. having the antidote Inderol on hand

    d. forcing fluids

24. The most common cause of intrapartum hemorrhage is

    a. placenta acreta

    b. placenta previa

    c. abruptio placentae

    d. uterine atony

25. The greatest risk of abruptio placentae to the fetus is

    a. Rh incompatibility.

    b. severe hypoxia.

    c. coagulopathy.

    d. renal failure.

26. Women at greatest risk for developing pregnancy-induced hypertension are

    a. employed full time.

    b. pregnant women who are anemic.

    c. teenagers of lower socioeconomic status.

    d. multigravidas.

CHAPTER 6

PAIN RELIEF

CHAPTER OBJECTIVE

After studying this chapter, the reader will be able to specify the causes of pain associated with labor and childbirth and indicate methods of pain relief that are most effective for women during labor and delivery.

LEARNING OBJECTIVES

After reading this chapter, the student will be able to

1. Identify the causes of pain during labor and delivery.

2. Recognize the effects of various pain-relief methods on the well-being of the fetus.

3. Select the advantages and disadvantages of the various methods of analgesia and anesthesia for use during labor and delivery.

4. Identify nonpharmaceutical methods of pain relief that are effective for laboring women.

5. Choose the appropriate nursing measures that should be implemented when assessing and alleviating pain in laboring women.

INTRODUCTION

Most women expect and experience pain in labor and childbirth, but pain is a subjective experience, and it is what-ever the patient says it is for her (Neeson, 1987; Martin, 1990). Labor pain is often described as the most intense ever experienced, and in many cases, it is the aspect of childbirth most feared by the expectant mother. Physical, psychological and cultural factors play an important role in the woman's response to childbirth, although the intensity of pain experienced varies a great deal from one woman to another.

Pain is managed in various ways, according to the following indicators: the frequency, duration, and intensity of uterine contractions; the character of labor; the patient's emotional behavior; her response to pain; the dilatation of the cervix; the condition of mother and fetus; the skill, experience, and attitude of the health care team; and the preferences of the woman and her family. Pain relief ranges from none or very mild sedation to regional anesthesia to heavy sedation and/or amnesic medication. When considering any form of analgesia or anesthesia, the safety of the mother and fetus are paramount.

Pain relief in labor presents unique problems. Sedatives and anesthesia cross the placenta and respiratory distress in the fetus can result. Unlike its use in surgery, which is brief, obstetrical analgesia may be needed for as long as 12 hours. And, more important, since labor begins without warning, the patient invariably has not had sufficient time to empty her gastric contents, leading to the threat of aspiration of vomitus. Therefore, the risks versus benefits of pain relief in labor and delivery must be carefully weighed, and any anesthetic given must be administered only by qualified personnel.

CAUSES OF PAIN

During the first stage of labor, pain is due to dilatation of the cervix, hypoxia of uterine cells during contraction, stretching of the lower uterine segment, and pressure on adjacent structures (Ladewig, London & Olds, 1990; Laff & Freisner, 1989). Initially, contractions are felt in the lower back, then progress to the lower torso in the back and abdomen.

In the second stage of labor, pain is due to hypoxia of the contracting uterine muscle cells, distention of the vagina and perineum, and pressure on adjacent structures.

During delivery there is often a decrease in pain, although many women describe the sensations of stretching, splitting, or burning. Most third-stage pain results from contractions and cervical dilatation as the placenta is expelled. After the third stage, anesthesia is needed primarily for episiotomy repair.

ANALGESICS AND ANESTHESIA

In our mothers' day, a delivery without analgesia or anesthesia was a rarity. Today, with family involvement in childbearing, the use of anesthesia and analgesia has diminished somewhat (Martin, 1990). With approaches to labor and delivery shifting from "always medicate" to "never or rarely medicate," obstetrics now takes a middle-of-the-road approach, and the value of anesthesia and analgesia is in the process of reevaluation. A subspecialty of obstetrical anesthesia now exists, and the maternal-child nurse now has far greater

knowledge and expertise, both of which have led to changes in approach.

Analgesics and Their Fetal and Maternal Side Effects

When cervical dilatation and uterine contractions cause pain, the use of a narcotic and a tranquilizer are usually indicated. Administration is either by intramuscular (IM) or intravenous (IV) route. The advantage of the IM or subcutaneous injection is that this is the fastest route in regard to nurse time and observation. The disadvantages include the length of time it takes for the drug to cause relief of pain, the danger of the drug crossing the placenta and affecting the fetus, and unequal absorption of the drug. The advantages of the IV route are prompt pain relief with predictable results and that small amounts can be given in equally divided doses. The disadvantage of IV administration is the possibility of bolus, but if given in the correct manner this is not of concern. Commonly used narcotic analgesics include the following:

Meperidine hydrochloride (Demerol) is typically administered IV in 12.5 to 25mg doses (with 50mg maximum), and IM in 75mg doses (with 100mg maximum). Pain relief usually occurs within 5 minutes after IV administration. Maternal side effects include central nervous system depression, especially respiratory; nausea, vomiting, and/or dry mouth; drowsiness; dizziness; flushing; transient hypotension; tachycardia; palpitations; and convulsions. Fetal/newborn side effects include neonatal hypotonia and lethargy; interference of thermoregulatory response for up to 72 hours after delivery; neonatal respiratory depression; neurologic and behavioral alterations for up to 72 hours postdelivery and depressed attention and social responsiveness for the first 6 weeks of life.

Fentanyl (Sublimaze) is given at a rate of 0.05mg (0.2mg maximum) by IV route only. It reaches its peak effect within two to five minutes, and lasts for 30 to 40 minutes. Chest wall rigidity can occasionally occur.

Butorphanol (Stadol) is a synthetic narcotic agonistantagonist analgesic that is thought to act on the subcortal portion of the central nervous system. The typical dose is 2mg IM every three to four hours. When given IV, lower doses are used. Its effects compare favorably to 40 to 60mg of meperidine, but care must be taken not to give the two drugs simultaneously or alternately, since butorphanol antagonizes the narcotic effects of meperidine Since it can cause respiratory depression, it is contraindicated in patients with respiratory disease. Other side effects include sedation, nausea, dizziness, a clammy, sweaty sensation, and a tendency to elevate cerebrospinal fluid pressure. Fetal side effects can include respiratory depression and a sinusoidal fetal heart rate pattern.

Nubain (nalbuphine) is frequently used in labor and delivery. It is also a synthetic narcotic agonist-antagonist, and its chief drawback is that it crosses the placenta and can cause respiratory depression in the fetus. It must be used with great caution if premature delivery is expected. Both Nubain and Stadol must be used with extreme caution in women who are addicted to drugs, since narcotic antagonists can induce acute withdrawal symptoms in the mother and fetus if the mother is addicted to heroin.

Assessment and Intervention

Nursing intervention in pain relief should start with nonpharmacological methods, which will be discussed later in this chapter. For some women, however, those methods will not bring adequate relief, and increasing discomfort will interfere with their ability to perform breathing techniques and maintain a sense of control.

Under these circumstances, pharmacological analgesics may be used to decrease discomfort, increase the patient's ability to relax, and reestablish her sense of control. But since analgesics will affect the mother, the fetus, and the contraction pattern, the nurse must first assess the woman's vital signs to determine that they are stable and must establish that the woman is willing to receive analgesia after being advised about its effects. She should understand the type of medication being administered, its route of administration, its expected effects, its implications for the fetus/neonate, and the safety measures required for its use. The fetus must also be assessed to determine that the FHR is between 120 and 160 beats per minute, with no late or variable decelerations present; short-term variability is present and long-term variability is average; normal movement and accelerations are present with fetal movement; the fetus is at term; and there is no meconium staining.

Labor assessment includes a well-established contraction pattern; cervical dilatation of four to five cm in nulliparas, and three to four cm in multiparas; engagement of the fetal presenting part; and progressive descent of the fetal presenting part with no complications existing.

When administering analgesic drugs, careful and continuous observation of maternal respirations and FHR are mandatory, with baseline FHR and maternal vital signs recorded on the monitor strip both before and after administration. The doctor's or nurse-midwife's written order is checked, and the drug is prepared and signed out on the narcotic or control sheet. The woman's armband is checked for identification, and she is again asked if she is allergic to any drug. The drug is administered by the route ordered, and the medication, time, dosage, route, and site of administration are charted on the nurse's notes and on the monitor strip. Safety precautions include side rails and continuous observation for nausea and vomiting, to prevent aspiration. While receiving analgesia, the woman should be in an individual birthing or labor room, with the environment free from sensory stimuli. She should be encouraged to empty her bladder before drug administration, and she should not be left alone.

ANESTHESIA

Regional

Regional anesthesia is the injection of local anesthetic agents that block transmission of painful stimuli from the uterus, cervix, vagina, and perineum to the thalamic pain centers in the brain. The methods most often used in labor are the pudendal block, the paracervical block, the peridural (lumbar, epidural, and caudal) block, subarachnoid or saddle block (spinal for cesarean birth, low spinal for vaginal delivery), and local infiltration (*see figure 6-1*). These blocks are accomplished by means of a single injection or continuously, by means of an indwelling plastic catheter. Paracervical and peridural blocks are used in the first stage of labor; during the second stage, pudendal peridural, or subarachnoid blocks are used.

Regional anesthesia has become increasingly popular due to its compatibility with the goals of psychoprophylactic preparation for childbirth. Its many advantages include the following: the area blocked is completely relieved from pain; depression of maternal vital signs is rare; aspiration of gastric contents is eliminated when no additional sedative is given; administration does not alter the course of labor; and the patient remains alert and able to participate in the birth.

The disadvantages of regional anesthesia include the high degree of skill required for its administration, the possibility of failure to adequately block pain, the side effects of some agents, and the possibility of systemic toxic reactions which can range from mild symptoms to cardiovascular collapse. Mild reactions include palpitations, vertigo, tinnitus, apprehension, confusion,

headache, and a metallic taste in the mouth. Moderate reactions include more intense degrees of the abovementioned mild symptoms plus nausea, vomiting, hypotension, and muscle twitching that can lead to convulsions and loss of consciousness. Severe reactions include loss of consciousness, coma, severe hypotension, bradycardia, respiratory depression, and cardiac arrest.

Because of the possibility of adverse reactions, regional anesthetics should always be used with an intravenous line in place. Except for nurse anesthetists or nurse/midwives, nurses may not legally administer anesthetic agents. This restriction includes the reinjection of agents through indwelling catheters. However, nurses with a knowledge of regional anesthesia can provide support, give reinforcing explanations to their patients, offer more efficient assistance to the administrator, and increase their patients' safety by recognizing complications and instituting proper interventions promptly.

Pudendal block consists of a local anesthetic agent injected around the pudendal nerve, which causes perineal analgesia. Used late in the second stage, just before spontaneous or low forceps delivery of the infant, it provides anesthesia for birth and for repair of the episiotomy It does not alter maternal or fetal respirations or other body functions, and does not affect uterine contractions. However, it may affect the woman's bearing down reflex and may cause broad ligament hematoma.

Paracervical block is accomplished by injecting a local anesthetic transvaginally, adjacent to the outer rim of the cervix. It may be administered during the active phase of labor, achieving rapid and complete relief of uterine pain during cervical dilatation. It does not anesthetize the lower vagina or the perineum and it does not interfere with the bearing-down reflex. However, it has several maternal disadvantages, including systemic toxic reaction and uterine vessel damage leading to

FIGURE 6-1
Spinal/Epidural Anesthesia

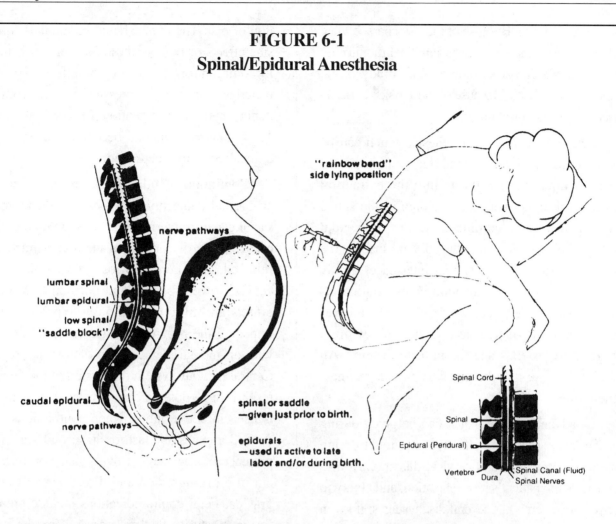

"rainbow bend"
side lying position

nerve pathways

lumbar spinal

lumbar epidural

low spinal
"saddle block"

caudal epidural

nerve pathways

spinal or saddle
—given just prior to birth.

epidurals
—used in active to late
labor and/or during birth.

Spinal Cord

Spinal

Epidural (Peridural)

Vertebre

Dura

Spinal Canal (Fluid)

Spinal Nerves

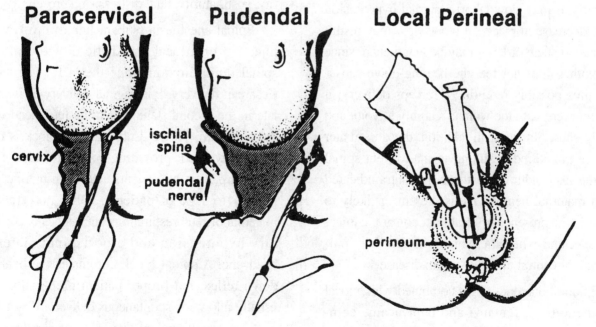

Paracervical

cervix

Pudendal

ischial
spine

pudendal
nerve

Local Perineal

perineum

severe hematoma. Because of the risks paracervical block poses to the fetus, electronic fetal monitoring is indicated. The risks include fetal bradycardia, acidosis, and death. Because of these risks, paracervical blocks are used infrequently.

Peridural (epidural) anesthesia, which can be used during the first or second stages of labor, consists of injecting anesthesia into the extradural space. It does not penetrate the dura or the spinal cord, and may be administered into the caudal space within the sacrum or the epidural space at the second, third, or fourth lumbar interspace. It may be given by a single injection or by continuous injection over many hours. A small amount relieves the discomfort of uterine contractions, while a larger dose extends anesthesia to the vagina. An additional dose may be given to provide perineal anesthesia.

Its advantages are that it can be given during active labor, providing effective pain relief during uterine contractions and cervical dilatation. It also enhances the patient's rest, relaxation, and ability to cope. However, it has several disadvatages: if given too early, it may slow labor; maternal hypotension and a decrease in placental blood flow may result; the second stage of labor may be lengthened, since the mother does not feel the bearing-down sensation, thus possibly requiring a forceps delivery; it may interfere with the woman's ability to void; and it may cause infection In addition, the dura mater may be punctured, resulting in inadvertent spinal anesthesia. Epidural anesthesia is contraindicated when maternal hemorrhage is present or likely to occur, in the presence of local infection at the injection site, and when the woman has cardiac, pulmonary, or central nervous system disease.

Epidural narcotics when combined with a local anesthetic (e.g., fentanyl and bupivacaine combined) have been shown to be effective pain relievers for late active labor. It has also been used during and after cesarean deliveries with effective reduc-

tion of pain The nurse should be familiar with the side effects of both of these medicines when used in combination; these include allergic reaction, maternal respiratory depression, nausea, vomiting, itching, and urinary retention (May & Mahlmeister, 1994). Naloxone should be immediately available to treat respiratory depression.

Continuous caudal block provides peridural analgesia by injection of a local anesthetic into the sacral canal in intermittent doses, with an epidural catheter. The discomfort of uterine contractions is relieved, and there is a loss of sensation in the cervix, lower vagina, and perineum. Maternal effects are minimal, although hypotension and impeding the progress of labor may result, along with an increased incidence of forceps delivery. Central nervous system depression of the fetus can result if large doses are administered. This method is used in active labor, when contractions occur every 3 minutes and last for 40 seconds, and in the presence of engagement, with dilatation of 5 to 6 cm in a primigravida and 4 to 5 cm in a multigravida. Fetal contraindications include prematurity, postmaturity, fetal distress, and breech.

Spinal anesthesia (subarachnoid) involves the injection of a local anesthetic directly into the spinal fluid, providing anesthesia for vaginal or Cesarean delivery. For vaginal delivery, it is given late in the second stage, when the fetal head is on the perineum. The midsubarachnoid block is most frequently used, providing complete relief from perineal pain in all patients, and from uterine pain in 90% to 95% of patients. It has no effect on maternal or fetal respirations but may cause temporary hypotension and a postspinal maternal headache. A spinal block eliminates the bearing-down reflex, but proper patient preparation will usually allow for spontaneous delivery. If not, forceps are easily applied due to perineal relaxation. Its advantages are simplicity, rapidity of action, high success rate, and a low incidence of maternal and fetal side effects. Contraindications include:

severe hypovolemia, central nervous system disease, infection at the puncture site, severe hypotension or hypertension, cephalopelvic disproportion, and fear of the procedure.

Nursing considerations during the administration of regional anesthesia include support for the laboring woman, encouraging her participation in decision making, and continuous monitoring of vital signs and fetal status. Also essential is a knowledge of medications, their proper dosages, their possible complications, early signs and symptoms of complications, and actions to initiate in the event of untoward reaction until the arrival of appropriate medical personnel.

Actions specific to blocks are as follows:

- **Paracervical:** Assess maternal blood pressure, pulse, and fetal heart rate; assure continuous FHR tracing; assess maternal bladder.

- **Epidural:** Initially, the nurse must assess maternal blood pressure and pulse and the fetal heart rate for baseline. An electronic fetal monitor must be used for continual tracing. Maternal blood pressure and pulse are assessed every one to two minutes during the first 15 minutes after the injection, and every 10 to 15 minutes until stable. Assess bladder at frequent intervals for distention past birth. Delay ambulation until all motor control has returned. Assess for orthostatic hypotension.

- **Spinal:** Assess maternal vital signs and fetal heart rate for baseline. Assist with positioning during administration. Assess for uterine contractions and inform anesthesiologist. Place wedge under patient's right hip to tip the uterus off the vena cava. Assess maternal blood pressure and pulse every two to five minutes until stable. Continue to monitor contractions. Provide safety and prevent injury when moving the patient. Provide bedrest for 6 to 12 hours following delivery.

- **Pudendal:** Provide support and assess for development of hematoma.

- **Local infiltration:** Provide support and assess for perineal trauma, such as swelling or bruising.

General Anesthesia

General anesthesia is inhalation anesthesia, which provides pain relief through the administration of a gaseous agent mixed with oxygen and inhaled until the patient becomes unconscious. Its advantages are that it produces overall relaxation, which is useful in difficult forceps deliveries, breech, and cesarean sections. The likelihood of convulsions in preeclamptic or eclamptic women is reduced when general anesthesia is administered, and perhaps its greatest advantage is that it can be administered rapidly in emergency situations when delivery must be immediate and pain relief is essential. However, among its disadvantages are that delivery must occur within five to seven minutes after administration, because inhalation anesthesia crosses the placenta quickly and can cause hypoxia and respiratory depression in the fetus. There is always a risk of maternal aspiration of gastric contents, which can result in pulmonary complications, and immediate postpartum recovery is more complicated due to the risks of nausea, vomiting, uterine atony, and postpartum hemorrhage. With this type of anesthesia the bearing-down reflex is stopped, and the mother cannot participate in the birth, nor can she interact with the baby immediately following birth.

General anesthesia is used today because of previous complications or high-risk problems due to pregnancy. Women whose regional anesthesia is ineffective, those with pregnancy-induced hypertension, prolapsed cord, severe bleeding, or fetal distress with a second twin may be candidates. Contraindications to general anesthesia are fetal prematurity or distress, and maternal upper respiratory infection, multiple births, or when the patient has eaten before administration.

The patient receiving general anesthesia requires preoxygenation, IV fluid loading, tracheal protection with cricoid pressure to prevent aspiration, and a pelvic tilt for maximum uterine circulation to the fetus. The nurse attending the patient under general anesthesia must observe the fetal heart rate constantly, while monitoring maternal vital signs and checking for uterine bleeding. Although it may slow down uterine contractions, general anesthesia can also relax perineal musculature and cause rapid expulsion of the fetus, for which the nurse must be alert.

TYPES OF GENERAL ANESTHESIA

Nitrous Oxide

Actually 40% nitrous oxide and 60% oxygen, this anesthetic is administered by face mask or inhaler. Its induction is fast and pleasant, and it is nonirritating, nonexplosive, and less disruptive of physiological function than any other general anesthetic. Its main use is in the second stage of labor; as an induction agent or as a supplement to more potent general anesthesia.

Halothane (Fluothane)

Not used as frequently as nitrous oxide, halothane nevertheless bears mention for obstetrical anesthesia. Its induction is rapid, predictable, and safe, since it causes little or no nausea or vomiting. It provides moderate-to-good uterine relaxation, although it may cause respiratory depression as well as irritability of cardiac tissue which can result in arrhythmia. It may also cause increased uterine contraction along with the risk of postpartum hemorrhage.

Methoxyflurane (Penthrane)

Administered by inhaler for analgesia, or in combination with other agents for anesthesia, methoxyflurane induction is pleasant but slower (as is recovery) than with gas agents. Uterine contraction may result from its use, and administration is restricted to low doses for short periods because of the risk of postpartum bleeding.

Thiopental Sodium (Pentothal)

This ultrashort-acting barbiturate is given intravenously and produces narcosis within 30 seconds. Induction and emergence are smooth, pleasant, with little nausea or vomiting. It is most frequently used for induction or as an adjuvant to more potent anesthetics.

Balanced Anesthesia

Today's trend is toward "balanced anesthesia" for both vaginal and cesarean births. This is achieved by giving several different agents by different routes, which increases effectiveness and safety. Because of the combined effect, smaller doses can be given of each agent than if given separately. For example, IV thiopental sodium may be given for sedation and induction, followed by halothane by face mask for analgesia and anesthesia.

Recovery

The recovery period from general anesthesia requires particular vigilance from the nurse. If the patient is conscious, her physiological and psychological well-being demand that she be with her baby and significant other. At the same time, the nurse must monitor temperature, blood pressure, pulse, and respiration while watching for bleeding, checking uterine tone, and observing bladder filling. Vital signs and observations of the uterus, bladder, and episiotomy or abdominal incision must be recorded every 15 minutes. The recovery period is generally two hours. During this time, the family can become acquainted with the baby while the mother is being closely monitored by the nurse.

NONPHARMACEUTICAL METHODS OF PAIN RELIEF

The Gate Control Theory

According to the gate control theory, pain is the result of interactions between several specialized neural systems. This theory postulates that a mechanism in the dorsal horn of the spinal column serves as a valve (or gate) that can increase or decrease the flow of nerve impulses from the periphery to the central nervous system. The gate mechanism is influenced by the size of the fibers that transmit impulses and by the impulses that descend from the brain. Pain perception and response may activate the gate system and may be influenced by psychological processes, including experiences, attention, and emotion. Therefore, according to theory, the gates can either be opened or closed by central nervous system activities such as anxiety or excitement, or through selective localized activity.

The gate control theory, as it applies to obstetrics, has vast implications. It suggests that pain can be controlled by tactile stimulation and can be modified by activities controlled by the central nervous system. These include backrub, sacral pressure, suggestion, distraction, and conditioning. Abdominal effleurage, a specific type of cutaneous stimulation, is used before the transitional phase of labor. It consists of light abdominal stroking and is used in the Lamaze method of childbirth preparation. It is particularly effective in relieving mild-to-moderate pain but is ineffectual for intense pain. The application of deep pressure over the sacrum is more effective for relieving back pain.

Other nonpharmaceutical methods of pain relief include biofeedback, acupuncture, acupressure, therapeutic touch, transcutaneous electrical nerve stimulation (TENS), bathing or showering, warmth, and positioning.

Biofeedback

Biofeedback is the use of monitoring equipment to detect and amplify internal physiological processes and feed them back to the individual in a comprehendable form. Then, the information fed back must reach the cortex of the brain and be understood by the woman, giving her the option to change her behavior or physiological response. The advantages of biofeedback are that no physician's order is needed, and, once a person is trained, no devices are required. However, in order to utilize biofeedback, the woman must locate a certified biofeedback trainer and invest a considerable amount of time and money learning the technique before going into labor.

Biofeedback approaches for pregnant women include the following: training in breathing, relaxation, focusing, and imagery skills to reduce fear and anxiety; appropriate labor positions to enhance the labor process and reduce pain; and stimulation of the parasympathetic nervous system and reduction in catecholamine production, which contributes to the maintenance of homeostasis. An informed nurse can ease the transition to the birthing agency of the woman who has mastered biofeedback and can help the patient increase the use and effectiveness of the technique during childbirth.

Acupuncture

Acupuncture bas been widely used in the Orient for many years, and there is increasing evidence that it may be an effective tool during labor. In some cultures, women have pressed combs into the palms of their hands to reduce the pain of contractions. Similarly, acupuncture involves the insertion and rotation of needles on specific points of the body, which is thought to produce analgesia and sedation through the release of betaendorphin. However, acupuncture is an invasive technique that may cause infection. In addition, finding a qualified professional to perform acupuncture during labor and/or delivery may pose problems.

Acupressure

Also long used in the Orient, acupressure is thought to activate the release of endorphins in the body. It is defined as finger pressure or massage over "pain prevention (or acupuncture) points," and is another form of touch therapy. Proponents of the gate control theory speculate that acupressure's pain-relieving qualities are based on blocking the gate at the level of the spinal cord. This technique is now taught in many childbirth education classes, but since some forms are thought to induce labor; instruction is limited to selected points.

Acupressure may be used to alleviate some of the common discomforts of pregnancy, such as dizziness, faintness, headache, or sciatic nerve pain and leg cramps. In labor, acupressure is used as part of a pain control routine that includes relaxation, concentration, and rhythmic breathing. Contraindications to this technique include any site where there is red, swollen, broken, or infected skin.

Therapeutic Touch

Throughout history, people have used touch (the ancient art of laying-on of hands) as a means of calming a person. Now, according to researchers, there is evidence of an actual transfer of energy taking place in some forms of touching, as evidenced in muscular relaxation. Therapeutic touch offers decided advantages. No devices are required, no physician's order is needed, the technique is noninvasive, and it incurs no cost since the technique is incorporated into nursing care. Indeed, there has been extensive research by nurses into the background and application of therapeutic touch, which was originally described by Dolores Krieger, a nurse. Unlike the laying-on of hands, the technique has no religious basis and does not require a declaration of faith from the subject in order to be effective. It does, however, require the conscious intent of the healer.

Therapeutic touch may offer a powerful means of enhancing relaxation, reducing anxiety, and controlling pain. It can be taught easily in childbirth education classes to the pregnant woman and her support network. It is particularly helpful for couples uncomfortable with physical touch, for it can help increase communication as well as alleviate the discomforts of pregnancy. During labor and birth it is used along with breathing and other relaxation strategies; and in the early months of parenting it is frequently used as a means of calming a crying baby, relaxing a distraught parent, or helping a woman through "postpartum blues." Not only the patient benefits from therapeutic touch. It also can enhance the healer's sense of inner harmony, well-being, and relaxation, enabling the healer to cope while healing. Touch is not just an end in itself. It is a means of making coping skills more powerful and effective.

Transcutaneous Electrical Nerve Stimulation (TENS)

This method of alleviating pain by electrical nerve stimulation generally requires the services of a physiologist or other professional. Although TENS is widely used outside obstetrics, its use in labor is questionable. It may interfere with continuous electronic fetal monitoring, since it must be applied constantly to gain relief. Moreover, it is most effective only if introduced before crisis. A TENS unit is costly, running between $200 and $500. However, many nonobstetrical patients, particularly those who cannot achieve pain relief by any other means, acquire the instrument and are taught how to use it themselves.

Bathing, Showering, Warmth

During the early stage of labor, bathing or showering may afford a measure of pain relief for the patient. No physician's order is needed for showering, but it is advisable that the nurse check institution protocol concerning tub bathing. Whichever method is employed, the nurse should remain in close attendance to avoid the possibility of accidents and hyperthermia. Of course, continuous electronic fetal monitoring is not possible when the patient is bathing. During labor, many women feel discomfort from cold feet. If they have not brought socks or slippers with them, the nurse can provide paper slippers to increase the patient's comfort. The nurse must also be alert to the patient's need for bodily warmth and should keep the room temperature at a comfortable level, providing blankets as needed, since the woman may be too absorbed in the process of labor to ask for help.

Positioning

The nurse should encourage the laboring woman to assume whatever position she finds most comfortable. However, any position used during labor and delivery should facilitate the alignment of the presenting part to the axis of the pelvis, and should also encourage the mother's efforts toward accomplishing delivery.

Babies have been born with their mothers in a variety of positions, including standing, squatting, kneeling, crouched on all fours, semi-sitting, and lying down on their sides or backs. Researchers have determined that in both the primipara and the multipara, labors are 25% shorter with the upright position employed, since standing is the most efficient position for dilating the cervix, and that contractions are stronger but less frequent when the woman is side-lying.

If the woman chooses a side-lying position in labor, she should be encouraged to make frequent position changes in order to achieve more efficient contractions. The nurse must observe the patient to assure that all body parts are supported, encouraging her to keep her knees slightly flexed. In the side-lying position, pillows may be placed against the woman's chest and under her upper arm, with a pillow or folded bath blanket placed between her knees to support her upper leg and to relieve muscle strain or tension. Additional support may be provided by placing a pillow at the patient's mid-back.

If the woman prefers to lie on her back, the nurse must elevate the head of the bed to lessen the pressure of the uterus on the vena cava. In this position, pillows should be placed under each arm and also under the knees for additional support. However, because pregnant women run a high risk of thrombophlebitis, the nurse must take care not to exert excessive pressure behind the knee and calf.

During delivery, the woman's position should be determined by her own wishes as well as those of her health care professional. The upright posture was considered normal in most societies until recent times, and only within the past two centuries has the recumbent (lithotomy) position been used, mainly for the convenience of the physician or nurse-midwife. Now alternative positions are accepted, based on the comfort of the laboring woman. These include sitting in a birthing chair, semi-Fowler's position, left-lateral Sims' position, squatting, and sitting in a birthing bed. When assisting in a birth using an alternative position, nursing implications are as follows:

Birthing chair: Encourage the woman to tilt the chair to increase her comfort. Assess for pressure points on her legs.

Semi-Fowler's: Assess that the upper torso is evenly supported. Increase support of the body by changing the position of the bed or by using pillows as props.

Left-lateral Sims: Adjust position so that the upper leg lies on the bed in scissor fashion or is supported either by the partner or by pillows.

Squatting: Help the woman maintain balance. Use a squatting bar if available.

Sitting in a birthing bed: Assure that legs and feet have adequate support.

SUMMARY

In helping the laboring woman to achieve pain relief, the nurse should focus on the body's natural resources and should emphasize supportive pain management techniques for labor and childbirth. For some women, however, mastery of childbirth on their own terms supercedes pain relief. The nurse must respect the patient's right to her feelings about pain, medication, and other aspects of labor and delivery. Most important is the assurance a nurse can give to the patient that using medication does not indicate guilt or failure on the woman's part. Couples must master the necessary skills to manage the pain and stress of labor and delivery with the dignity and comfort that they want, while remaining flexible to cope with whatever situation arises. The nurse must attempt to convey a realistic picture of the childbirth pain experience, assist the couple in their efforts to manage pain, and bolster their confidence so they can cope with the experience of childbirth.

EXAM QUESTIONS

CHAPTER 6
Questions 27–33

27. Pain during labor and childbirth is primarily caused by

    a. dilatation of the cervix and uterine cell hypoxia.

    b. pressure on the bladder.

    c. stretching of the pelvis.

    d. increased levels of endorphin.

28. Maternal side effects from intravenous meperidine hydrochloride (Demerol) include

    a. respiratory depression and tachycardia.

    b. hypertension and decreased pulse rate.

    c. agitation and hypertension.

    d. dehydration and neonatal hypotonia.

29. Before administering a narcotic analgesic to a woman in labor, the nurse should

    a. discourage the patient from taking it.

    b. verify that the patient is soon to deliver.

    c. assess maternal respirations, fetal heart rate, and labor progress.

    d. notify the anesthesiologist.

30. The injection of a local anesthetic agent to block transmission of painful stimuli from the uterus, cervix, vagina, and perineum is classified as

    a. general anesthesia.

    b. regional anesthesia.

    c. local anesthesia.

    d. regional analgesia.

31. The major side effects of epidural anesthesia are

    a. hypertonus and fetal arrhythmia.

    b. hypertension and increased placental blood flow.

    c. hypotension and urinary retention.

    d. dehydration and rapid delivery.

32. Two hours after receiving meperidine (Demerol) IV, the patient progresses to complete dilation and delivers. The nurse must be aware of the potential for

    a. maternal hypertension.

    b. neonatal respiratory depression.

    c. postpartum hemorrhage.

    d. jaundice in the newborn.

33. Nursing care of the patient who has received epidural anesthesia includes which of the following?

    a. Monitoring maternal blood pressure.

    b. Monitoring maternal temperature.

    c. Monitoring maternal respiratory rate.

    d. Monitoring PO fluid intake.

CHAPTER 7

ASSESSMENT OF FETAL WELL-BEING

CHAPTER OBJECTIVE

After studying this chapter, the reader will be able to identify methods of assessing fetal well-being during the last trimester of pregnancy and during labor and delivery, and be able to direct nursing care toward the goal of delivering a viable infant.

LEARNING OBJECTIVES

After studying this chapter, the student will be able to

1. Identify the rationale for assessing fetal well-being during labor and delivery.

2. Indicate the sources of fetal oxygenation and select situations and conditions that may impair fetal oxygenation during pregnancy, labor, and delivery.

3. Choose nursing strategies for intervention when fetal monitoring indicates that a deviation from normal exists.

4. Recognize results of fetal monitoring that indicate the fetus is stressed or fetal well-being is in jeopardy.

5. Specify nursing responsibilities when monitoring fetal well-being.

INTRODUCTION

This chapter focuses on the evaluation of fetal well-being late in pregnancy and during labor and delivery. (Chapter 3 discusses fetal surveillance during the remainder of the antepartal period.) Assessment of fetal well-being is a critical part of obstetrics because maternity nursing is directed toward delivering a viable fetus while supporting the mother. Assessment of fetal well-being also is an integral part of maternity care because obstetrics historically is a high-risk field for malpractice actions. Any such actions will inevitably focus on the well-being of the fetus during the last trimester of pregnancy or during labor and delivery. If fetal well-being is challenged, fetal distress may result. That is why a knowledge of fetal well-being evaluation techniques is crucial to the maternity nurse. Topics covered in this chapter include a review of fetal circulation and oxygenation, since those are the factors commonly measured in assessments of fetal well-being; factors involved in fetal distress; the consequences of fetal asphyxia; monitoring fetal well-being; interpreting the results of fetal heart rate monitoring; and nursing strategies for the patient undergoing fetal monitoring.

FETAL CIRCULATION AND OXYGENATION

Any assessment of fetal well-being will involve evaluating the status of the fetal circulation, including the placenta and umbilical cord, the fetus, and the uterus, because impairment of one or more of these may compromise the fetus. Many measures of fetal well-being performed late in pregnancy or during labor or delivery are designed to evaluate fetal circulation and oxygenation. The information gleaned from the assessment of fetal well-being will be used to make determinations on medical, surgical, or nursing intervention. So it is essential that nurses have an understanding of fetal circulation and oxygenation if they are to care for the pregnant patient.

Fetal Circulation

Connected to the mother by the umbilical cord, the fetus is dependent upon its mother for nourishment, circulation, and gas (oxygen, carbon dioxide) exchange. This is accomplished through the placental and fetal circulation. The mother's body delivers oxygenated blood to the fetus and removes carbon dioxide from the blood that is returned to the maternal circulation. This blood flow is conducted through the umbilical cord, which normally consists of two arteries and one vein. Blood leaving the fetus courses through the umbilical arteries; blood running to the fetus travels through the umbilical vein. Covered by a gelatinous material known as Wharton's jelly, the umbilical cord connects to the placenta, where the exchange of gas and nutrients takes place. The placenta also serves to block some noxious substances from the fetus. As in adults, fetal circulation consists of the systemic and pulmonary circuits, but the fetus also has a third circuit, the placental circulation *(see figure 7-1)*.

Korones (1986) gives an overview of fetal circulation:

Pulmonary circulation begins at the pul-monic valve at the origin of the main pulmonary artery, which arises from the right ventricle. It continues through the lungs and terminates at the pulmonary vein orifices in the wall of the left atrium. The systemic circulation includes all other arterial and venous channels elsewhere in the body. The placental circuit is composed of the umbilical and placental vessels… Fetal circulation differs from the neonatal or adult pattern in three major respects: (1) presence of anatomic shunts, one within the heart at the foramen ovale, one immediately outside the heart in the ductus arteriosus, and another at the juncture of the ductus venosus and the inferior vena cava; (2) presence of a placental circulation; and (3) minimal blood flow through the lungs (3% to 7% of cardiac output).

Although the ductus venosus and the ductus arteriosus are seldom factors in fetal distress, they are briefly reviewed here to enhance your understanding of fetal circulation. The ductus venosus links portions of the gastrointestinal and hepatic circulation to the inferior vena cava; it generally closes by the end of the first week of life and seldom presents any difficulty. The ductus arteriosus serves to help bypass the lungs in the fetus, since the lungs are not functioning as organs of respiration and need only a limited amount of blood for growth and development. Yet the ductus arteriosus may fail to close normally after birth, especially in the pre-term infant. Because the ductus arteriosus links the aorta and pulmonary artery, a flood of blood flow to the lungs can lead to pulmonary edema and reduce the amount of blood available to circulate to other vital organs.

Fetal Oxygenation

Critical components in fetal circulation and oxygenation: According to Korones (1986), alteration of uteroplacental blood flow is the

FIGURE 7-1
Fetal Circulation

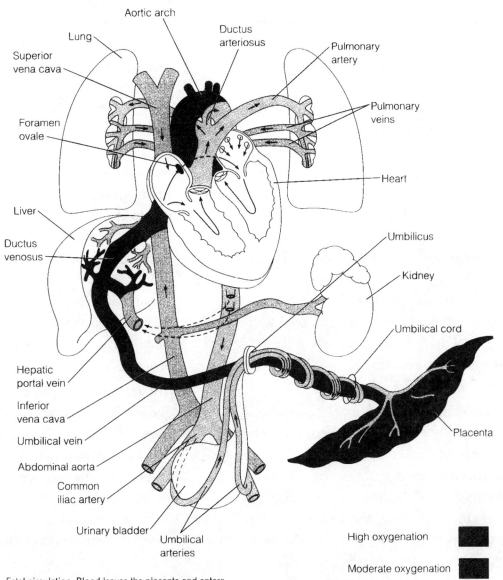

Fetal circulation. Blood leaves the placenta and enters the fetus through the umbilical vein. After circulating through the fetus, the blood returns to the placenta through the umbilical arteries. The ductus venosus, the foramen ovale, and the ductus arteriosus allow the blood to bypass the fetal liver and lungs.

Source: *Maternal Newborn Nursing Care,* 4th ed., Ladewig, P.W., London, M.L. & Olds, S.B., 1998, Addison-Wesley, Longman, Inc. New York, NY.

most frequent cause of fetal hypoxia. When the fertilized egg (trophoblast) implants in the wall of the mother's womb during the first days of pregnancy, vascular protrusions called villi sprout from the trophoblast. The trophoblast is then called the chorion and the villi are referred to as chorionic villi. These vascular protrusions form the foundation of the placenta. Oxygen from the mother's blood diffuses across the membranes of the intervillous spaces formed by the placenta. This diffusion oxygenates the fetal blood, which is then carried by the umbilical vein to the fetus, where it is extracted for use. Carbon dioxide, a by-product of metabolism, is returned to the placenta via the umbilical arteries. Korones notes that the most common cause of fetal asphyxia is impairment of maternal blood flow through the intervillous space. Thus, oxygenation is a critical factor in fetal well-being; fetal mortality and morbidity are associated with a decrease in fetal oxygenation *(see figures 7-1 and 7-2).*

Umbilical cord: As noted above, the umbilical cord normally contains two arteries and one vein. The umbilical cord is flexible and may be compressed during labor or delivery. Compression will impede the flow of blood through the cord; it may also compromise fetal circulation and reduce fetal oxygenation. Maintenance of fetal well-being is therefore heavily dependent upon an intact and functioning cord. Sometimes during pregnancy the cord will become loosely knotted or wrapped around a fetal part; this does not usually compromise the fetus unless circulation through the cord is impeded or halted by a tight knot or kink in the cord. The average length of the umbilical cord is 53 cm (21 inches) at term.

Placenta: Because the fetus cannot breathe in the amniotic fluid, the placenta takes over the respiratory functions of the fetus. The placenta is a structure that imbeds into the wall of the uterus

and functions to exchange oxygen and carbon dioxide and nutrients with the fetus. The maternal and fetal circulations are separated only by a thin membrane at the microscopic levels of exchange. (Korones, 1986). Adequate structure and proper functioning of the placenta are therefore essential to fetal well-being; alterations or pathology in the placenta will threaten fetal well-being. Some of these conditions include a placenta that is abnormally implanted in the uterine wall, one that separates prematurely, or one that develops abnormally. During labor, uterine contractions will impede placental blood flow, but normally this is not sufficient to jeopardize the fetus. However, in certain conditions, such as maternal hypertension, this margin of safety is reduced. Flow through the placenta can also be reduced by maternal hypotension or hemorrhage and by some drugs administered to the mother *(see Figure 7-2).*

Uterus: The developing fetus requires a safe structure in which to grow, and a source of nourishment, circulation, and oxygenation. The uterus and placenta function to meet these needs. Any factors that reduce uterine or placental capacity can negatively affect the fetus, leading to fetal distress; some of these conditions will be reviewed in greater detail later in this chapter.

FACTORS INVOLVED IN FETAL DISTRESS

According to Korones (1986), intact fetal survival during labor depends on a balance between the forces generated by uterine contractions to expel the fetus and the extent to which placental blood and oxygen transfer is interrupted by these forces. Korones further indicates that the principal stress exerted by labor on a fetus is interference with placental perfusion. As already discussed, fetal circulation and oxy-

FIGURE 7-2
Placental Circulation

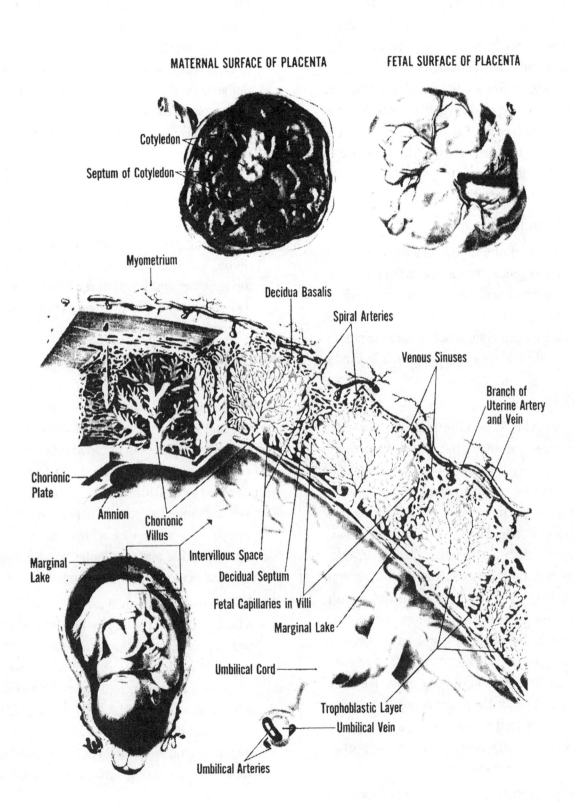

MATERNAL SURFACE OF PLACENTA

FETAL SURFACE OF PLACENTA

Cotyledon

Septum of Cotyledon

Myometrium

Decidua Basalis

Spiral Arteries

Venous Sinuses

Branch of Uterine Artery and Vein

Chorionic Plate

Amnion

Chorionic Villus

Marginal Lake

Intervillous Space

Decidual Septum

Fetal Capillaries in Villi

Marginal Lake

Umbilical Cord

Trophoblastic Layer

Umbilical Vein

Umbilical Arteries

genation must be adequate if the normal fetus is to remain viable. Some factors that result in nonviable or abnormal infants may play a role in fetal distress, but they are in general due to the anomaly and not factors that interfere with fetal circulation and oxygenation. The focus of this section is the fetus that falls victim to distress during the late stages of pregnancy or during labor and delivery. The factors involved in causing fetal distress can often be traced to disruptions in the structure or functioning of the placenta, the umbilical cord, the uterus, or the maternal circulation.

Placental Factors

As mentioned above, the placenta serves to nourish and oxygenate the fetus. Anything that disrupts the placenta will also disrupt the flow of nutrients and oxygen to the fetus. Some conditions that may disrupt placental function include premature separation of the placenta, abnormal implantation of the placenta, and an abnormality in the placenta itself.

Placenta previa: While the placenta normally embeds into the wall of the upper portion of the uterus, it may implant lower, in some cases even covering the internal os, the opening of the uterus to the cervix. As the pregnancy approaches term, the stretching of the lower uterine segment can cause the placenta to slowly separate. Painless vaginal bleeding, a cardinal sign of placenta previa, may result. Blood loss is usually minimal at first, but increases as the pregnancy progresses. Because placenta previa can compromise fetal circulation and oxygenation, it may cause fetal distress. However, since placenta previa can most often be detected by ultrasonography and the bleeding generally develops slowly, it is often manageable if recognized early.

Abruptio placentae: When the placenta separates from the wall of the uterus before the delivery of the fetus, an obstetric emergency exists.

Unless the fetus is delivered within minutes of the time the placenta separates, fetal death is likely. Maternal mortality is also high, because hemorrhage into the uterus may be significant. The outcome is generally based on the length of time between separation of the placenta and delivery of the infant. Symptoms of abruptio placentae in the pregnant patient include the sudden onset of abdominal pain and vaginal bleeding.

Placental insufficiency: Women with diabetes, hypertension, thyroid disorders, or other chronic medical disorders have a higher risk of developing placental insufficiency. In this condition, the placenta lacks (to varying degrees) the structure and function necessary to nourish and support the fetus. Impairment of fetal circulation and oxygenation result.

Umbilical Cord Factors

The umbilical cord is flexible and compresses easily. It also serves as the vital conduit between mother and child. Anything that compresses the cord or obstructs the flow of blood between mother and child can result in a decrease in fetal circulation and oxygenation. And because the flow through the umbilical cord is not just occluded in one direction, there may be a build-up in the fetus of carbon dioxide and metabolic waste products, causing fetal acidosis and hypercapnia.

Nuchal cord: As mentioned earlier, sometimes the umbilical cord is knotted in one or more places, or wrapped around the infant's neck. This is generally innocuous; it is only when this knot, wrap, or kink obstructs the flow of blood that fetal distress may result. Unfortunately, however, fetal death in the antepartal period is sometimes the result of a nuchal cord, which is an umbilical cord wrapped around the fetal neck.

Prolapsed cord: Sometimes the umbilical cord is caught between the presenting part and the mother's body structures, causing a situation known as a prolapsed cord. This most commonly occurs when the amniotic membranes rupture, the fetal presenting part is not engaged in the pelvis, and the cord follows the flow of fluid down the birth canal. This is a serious obstetric emergency that will result in severe fetal distress or death if the occlusion of the cord is not promptly relieved. Fetal hypoxia will develop within two or three minutes under these circumstances.

Uterine Factors

The uterus is a muscular structure; it contracts and relaxes in an effort to move the fetus down into the pelvis and out the vagina. The relaxation between contractions is essential to fetal well-being since it allows the fetus to recover from the decreased placental blood flow that occurs during the contraction. In general, contractions last about one minute, and occur in a crescendo-decrescendo manner. As labor progresses, the interval between contractions shortens to about one to two minutes. Intrauterine pressure rises up to 50 torr or even higher when the mother bears down with the contraction, and placental blood flow naturally decreases.

Effective uterine contractions are obviously essential to the delivery of the fetus but must not be so strong or so frequent that the fetus is threatened. Uterine factors that can alter fetal outcome include the following:

Hypertonic uterus: This condition may be iatrogenic, which means it is caused by the medical team in treating the patient. If iatrogenic, it generally occurs following the administration of agents such as oxytocin, which stimulate uterine contractions. Because the potential for hypertonic contractions or uterine tetany exists with the administration of such drugs, uterine pressure and fetal heart rate must be carefully monitored in the mother receiving uterine stim-

ulants. Hypertonic contractions will reduce the placental blood flow to the fetus.

Uterine rupture: In women receiving uterine stimulants such as oxytocin, or those who have previously had a Cesarean section, the uterus may rupture. Although this complication is rare, it is generally rapidly fatal due to maternal blood loss; the fetus often is lost also.

Maternal Factors

Because the fetus depends upon the mother for all life support, anything that compromises the mother's condition will also compromise the baby's condition. As mentioned earlier, this can include chronic medical conditions such as hypertension or diabetes. Since fetal circulation and oxygenation are dependent upon maternal circulation and oxygenation, anything that affects the mother will, in general, affect the child. Anytime maternal circulation or oxygenation is impaired by medical disorders, trauma, hemorrhage, or other serious conditions, it is only reasonable to expect that the fetus is impaired also. Therefore, it is essential to treat the mother for hypoxia or hypotension immediately in order to offer the fetus the best chance of survival.

Fetal Factors

Normally developed, full-term infants in general have the best hope of survival and avoidance of fetal distress. As mentioned earlier, the fetus with congenital anomalies may suffer unavoidable fetal distress as it attempts the transition to extrauterine life. Pre-term and post-term infants increase the risk of fetal distress because they are not in optimal condition to withstand the rigors of labor and delivery.

CONSEQUENCES OF FETAL ASPHYXIA

When the human body does not receive enough oxygen and is unable to excrete its waste product, carbon dioxide, a condition known as asphyxia develops. Asphyxia usually results when a person's airway is occluded, halting the free exchange of air between the lungs and the environmental air. Left untreated, asphyxia will cause hypoxia, hypercapnia, acidosis, and death. The fetus, of course, doesn't actively exchange air with the environment. It relies on its mother, the uterus, the umbilical cord, the placenta and its circulation for respiration.

If any of these factors is impaired to the degree that it interferes with fetal circulation and oxygenation, fetal distress may result. The consequences of fetal distress and asphyxia are multiple and serious.

Neurologic: The effects of hypoxia on the brain are well known to all healthcare professionals. Profound, devastating, and irreversible brain damage may occur. Seizures, brain hemorrhage, and other major neurologic catastrophes can be a direct result of fetal asphyxia. Death can result from neurologic insult.

Cardiovascular: Fetal asphyxia may result in failure of the fetal blood flow to assume the normal neonatal pattern after birth; this phenomenon is referred to as "persistent fetal circulation" (Korones, 1986). The heart and vasculature may also suffer insults as a result of fetal asphyxia; the acidosis that accompanies asphyxia can damage the cardiovascular system.

Respiratory: Asphyxia amplifies and complicates lung disorders such as respiratory distress or meconium aspiration that may develop in the distressed newborn. Meconium (a thick, sticky brown or green stool passed by the full-term infant) may be passed in utero in response to asphyxia. With its first breath, the baby may inhale meconium into the lungs, causing a severe pneumonia known as meconium aspiration. Fetal asphyxia may also result in persistent fetal circulation or a patent ductus arteriosus, which can result in respiratory distress. And of course, fetal distress may force pre-term delivery of an infant with immature lungs.

Metabolic: Acid-based disturbances accompany hypoxia and asphyxia, and the fetus or newborn are no exception. Disturbances in glucose and calcium metabolism are relatively common if the fetus suffers asphyxia.

Renal, hepatic, and gastrointestinal: Each of these body systems will be negatively influenced by hypoxia and fetal asphyxia. Kidney function may shutdown. The intestines may become necrotic. Liver function can be severely compromised by fetal asphyxia, and since the liver plays a vital role in the metabolism and daily functioning of the body, severe impairment can prove fatal.

MONITORING FETAL WELL-BEING

It becomes quite obvious at this point that the transition to extrauterine life is riddled with hazards and hurdles for the fetus. Yet nature, aided by nurses and other healthcare professionals, manages to ensure that the overwhelming majority of infants are born healthy and viable.

Modern healthcare has made significant strides in fetal and maternal monitoring in the last two decades, but not everyone agrees that these advances have been worthwhile or in the best interests of the mother. Some assert that routine fetal and maternal monitoring only contribute to a high Cesarean section rate, especially if the results of such monitoring are misinterpreted by the professionals caring for the mother. Indeed, nursing the numbers generated by the monitor or nursing the monitor itself rather than the patient is a serious pitfall of which all professional nurses should be aware.

However, the benefits of fetal monitoring and other assessments of fetal well-being, when used in conjunction with skilled nursing care and correlated with the patient's clinical condition, can be invaluable in preventing a tragedy. Moreover, the litigious nature of obstetrics in our country almost mandates that some type of monitoring for fetal well-being be employed late in the antepartal period and during labor and delivery. In any event, it is imperative that fetal well-being be established and documented as the pregnancy progresses to term and the newborn is delivered. This section reviews common methods of monitoring fetal well-being as the pregnancy nears term, and during labor and delivery. Many of these methods involve assessment of the fetal heart rate.

The heart rate in human beings is an indicator of stress and distress. Stress stimulates the release of fight-or-flight hormones that initially increase the heart rate. In extreme cases such as asphyxia, this stress can cause hypoxia that will eventually result in bradycardia as the myocardium reacts to the reduced oxygen supply. It is not surprising then, that an assessment of fetal well-being is largely based on the fetal heart rate and the status of the uterine contractions that come to bear on the fetus. Indeed, the overwhelming number of labor and delivery facilities either measure or maintain the capacity to measure the fetal heart rate. Some tests of fetal well-being are invasive, others noninvasive. In any case, Korones (1986) notes that electronic heart rate monitoring reveals the cardiac responses that are characteristic of hypoxic stress and thus identifies the fetus in jeopardy. It is important to note that when the fetal heart rate is normal on these measures, there is a high degree of correlation with a healthy fetus. However, if the result of fetal heart rate monitoring is abnormal or questionable, the results are not so clear-cut and further investigation is often indicated. The following is a review of both internal and external methods of monitoring fetal well-being. It is not a complete list but rather a review for the nurse who wishes to know more about common methods of fetal monitoring. And, as always, advances in modern medicine mean that fetal surveillance will become increasingly sophisticated, perhaps outdating some of these methods.

External Monitoring for Fetal Well-Being

Some of the common methods of assessing fetal well-being without invading the uterine cavity are discussed below.

Fetoscope: The fetoscope is a special stethoscope that aids auscultation of the fetal heart tones because it has a special headpiece that conducts sound through bone. It is used in the routine assessment of fetal heart sounds. In many cases, the fetal heart sounds can be detected with the fetoscope around the 20th week of gestation.

Doppler ultrasonic fetal heart rate monitoring: Many nurses are familiar with this common technique which is used in a variety of health care settings to detect blood flow. A simple and easy technique, doppler monitoring of fetal heart tones makes the fetal heart sounds audible to the examiner and to the mother or others present in the room. A small sensor is placed over the mother's abdomen and manipulated until the fetal heart tones are heard clearly *(see figure 7-3)*. The technique is painless and is not believed to be harmful to the fetus. The nurse must be cautious that he or she doesn't mistake the sound of maternal blood flow for the fetal heart sounds; the maternal pulse is normally around 80 beats per minute (bpm), whereas the fetal heart rate should be 120 to 160 bpm. This type of monitoring for fetal well-being may be formed at intervals throughout pregnancy, labor, and delivery.

Sonography: The use of sound waves to generate computerized images of the fetus became popular in the 1970s and is considered a safe and fairly accurate method of assessing fetal well-being. In addition to detecting some congenital abnormalities, a sonogram can show fetal cardiac action, fetal position, size and number, placental size and location, and amount of amniotic fluid. This test is generally performed by a technician trained in it and interpreted by a radiologist, obstetrician, or in some cases, a nurse midwife. This painless test involves moving a lubricated transducer over the maternal abdomen until accurate images are obtained. In some cases a vaginal probe may be used to obtain more direct images. The test takes about 10 to 20 minutes. It is often performed at 20 weeks gestation to assess the fetus and placenta; it may also be performed during labor.

Uterine contraction and fetal heart rate monitoring: During pregnancy or after labor is established, the obstetrician or nurse midwife may elect to begin external monitoring of uterine contractions and the fetal heart rate. In many health institutions, this monitoring is routine for all patients in labor. These two types of monitoring are also an integral part of certain tests for fetal well-being. To initiate uterine and fetal heart rate monitoring, the nurse applies an external uterine pressure monitor (tocodynamometer) over the mother's upper abdomen and a fetal ultrasound transducer over her lower abdomen. Both of these devices are secured by means of belts around the maternal abdomen. The signals transmitted by these monitors are translated into data displayed on a continuous strip of paper. The nurse makes notations on this paper indicating when treatments were performed, when the patient was out of bed and off the monitor, when medications were given, and other nursing activities or medical interventions. This monitor strip and the notations made by the nurse are an essential part of the patient medical record and will no doubt be carefully scrutinized should litigation result after the delivery. This type of external fetal monitoring is believed to be safe and is generally painless, although some patients will complain that the straps securing the monitors are too tight or confining. This monitoring is also used in patients who are at high-risk for preterm labor, since it affords early detection of uterine activity.

Nonstress test (NST): This test measures changes in the fetal heart rate observed in response to spontaneous or evoked fetal movement. It is based on the presumption that a fetus that elevates its heart rate in response to movement is believed to be in good condition. The NST is generally employed late in pregnancy to assess fetal well-being. To perform this test, the nurse applies a tocodynamometer and a fetal ultrasound transducer as mentioned above. The patient then indicates when she feels fetal movement, and the changes in the fetal heart rate in response to that movement are noted. If the fetal heart rate increases a certain degree in response to the fetal movement, the test is termed reactive, and there is some assurance that fetal well-being is not compromised. A reactive nonstress test is often defined as a minimum of two fetal movements within ten minutes with the fetal heart rate accelerations at least 15 beats per minute above the baseline that last for 15 seconds at that rate (Afrait, 1989). A nonreactive test indicates further investigation may be necessary to evaluate fetal well-being. If results are equivocal or unconvincing, further investigation may be indicated. The nonstress test is generally performed by a nurse. It usually takes about 20 to 40 minutes and is painless.

Contraction stress test (CST): Also known as the oxytocin challenge test (OCT), this test is not as popular today as it has been in the past, having been supplanted by other techniques that are believed safer. It may be performed when other measures of fetal well-being, such as the NST, indicate the fetus may be compromised. This test is usually performed late in pregnancy to assess fetal well-being; it involves the intravenous administration of oxytocin, a uterine stimulant. The purpose of the infusion is to induce uterine contractions and then measure the response of the fetus to those contractions. If the fetal heart rate decelerates as the contraction recedes, the test is positive (abnormal). A positive contraction stress test is often defined as a test which results in late decelerations accompanying each uterine contraction of equal duration and intensity (Afriat, 1989). This indicates that the uterine contraction has slowed blood flow through the placenta to the extent that the fetus is stressed and its heart rate drops in response to the lowered delivery of oxygen during the contraction. The patient with an abnormal test should be evaluated by the obstetrician or nurse-midwife, since delivery

may be necessary to prevent further compromise of the fetus. Because it involves the intravenous administration of a uterine stimulant that can initiate labor or cause uterine tetany or rupture, this test requires meticulous nursing care. Most childbirth institutions have protocols that the nurse must follow when performing this test, which may take 20 to 60 minutes or longer.

Nipple stimulation test: This is another test performed late in pregnancy to assess fetal well-being. Nipple stimulation can cause the release of oxytocin from the pituitary; oxytocin can cause uterine contractions. These contractions (if they are of sufficient intensity) and the fetal response to them can be measured as in the OCT. The fetal heart rate and uterine contraction monitors are generally applied as noted above. The patient stimulates her nipples by manipulating them gently, while the nurse monitors for contractions and the fetal heart rate response. The test may take 20 to 40 minutes, is considered relatively safe and painless, and is generally performed by the nurse. If the results do not strongly indicate fetal well-being, or if the stimulation does not produce sufficient uterine contractions, then other methods of evaluation may be employed.

Internal Monitoring for Fetal Well-Being

Once labor is established and the membranes are ruptured, there are several internal monitoring methods useful in assessing fetal well-being. Some are used in conjunction with external fetal monitoring, which includes the tocodynamometer and fetal heart rate monitor described above. Internal methods require some degree of dilation of the cervix in order to gain access to the uterine cavity. All pose certain hazards due to the invasive nature of the monitoring.

Fetal scalp monitor: If the membranes are ruptured, then an electrode can be attached to the fetal scalp. This electrode can transmit the fetal heart rate or even the fetal electrocardiogram to the monitor. It is essential that the presenting part of the fetus be clearly and confidently identified before the electrode is attached; misplacement of the electrode on a part other than that intended can have disastrous consequences. And because the electrode involves invading the uterine cavity and penetrating the fetal scalp, this monitoring technique also opens the way for both maternal and neonatal infection.

Intrauterine pressure monitor: A catheter can be placed into the uterus to measure intrauterine pressure during labor. This of course requires that the membranes be ruptured, and does risk the possibility that the uterus could be perforated during insertion. It also forms a tract for harmful organisms to enter the uterine cavity. Because of these risks, many healthcare professionals rely on indirect extrauterine rather than direct intrauterine pressure monitoring.

Fetal scalp pH sampling: When the fetal heart rate monitoring indicates the fetus may be compromised, fetal scalp blood is obtained for pH measurement by inserting an endoscopic tube vaginally, making a small incision in the fetal scalp and using a capillary tube to draw the sample. While the oxygen and carbon dioxide can also be measured from this sample, it is the pH that has proved most useful in assessing fetal well-being. When fetal well-being is compromised, hypoxia and hypercapnia inevitably result in an acidosis that reduces the fetal pH from its normal 7.25–7.35. A pH below 7.20 generally indicates the fetus is experiencing distress. The sampling may need to be repeated and is usually correlated with other measurements of fetal well-being before intervention is undertaken.

INTERPRETING THE RESULTS OF FETAL HEART RATE MONITORING

Nurses must have an understanding of the results generated by the monitors that assess fetal well-being, for they are the ones at the patient's side throughout labor and delivery. When the monitor indicates that fetal well-being is in jeopardy, immediate intervention may be necessary to avert disaster or maximize the infant's potential for survival. Although a nurse certainly does not perform a Cesarean section, there are a number of nursing interventions that can help salvage the fetus while awaiting medical or surgical intervention *(see table 7-1)*. Fetal monitoring, combined with astute and skilled obstetric nursing care, can mean the difference between life or death for both mother and child. There are few other nursing specialties that can make this claim. Because there are two lives at stake instead of one, it is important that nurses seek advice and consultation whenever there is any question about interpreting the results of fetal monitoring.

This section focuses on the fetal heart rate, since, as mentioned earlier, it is an indicator of fetal distress. In general, there are three areas in which the heart rate is evaluated: *acceleration, deceleration, and variability.* These three variations are generally considered in context of the uterine contractions, since that gives an idea of how the fetus is withstanding labor.

Acceleration

As the fetus matures, its nervous system demonstrates increasing control over the fetal heart rate. The fetal heart rate begins to accelerate in response to stress or lowered oxygen availability. This healthy response allows the fetus to take up more oxygen, because more is delivered to the fetus with the increased heart rate. The fetal heart rate should also increase with fetal movement. The

TABLE 7-1 *(1 of 2)*
Nursing Guidelines for Intervention for Fetal Heart Rate Patterns

I. *Periodic changes—uniform decelerations*

A. Early decelerations

Description: FHR begins to slow with the onset of the uterine contractions and returns to baseline when the contraction is over.

Pathophysiology: Head compression

Nursing Intervention	*Rationale*
1. Be aware that the FHR slows with a contraction.	Fetal head compression associated with the contraction, resulting in a parasympathetic discharge mediated by the vagus nerve. Parasympathetic stimulation results in slowing of the FHR. This pattern represents normal response of the fetus to this stimulus and is associated with a good outcome.
2. Chart descriptive note or chart on flow sheet according to institutional practice.	

B. Late decelerations

Description: FHR begins to fall at height of contraction and returns to baseline after the contraction has ceased. Usually the FHR remains within the normal range. Decelerations may be subtle but still ominous.

Pathophysiology: Uteroplacental insufficiency

Nursing Intervention	*Rationale*
1. Recognize the pattern on the tracing as well as be alert for audible changes in the rhythm of the FHR.	Nursing personnel must have knowledge and experience in FHR monitoring.
2. Follow institution policy: do you assess and wait for next deceleration to occur before notifying physician or proceed to intervention #3?	Effective nursing and physician management to provide for safe labor and delivery for mother with an uncompromised infant; compliance with institution policies is important.
3. Turn client to her left side and give oxygen by mask @ 10 liters/min.	Changing position relieves aorta or vena cava pressure. Hypotension, hyperstimulation or conduction anesthesia may also be the cause and need to be addressed by nurse and physician.
4. Chart a descriptive note or chart on flow sheet.	Nursing management is dictated by institution policies.

II. *Non-uniform Decelerations*

A. Variable decelerations

Description: A slowing of the FHR either with a contraction or between contractions. The pattern of the deceleration is often either a U or V shape that drops suddenly from the baseline and returns abruptly to the baseline.

Pathophysiology: Cord compression

Nursing Intervention	*Rationale*
1. Recognize the pattern and assess the frequency, depth, and duration of the deceleration.	There is correlation between the severity of the variable deceleration and fetal condition.
2. Follow institution policy: do you assess before notifying the physician and carrying out the interventions of #3?	Some institutions have 24-hour physician coverage on the unit; in other institutions the nurse must inform the physician by phone, since they have standing orders.
3. Turn client to her left side or to knee -chest position and give oxygen by mask @ 10 liters/min.	Changing position may help to remove the pressure on the cord. If this is not effective, physician may attempt upward displacement of presenting part.

TABLE 7-1 *(2 of 2)*
Nursing Guidelines for Intervention for Fetal Heart Rate Patterns

III. Baseline changes

A. Tachycardia

Description: A baseline FHR of more than 160 bpm persisting 10 to 15 minutes
   Mild: 160–179 bpm
   Marked: 180 or more bpm
Pathophysiology: Fetal hypoxia, maternal fever, idiopathic maternal anxiety, prematurity, drug related, fetal arrhythmia

Nursing Intervention	*Rationale*
1. Confirm by auscultating FHR.	Confirm that monitor is operating properly and FHR has increased. Tachycardia may be in response to fetal movement.
2. Monitor maternal vital signs.	Tachycardia may be due to maternal fever.
3. Monitor contractions.	FHR may increase in response to excessive contractions.
4. Change maternal position.	Aortoiliac compression is alleviated.
5. Continue to watch closely by reviewing tracings for changing patterns.	Etiologic factors might be identified. Tachycardia may be a sign of fetal distress; arrhythmias may be identified by fetal EKG.
6. Chart descriptive note or chart on flow sheet.	Nursing management is dictated by institution policies.

B. Bradycardia

Description: A FHR of less than 120 bpm persisting 10 to 15 minutes
   Mild: 100–119
   Marked: Less than 100

Nursing Intervention	*Rationale*
1. Change maternal position.	Changing position alleviates uterine pressure on the aorta and vena cava.
2. Give oxygen by mask @ 10 liters/min.	Baby may have congenital heart abnormality.
3. Continue to watch closely for:	Ominous signs indicate fetal distress, even impending death.
• Marked bradycardia with loss of variability and late decelerations	This is a sign of fetal distress.
• Mild bradycardia with good FHR variability and absence of late decelerations	This is generally not a sign of fetal distress.
• Bradycardia due to heart block	This is not a sign of acute fetal distress.
4. Chart descriptive note or chart on flow sheet.	Nursing management is dictated by institution policies.

C. Variability

Description: A variation of the resting FHR
   Average: 6–10 bpm
   Minimal: 3–5 bpm
   None: 0–2 bpm
Pathophysiology: Maternal medication, fetal acidosis, fetal neurologic immaturity.

Nursing Intervention	*Rationale*
1. Observe variability of the FHR.	Variability is an indication of normal neurologic control of heart rate and a measure of fetal reserve.
2. Increased variability requires no nursing intervention.	This may be due to external uterine palpitation, UC, fetal activity, or maternal activity.
3. Decreased variability: follow physician's order based on cause.	Possible causes include prematurity, drugs, hypoxia and acidosis, fetal sleep, fetal cardiac arrhythmias.
4. Chart descriptive note or chart on flow sheet.	Nursing management is dictated by institution policies.

Source: *Maternity Nursing,* 16th ed., Reeder, S. J. & Martin, L. L., 1987, J. B. Lippincott, Philadelphia, PA.

normal rate is between 120 and 160 bpm when the uterus and fetus are both quiescent. Increases above 160 bpm can, however, indicate pathology such as fetal heart disease. It is also important to note that while the fetal heart rate normally increases in response to hypoxia, it will inevitably decrease and finally stop if the hypoxia continues. In general, increases in the fetal heart rate with contractions and with fetal movement are reassuring signs of fetal well-being, especially when correlated with the mother's clinical condition and other indicators of fetal well-being *(see figure 7-4).*

Deceleration

The fetal heart rate may decrease in response to stress, and the assessment of the implications of the decelerations depends upon when they occur.

Early deceleration: When the fetal heart rate slows as a uterine contraction peaks, it is seen on the monitor tracing paper as a mirror image of the contraction. Commonly associated with compression of the fetal head, early decelerations are believed to result from vagal stimulation. Early decelerations are not generally considered pathological, but a normal response to labor *(see figure 7-5).*

Late deceleration: When the fetal heart rate slows after the contraction peaks it is called a late deceleration. Commonly considered an indication of fetal distress, late decelerations can indicate fetal hypoxia. Sometimes late decelerations may be observed in response to clinical events such as maternal hypotension, which when corrected alleviate the condition. Uteroplacental insufficiency is also commonly linked with late decelerations. Whatever the presumed cause, late decelerations warrant further investigation. An emergency Cesarean section may be necessary to salvage the fetus *(see figure 7-6).*

FIGURE 7-4
Fetal Heart Rate Acceleration

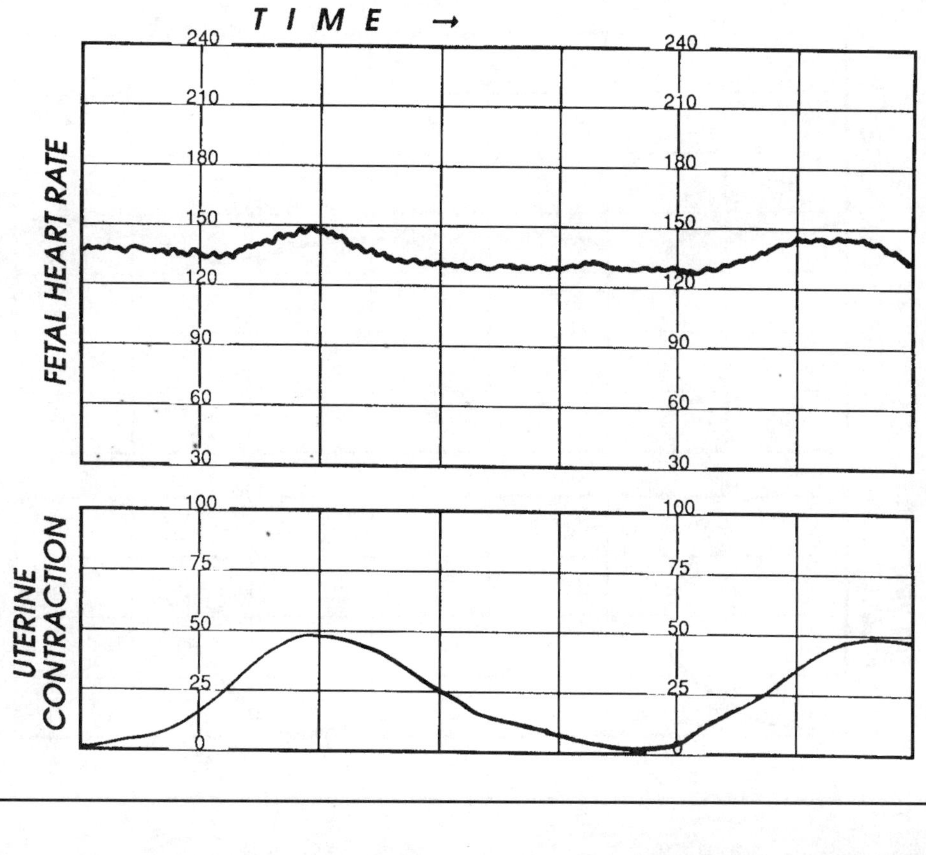

Variable decelerations: With decelerations and accelerations, the fetal heart rate waveform on the monitor tracing paper will generally appear uniform. But with variable decelerations, the waveform is just that: variable. Mild variable decelerations are common during labor and believed to be a result of reflex vagal stimulation. Variable decelerations should be considered in light of clinical events and along with other indicators of fetal well-being. Mild variable decelerations may be innocuous but warrant continued observation and follow-up *(see figure 7-7).*

Variability

The normal fetus will demonstrate variability in its heart rate as the autonomic and sympathetic nervous systems mature. The heart rate may vary from 5 to 10 bpm with contractions and fetal or maternal movement. The absence of variability in the fetal heart rate may be an ominous indicator of fetal distress, depression, or hypoxia *(see figure 7-8)*.

NURSING STRATEGIES FOR THE PATIENT UNDERGOING FETAL MONITORING

This section offers an overview of common nursing strategies that may be useful when caring for the laboring or near-term pregnant patient. Nursing strategies for assessing and monitoring fetal well-being are also presented. Because obstetric nursing is a complex and demanding specialty, this information is presented only as a review of nursing care for the pregnant patient; it is not a complete guide to maternity nursing. The Nurses Association of the American College of Obstetricians and Gynecologists (NAACOG) should be contacted for detailed standards on maternity nursing care. Advanced training, knowledge, and skills are generally necessary to provide nursing care to obstetric patients, since this is an increasingly complex field and two lives, not just one, are at stake. As always, nursing care and nursing actions should be within the scope of the institution's practice guidelines and/or the state's Nurse Practice Act and commensurate with the nurse's skills and training.

Nursing Strategies

• Determine which physician or nurse midwife is "on call" and responsible for the management of the laboring patient before you assume responsibility for the patient's nursing care. This can save precious moments in the event of an emergency.

• Know the location of emergency equipment such as the cardiac defibrillator, emergency drug cart, and emergency supplies before starting duty in labor and delivery. Note also the location of a fire extinguisher and how to alert authorities of a fire. Memorize or carry the telephone or pager numbers of the emergency

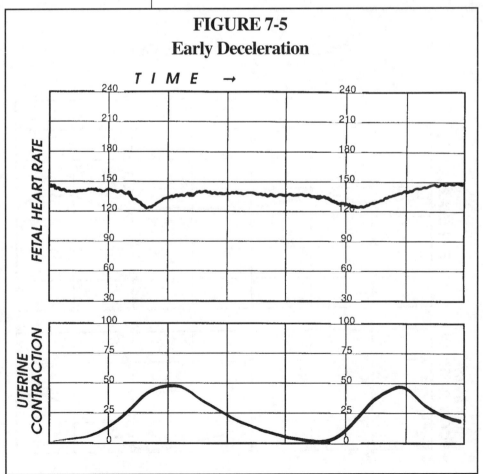

FIGURE 7-5
Early Deceleration

team. Knowledge and preparation can save valuable minutes if an emergency arises.

• Determine that an operating room with a Cesarean section setup is available before assuming responsibility for the nursing care of the laboring patient. Such a setup should be in place, because there can be no waste of time if the fetus or mother suffers untoward events during labor.

• Check the labor room for essential supplies before accepting responsibility for the patient. In the labor room, some essential supplies include equipment for monitoring maternal blood pressure, an oxygen regulator and oxygen face mask, and a suction canister with tubing and suction catheters. This equipment must be at hand, since any time spent searching for and setting it up in an emergency would be precious moments stolen from the mother and child. In addition, many institutions require that a box of emergency drugs and airway management equipment be available at the bedside of the patient receiving regional anesthesia.

• Be aware of self limitations when it comes to interpreting tests of fetal well-being. If in doubt, ask the obstetrician or nurse midwife to evaluate the results on the unit and correlate them with the patient's clinical condition. This can help avert tragedy.

• Explain to the mother and her support person that fetal monitoring is routine in many institutions and does not necessarily indicate that anyone believes the fetus is in danger. Also, explain the purpose and rationale for fetal monitoring. Answer any questions and, if the institution requires it, obtain consent for the monitoring. An understanding of fetal monitoring should reduce the expectant mother's anxiety and therefore help reduce the potential for complications associated with maternal stress.

• Treat the patient, not her numbers; avoid fixating on the monitors and ignoring the patient to which the monitors are connected. It is also essential to correlate data generated by the monitors with the patient's clinical status. Doing so will help avoid false-positives and a rush to intervene in a situation that doesn't require it. However, do not ignore monitor-generated data, as that is the purpose of monitor-

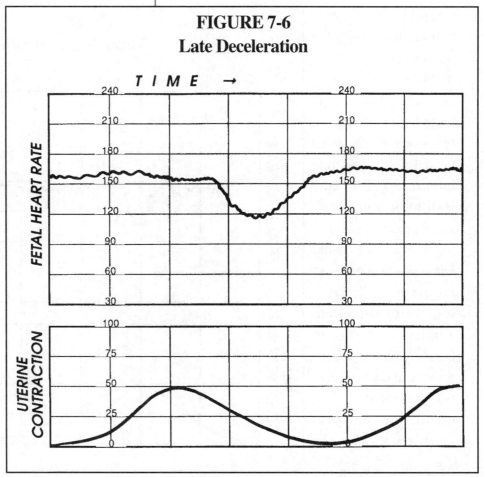

FIGURE 7-6
Late Deceleration

ing, to generate data about the condition of the mother and the fetus.

- Investigate all complaints of a sudden change in degree of pain by the laboring patient. Rupture of the uterus and abruptio placentae are just two of several conditions that may result in sudden, severe abdominal pain and threaten fetal and maternal survival.

- Apply oxygen via face mask 8–10 liters per minute to the pregnant patient who appears in distress or when fetal monitoring indicates the fetus may be compromised. Stay with the patient and ask a colleague to stat-page the obstetrician or nurse midwife. Brief oxygen administration will not harm mother or child, and it may be beneficial if a serious complication is developing. If oxygen administration is to continue, secure an order for it, since it is considered to be a drug.

- Since an emergency Cesarean section may be indicated, notify the obstetrician or nurse midwife immediately if late decelerations, fetal bradycardia, or absence of variability are noted on the fetal heart rate monitor. Follow the institution's protocol, which may include turning the patient on her left side and administering oxygen while awaiting their evaluation. Turning the patient to her side will help reduce aortocaval compression, which can reduce fetal circulation and oxygenation. Oxygen

administration will help increase the amount of oxygen delivered to the fetus.

- Consider the strips produced by the fetal and uterine contraction monitors to be a critical part of the patient's medical record and safeguard these accordingly. Make notations clearly and legibly on the paper, because this may be an essential part of reconstructing events should the care be challenged in court.

- Although some medications do not cross the placental barrier, always assume that a drug administered to the mother will pass to the fetus. With this in mind, increase the level of vigilance of the mother and fetus after a drug is administered. Document on the chart and on the monitor strip the medication administered and the response to it.

- Follow the institution's policy on a patient's oral intake during labor. Many institutions

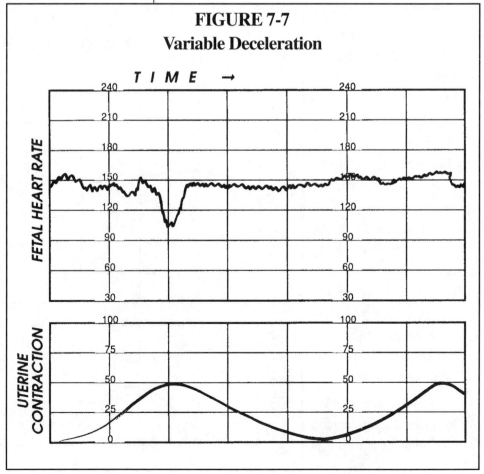

FIGURE 7-7
Variable Deceleration

require the patient to be NPO due to the high risk of aspiration, a condition to which the pregnant female is especially vulnerable. This is especially critical if an emergency Cesarean section must take place. Some institutions allow the patient to have ice chips. In no case should the patient in active labor be allowed to eat; to do so risks fatal aspiration.

- Monitor the fetal heart rate continuously or every 1 to 2 minutes for about 10 minutes (or until stable) after the membranes rupture, because this is a time that umbilical cord prolapse may occur and prompt intervention may be necessary to avert tragedy.

- Know the institution's policy on nursing actions to take if there is a drop in fetal heart rate after the membranes rupture. In most cases, while putting the patient into a knee-chest position to help relieve pressure on the umbilical cord and thereby reducing fetal asphyxia, the obstetrician or nurse-midwife must be called.

- Check the odor and consistency of the fluid after the membranes rupture, and document the findings. The presence of meconium is considered to be a sign of some degree of fetal distress.

- Be aware that vaginal bleeding after the placement of a fetal scalp electrode can be caused from fetal scalp hemorrhage; notify the obstetrician or nurse midwife if this occurs.

- When an infant has had a scalp electrode placed, the site needs to be monitored closely for bleeding or infection.

- In the event of an emergency, explain to the mother what is happening as she will inevitably be anxious about her safety and the baby's welfare.

- Follow the institution's policy when administering a uterine stimulant such as oxytocin, because this powerful drug can cause uterine rupture and subsequent maternal and fetal demise.

- Do not perform vaginal examinations on the laboring patient without special training in obstetric nursing. Multiple vaginal examinations increase the risk of maternal and neonatal infections and in some cases can precipitate maternal hemorrhage.

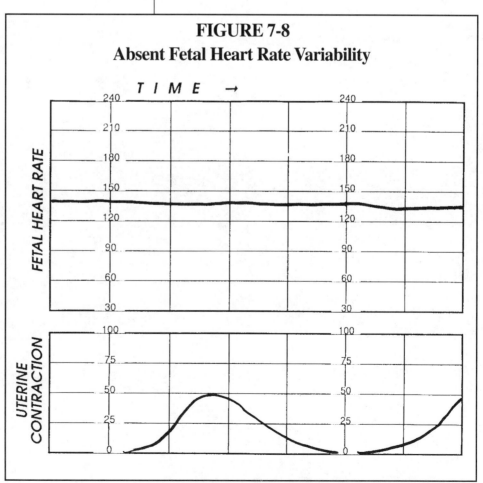

FIGURE 7-8
Absent Fetal Heart Rate Variability

EXAM QUESTIONS

CHAPTER 7
Questions 34–48

34. The fetal circulation consists of three circuits; the systemic, pulmonary, and

    a. cardiac.

    b. renal.

    c. placental.

    d. mesenteric.

35. The part of the fetal circulation that directs most blood flow to bypass the lungs is the

    a. aortic valve.

    b. ductus arteriosus.

    c. umbilical cord.

    d. ductus venosus.

36. The most common cause of fetal hypoxia is an alteration in

    a. uteroplacental blood flow.

    b. maternal glucose levels.

    c. fetal anatomy.

    d. maternal position.

37. In beats per minute, the normal fetal heart rate is

    a 80–120.

    b. 100–120.

    c. 140–180.

    d. 120–160.

38. Abdominal pain and vaginal bleeding in the pregnant patient may indicate

    a. abruptio placentae.

    b. nuchalcord.

    c. uteroplacental insufficiency.

    d. placenta previa.

39. Persistent fetal circulation is a condition that may develop after

    a. fetal asphyxia.

    b. maternal hypercalcemia.

    c. fetal aldosteronism.

    d. maternal hypothyroidism.

40. Fetal scalp sampling indicates the fetus blood pH is 7.33. How should this be interpreted?

    a. The fetus is not compromised.

    b. The test should be repeated in 10 minutes.

    c. The fetus needs to be delivered soon.

    d. The fetus is not tolerating labor well.

41. A test of fetal well-being that involves evaluating fetal movement and changes in the fetal heart in response to that movement is the

    a. oxytocin challenge test.

    b. nonstress test.

    c. contraction stress test.

    d. fetal scalp pH test.

42. The initial fetal response to hypoxia is generally

    a. a decreased heart rate.

    b. an increased heart rate.

    c. an increase in movement.

    d. a decrease in movement.

43. A test for fetal well-being that involves the intravenous administration of a uterine stimulant is the

    a. nipple stimulation test.

    b. nonstress test.

    c. fetal scalp pH test.

    d. contraction stress test.

44. A fetal heart rate tracing associated with compression of the fetal head during a contraction is

    a. late decelerations.

    b. early decelerations.

    c. early accelerations.

    d. variable decelerations.

45. A fetal heart rate tracing seen commonly during labor is

    a. late decelerations.

    b. variable decelerations.

    c. early accelerations.

    d. early decelerations.

46. Late decelerations noted on the fetal heart monitor require

    a. immediate and further assessment of fetal well-being.

    b. no intervention.

    c. turning the mother on her back.

    d. putting the mother in a semi-Fowler's position.

47. The absence of variability in the fetal heart rate generally indicates that the fetus is

    a. in good condition.

    b. in distress.

    c. dead.

    d. not ready for delivery.

48. The nurse is caring for a labor patient when fetal bradycardia suddenly develops. What should the nurse do?

    a. Race from the room in search of assistance.

    b. Sit the mother up in bed, ask her to pant, and reassure her the baby is thriving.

    c. Turn the mother on her left side, apply an oxygen mask, and call for assistance.

    d. Turn the mother on her right side and perform a pelvic examination.

CHAPTER 8

DELIVERY MANAGEMENT

CHAPTER OBJECTIVE

After studying this chapter, the reader will be able to identify the principles of delivery management for both vaginal and cesarean births, and specify appropriate nursing assessment and intervention strategies for the immediate care of the newborn.

LEARNING OBJECTIVES

After studying this chapter, the student will be able to

1. Select the cardinal movements of the fetus during vaginal delivery.

2. Indicate the risks of and indications for cesarean delivery.

3. Specify appropriate nursing assessment criteria on the newborn immediately following birth.

4. Recognize standards for resuscitation of the newborn in the delivery room.

5. Identify the critical areas in the newborn that need to be assessed during the stabilization period.

VAGINAL DELIVERY

Cardinal Movements

The cardinal movements of labor are a predictable sequence that a fetus in the vertex position will go through during labor and childbirth. The six movements are descent, flexion, internal rotation, extension, external rotation, and expulsion (see figure 8-1).

Descent occurs as the fetus moves down through the maternal pelvis. The progression of the fetus is evaluated according to the relationship of the presenting part to the pelvis. The presenting part is the part of the fetus that enters the pelvis first, vertex (head) or breech (buttocks). When the presenting part is above the pelvic inlet, the fetus is considered to be "floating." The fetus is "fixed" when the presenting part has entered the pelvic inlet but is not yet engaged. During "engagement," the widest part of the presenting part is level with the ischial spines. When the presenting part is halfway to the pelvic floor, it is considered in the midpelvis; it is considered on the pelvic floor when it has descended to the perineum.

Flexion occurs when the fetal chin rests against the chest. In this position, the smallest diameter of the head enters the pelvis. Factors that contribute to flexion include resistance from the cervix, pelvic walls, or floor.

Internal rotation occurs when the anteroposterior diameter of the fetal head comes in line with the anteroposterior diameter of the pelvic outlet. The head rotates approximately 45 degrees when it meets resistance from the pelvic floor. During this movement the shoulders do not move; only the neck is twisted. Following internal rotation, the majority of fetuses assume an occiput anterior position (the fetal occiput faces the anterior maternal pelvis). A prolonged labor may result if the fetus assumes an occiput posterior or occiput transverse position, due to the inability of the occiput to adequately fill the pelvic cavity or exert equal pressure around the cervical os.

Extension occurs when the fetal head extends after passing under the symphysis pubis. Factors contributing to this extension include pressure from uterine contractions, resistance from the pelvic floor, and intra-abdominal pressure from the woman's bearing-down efforts.

External rotation, also called restitution, occurs as the head again rotates 45 degrees, back to the position assumed before internal rotation. The fetus then rotates an additional 45 degrees in order to position the shoulders in an anteroposterior position in the pelvis. Generally, the anterior shoulder appears under the symphysis pubis first, followed by the posterior shoulder.

Expulsion occurs as the trunk of the body is pulled upward and away from the perineum.

Principles of Management

Management of the patient in labor centers on ensuring maternal and fetal well-being. Nursing interventions include the following:

- Providing emotional support to the patient and coach. All procedures must be explained to reduce anxiety and enhance cooperation. The patient's progress in labor dilation, station, effacement and fetal status must be continually updated.

- Monitoring and recording the frequency, duration, and strength of contractions.

- Monitoring and recording fetal heart rate during and between contractions, noting rate, accelerations, decelerations, and variability.

- Monitoring and recording intravenous fluid intake and output.

- Monitoring and recording maternal vital signs according to hospital policy.

- Assessing the need for and effectiveness of analgesia.

- Maintaining patient comfort through frequent position change, mouth care, providing ice chips, and changing bed linen as needed.

- Teaching and reinforcing the use of relaxation techniques.

- Encouraging rest between contractions.

- Monitoring and recording rupture of membranes (ROM), noting the time, color, amount,

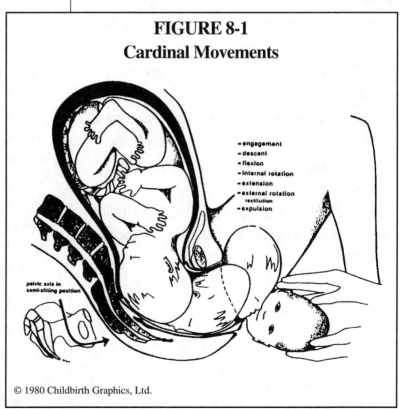

FIGURE 8-1
Cardinal Movements

- engagement
- descent
- flexion
- internal rotation
- extension
- external rotation restitution
- expulsion

pelvic axis in semi-sitting position

© 1980 Childbirth Graphics, Ltd.

FIGURE 8-2

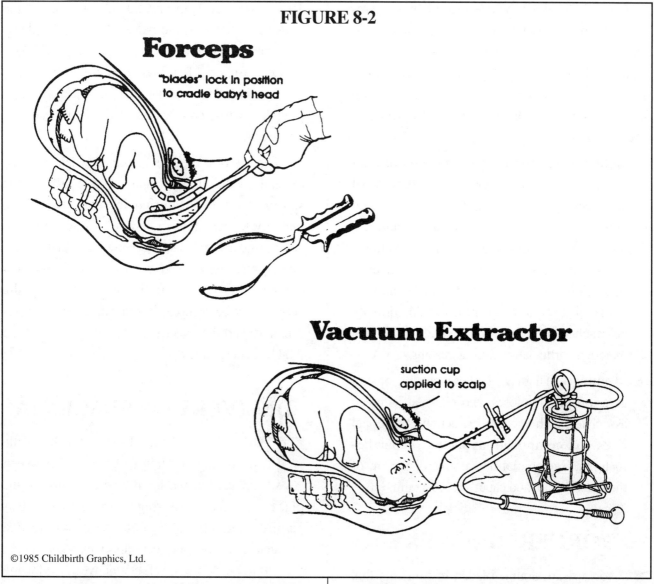

Forceps

*"blades" lock in position
to cradle baby's head*

Vacuum Extractor

*suction cup
applied to scalp*

©1985 Childbirth Graphics, Ltd.

odor, and consistency of the amniotic fluid. The fetal heart rate and possibility of cord prolapse must be assessed immediately following ROM.

• Assessing the patient for signs of imminent delivery, e.g., bulging of the perineum and an urge to push.

Vacuum Extraction

In order to facilitate descent of the fetal head, vacuum extraction is an alternative delivery tool in lieu of forceps. After a vacuum cup is applied close to the fetal occiput, negative pressure is exerted, resulting in the scalp tissue being drawn up into the cup *(see figure 8-2)*. The scalp beneath the cup

becomes edematous, with fluid forming the characteristic "chignon" or knot within 5 to 10 minutes in the cavity of the vacuum cup. This collection of fluid under the scalp begins to disappear soon after delivery and is generally gone within several days. During contractions and in conjunction with the mother's pushing efforts, traction is applied to the fetal head and the fetus is drawn through the birth canal. This technique can also be used to deliver the head during a cesarean birth.

Indications for use include failure to rotate, prolonged second stage of labor, fetal distress, maternal cardiac or respiratory disease, and hypertension.

Contraindications include face or breech presentation, malpresentation, cephalopelvic disproportion (CPD), and prematurity. Use of vacuum extraction before 36 weeks gestation is not recommended because of the increased incidence of scalp damage and intracranial injuries in pre-term infants.

Advantages: Because the vacuum cup does not occupy any additional space in the birth canal as forceps do, little discomfort is associated with its use. Additional advantages include a lower incidence of cervical, vaginal, and third- and fourth-degree lacerations; lower incidence of episiotomies; the ability to utilize the vacuum cup at stations higher than could normally be reached by forceps; and continued active maternal participation during pushing.

Disadvantages: There is a higher incidence of skin abrasions, ecchymoses, and neonatal jaundice associated with vacuum extraction. Additional risks and complications include cephalhematoma, intracranial hematoma, distortion of the fetus's head, and caput succedaneum.

FORCEPS DELIVERY

Forceps are double-bladed instruments that are used to rotate the fetus and/or shorten the second stage of labor *(see figure 8-2)*. The type of forceps selected depends upon the fetus's station and condition. If the fetal head is visible on the perineum (+2 station), low or outlet forceps are used (e.g., Elliot, Simpson, or Tucker-McLean). A low or outlet forceps delivery is considered safe with possible complications limited to minor vaginal, perineal, or cervical trauma and fetal head bruising. The use of mid forceps (head is engaged but not visible on the perineum) is considered dangerous due to the increased incidence of skull fracture, maternal blood loss, and third-degree perineal lacerations. When used to deliver pre-term infants, the solid blades of the Tucker-McLean help prevent head trauma. If the fetus needs to be rotated before delivery, the physician may select either Kjelland, Barton, or Tucker-McLean forceps. If a breech vaginal delivery is attempted, the curved shank of Piper forceps helps provide traction and flexion of the fetal head *(see figure 8-3)*.

The use of forceps is indicated when maternal or fetal conditions exist that could jeopardize the safety of either. Maternal indications include inability to push due to cardiac disease, regional anesthesia, and exhaustion. The major fetal indication is fetal distress and the need for an expedient delivery. Before the application of forceps, the cervix must be completely dilated, the membranes ruptured, and the exact position and station of the fetal head determined.

DELIVERY OF PLACENTA

The delivery of the placenta concludes the third stage of labor, the period between delivery of the infant and expulsion of the placenta. During this stage, strong though less painful contractions continue every one to five minutes. The placenta generally is expelled within 5 to 30 minutes of the infant's delivery. Following delivery, the uterus firmly contracts, thus decreasing its capacity and placental attachment surface area. As the surface area decreases, the placenta begins to separate, causing the formation of a retroplacental hematoma and further separation from the uterine wall. If the uterus is relaxed or boggy, the placenta will not easily separate because the attachment site cannot sufficiently decrease in size. Signs of placental separation include a sudden gush or trickle of dark blood from the vagina, lengthening of the umbilical cord, a change in uterine shape from discoid to globular, and possibly a subjective feeling of vaginal fullness. The woman should be encouraged to aid with the expulsion process once these signs of separation occur. If the fundus is

FIGURE 8-3

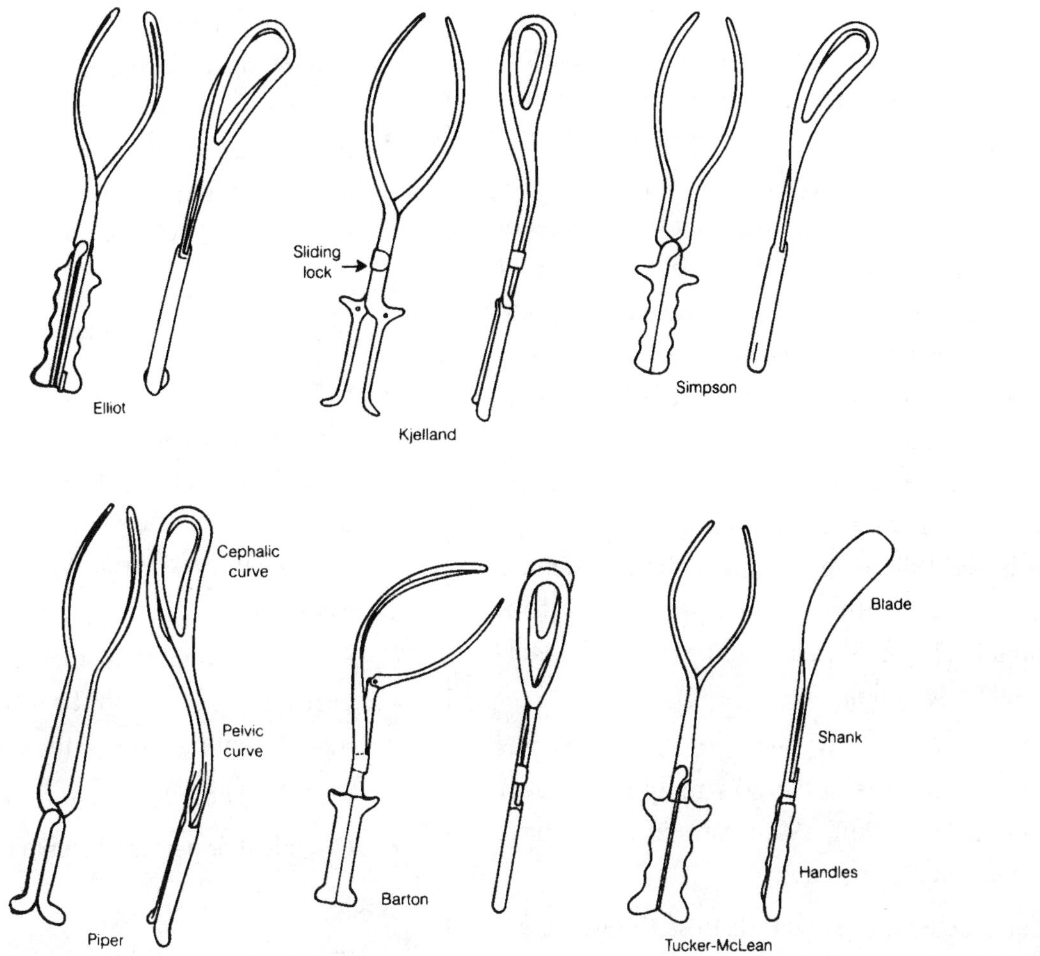

Forceps are composed of a blade, shank, and handle and may have a cephalic and pelvic curve. (Note labels on Piper and Tucker-McLean forceps). The blades may be fenestrated (open) or solid. The front and lateral views of these forceps illustrate differences in blades, open and closed shank, and cephalic and pelvic curves. Elliott, Simpson, and Tucker-McLean forceps are used as outlet forceps. Kjelland and Barton forceps are used for midforceps rotations. Piper forceps are used to provide traction and flexion of the aftercoming head of a fetus in breech presentation.

Source: *Essentials of Maternal-Newborn Nursing,* Ladewig, P. W., London, M. L. & Olds, S. B., 1990, Addison-Wesley, New York.

contracted, the birth attendant can apply firm, gentle traction to the cord to aid with the expulsion. The placenta is expelled by either the Schultze's ("shiny Schultze") or Duncan's ("dirty Duncan") mechanism. In the former, the central portion of the placenta separates from the uterine wall, away from the retroplacental hematoma. When delivered, the fetal or shiny side of the placenta is delivered. During Duncan's mechanism, the outer edges of the placenta separate before the central portion. The placenta rolls up sideways so that the rough-surfaced maternal side is delivered. There is a higher incidence of retained fragments and increased maternal blood loss in Duncan's mechanism. No matter how the placenta is expelled, it must be carefully evaluated for completeness and the woman assessed for excessive bleeding or uterine relaxation. Some physicians may order the addition of oxytocin to a patient's hydration bottle following delivery of the infant to induce uterine contractions and placental expulsion.

CESAREAN DELIVERY

During a cesarean delivery, the surgeon delivers the infant either through a transverse or low vertical abdominal incision. The preferred incision is transverse, at or just below the pubic hairline. The advantages of this type of incision include decreased incidence of peritonitis and postoperative adhesions, ease of repair, barely visible scar, decreased incidence of scar rupture during subsequent pregnancies, and minimal blood loss. The disadvantages of the transverse incision are the extra time needed to remove the fetus and the possible extension of the incision laterally into the major uterine vessels. Though performed less often, a low vertical incision may be made in the following cases: an obese patient; a macrosomic fetus; multiple gestation; maternal/fetal distress; placenta previa; and abnormal fetal presentation.

The incidence of cesarean deliveries has increased from 5% in the 60's to approximately 20% in the 90's (Neff, 1996). Several factors have contributed to this increase:

- Early detection of fetal distress through electronic fetal monitoring.

- Advances in surgical technique, anesthesia/analgesia, and technology that make the procedure safer.

- Reduced risks from surgery due to improved pharmacologic and parenteral fluid therapy.

- Decreased risk to fetus as compared to high or mid forceps delivery.

- Reluctance to vaginally deliver a fetus in a breech presentation.

Indications

General indications for a cesarean delivery include the following:

- A previous cesarean delivery (see "Vaginal Birth after Cesarean," page 143).

- Dystocia: a difficult labor due to either mechanical and/or functional factors. Examples of maternal mechanical factors include contracted pelvis and obstructive tumors; fetal mechanical factors include malpresentation and congenital malformation. Dysfunctional uterine patterns (e.g. hypertonic and hypotonic contractions) are examples of functional factors leading to dystocia.

- The fetus is in a breech presentation or malpresentation, i.e. transverse.

- Fetal distress.

- The presence of an infectious process that could be potentially dangerous if transmitted to the fetus during a vaginal delivery: e.g. HIV, herpes simplex virus type 2 or condylomata acuminata.

- Preexisting maternal medical condition (e.g. cardiac disease) that would preclude the mother's going through the stresses of labor.

- Prolapsed umbilical cord.

- Complete or partial placenta previa.

Risks

The mortality and morbidity rates associated with a cesarean delivery are both higher than those for a vaginal delivery (Petitti, 1985). The two to four times greater mortality rate most often results from anesthesia difficulties and/or underlying medical conditions such as severe pregnancy-induced hypertension (PIH), cardiac or renal disease, and diabetes. The five to ten times higher morbidity rate results from infection, hemorrhage, blood clots, and injury to the bladder or intestines during surgery (Gibbs, 1985).

VAGINAL BIRTH AFTER CESAREAN (VBAC)

Cesarean deliveries became the most frequently performed major operation in the United States in 1981 (Flamm et al., 1990). In 1982 the American College of Obstetricians and Gynecologists (ACOG) released its original guidelines regarding vaginal births following a previous cesarean, with revisions published in 1984 and 1988. Despite the lifting of several original VBAC restrictions put forth in 1981, the rate of cesarean deliveries continues to rise, with 49% of the rise between 1980-1985 resulting from repeat cesareans. It is estimated there will soon be one million cesarean deliveries in the United States annually. One study (Flamm et al., 1990) suggests over 200,000 cesarean deliveries could be eliminated yearly, if all eligible women were allowed to have VBAC. A history of a cesarean delivery is the most frequent cause (33%) of the operation. Originally, the reluctance to attempt a VBAC was based on a fear of uterine rupture in subsequent labors. Currently, however, the majority of cesareans involve low transverse as compared to low vertical uterine incisions. The latter type of incision was associated with rupture and maternal shock. While low transverse incisions carry a 0.25 to 0.5% rupture rate, approximately 90% of these only involve separation of the myometrium (Cohen et al., 1991).

Approximately 60% of women who had previous cesarean deliveries may desire to attempt a VBAC; the majority of these women will go on to deliver a future child vaginally. The reason for a previous cesarean must be known to determine whether it is still a valid reason to perform a Cesarean (e.g. cardiac history) or whether a vaginal delivery can be attempted (e.g. fetal distress). In addition to decreased morbidity and mortality rates, VBAC's result in less discomfort and recovery time and lower costs. In addition, some couples may desire a vaginal delivery because they see it as a more natural experience.

Criteria for attempting a VBAC includes a previous low transverse incision, availability of a physician during labor; ready availability of surgical personnel/equipment should a cesarean be necessary, the woman's desire for a vaginal delivery, and the absence of medical problems that would contraindicate a VBAC. Contraindications for attempting a VBAC include a previous vertical incision and multiple gestation. Though current ACOG guidelines allow oxytocin augmentation and epidural anesthesia in trial-of-labor patients, caution is still suggested when estimated fetal weight is 4,000 grams. Additional areas requiring further research include the possible increased risk of uterine rupture if the patient attempts a VBAC after having had more than one cesarean and whether a woman with a history of cephalopelvic disproportion should ever be allowed to attempt a VBAC.

Immediate Newborn Care

- Immediately following delivery, the infant should be transferred to a preheated radiant warmer in a flat, single lateral position to promote drainage of secretions. Drying the infant with a warm blanket helps prevent heat loss through evaporation, it also provides tactile stimulation that helps establish respiration. Through oral and then nasal suctioning, a patent airway is provided. Following initial drying, positioning, and suctioning, the infant is assessed for gross abnormalities and/or clinical manifestations of abnormalities. The nurse should continue to assess the five parts of the Apgar score even after the 5-minute score is obtained.

- Proper identification is vital, and unless the infant's condition precludes it; this must be completed before the infant is transferred from the delivery room. Identification bands with matching numbers must be placed both on the infant (two bands) and mother (one band). Clear and complete footprints of the infant and fingerprints of the mother must also be obtained.

- The occurrence of infant voiding or stooling must be noted and recorded.

- The cord clamp is applied and the cord assessed for three vessels (two arteries and one vein) and abnormal bleeding.

- Infant/parental bonding can be initiated immediately after delivery and the mother can attempt to breastfeed the infant, if her and her baby's condition permit.

- Additional newborn care will be provided according to hospital policy. The infant is weighed, vital statistics (length, head, chest, and abdominal circumferences) obtained, vital signs monitored, Aquamephyton (Vitamin K) administered, and prophylactic eye treatment performed with 0.5% erythromycin ointment, 1% tetracycline ointment, or 1% silver nitrate ophthalmic solution.

ADAPTION TO EXTRAUTERINE LIFE

Neonatal Circulation/Changes from Fetal Circulation

There are five structures that differentiate fetal from neonatal circulation: two umbilical arteries, one umbilical vein, the ductus venosus, ductus arteriosus, and foramen ovale. The umbilical arteries carry deoxygenated blood from the fetus back to the placenta, while the umbilical vein carries oxygenated blood to the fetus from the placenta. The foramen ovale, which means open window, is a septal opening that allows for the movement of oxygenated blood from the right to left atrium. The ductus venosus, which bypasses the liver; carries oxygenated blood from the umbil-

ical vein to the inferior vena cava. The ductus arteriosus, a connection between the pulmonary artery and aorta, allows blood to shunt around the fetal lungs. Following delivery, these five structures are no longer needed.

Once the umbilical cord is clamped and cut, the umbilical arteries and vein are obliterated. Within one to two hours following delivery, the foramen ovale closes, though permanent closure takes several months. Closure of the foramen ovale is dependent upon pressures within the atria. During fetal existence, higher pressure within the right atrium allows for the right-to-left movement of blood through the foramen ovale Following delivery, decreased pulmonary resistance and increased pulmonary blood flow cause the pressure in the left atrium to increase, thus causing the foramen ovale to close. Any increase in pulmonary resistance following delivery may result in a right-to-left shunting, which results in the mixing of oxygenated blood in the left atrium with deoxygenated blood from the right atrium. Increased pulmonary resistance is due to hypoxia caused by factors such as suctioning, respiratory distress, and hypothermia.

While functional closure of the ductus arteriosus occurs within 15 hours of delivery, fibrosis takes up to 3 weeks. Closure of the ductus arteriosus results from increasing blood PO_2 levels and decreasing levels of prostaglandins. Increasing blood oxygen levels generally cause pulmonary vasodilation, but they have the opposite effect on the ductus arteriosus, causing vasoconstriction. Ductus vasodilation results from the effects of prostaglandins from the placenta during pregnancy. Once the placenta is gone and prostaglandin E2 levels drop, the ductus arteriosus constricts. Closure of the ductus venosus is believed to be related to the mechanical pressure changes resulting from cord severing, redistribution of blood, and increased cardiac output. The ductus venosus undergoes fibrotic closure within three to seven days following delivery.

Thermoregulation

The maintenance of a stable body temperature (thermoregulation) is vital for successful adaptation to extrauterine existence. Thermoregulation is the prevention of heat loss, or the regulation of the newborn's environment to prevent hypo/hyperthermia, conditions that can result in serious adverse effects for the newborn if left untreated. Hypothermia increases oxygen consumption, metabolic processes, and caloric consumption, and stimulates the release of norepinephrine, a catecholamine that leads to pulmonary vasoconstriction. The increased pulmonary vascular resistance from this vasoconstriction can cause a right-to-left shunt through the foramen ovale. The mixing of the oxygenated and deoxygenated blood leads to hypoxia, anaerobic metabolism, increased acidosis, and, if untreated, death. Hypothermia also results in peripheral vasoconstriction which adds to the acidotic state. Characteristics of newborns that increase their chances of hypothermia include a large body surface in relation to body mass, a limited amount of subcutaneous fat, vasomotor instability, and limited metabolic capacity. Newborns can lose body heat through four mechanisms: evaporation, radiation, conduction, and convection.

Evaporation—Loss of body heat when a liquid on the body surface is changed to a vapor.

Examples:

- Infant covered with amniotic fluid immediately following delivery is not promptly dried off.

- Routine bath is not done in an organized, timely fashion.

Radiation—Loss of body heat to a solid cold object without direct contact.

Example:

- Bassinet or single-walled isolette is placed close to cold exterior wall of building.

Conduction—Loss of body heat to a solid cold object through direct contact.

Examples:

- Infant is placed on unpadded scale for weighing;

- Infant is placed on unpadded metal table for examination;

- Cold stethoscope is placed on infant.

Convection—Loss of body heat to cooler ambient air.

Examples:

- Infant positioned near drafts or open windows.

- Portholes on isolette are frequently opened.

The newborn's most efficient method of heat production is nonshivering thermogenesis. Heat is produced through lipolysis of brown fat, a type of adipose tissue that makes up 1.5% of a full-term infant's weight. Brown fat, which gets its color from a rich vascular supply, dense cellular content, and multiple nerve endings, is located around the head, heart, neck, great vessels, kidneys, and adrenal glands, between the scapula, behind the sternum, and in the axilla. When heat loss occurs, norepinephrine is released from sympathetic nerves. Norepinephrine stimulates the oxidation of brown fat, thus causing heat production. This heat is then distributed throughout the body by the blood, which has absorbed heat as it flowed through fatty tissue.

The newborn also defends against heat loss through vasomotor control, thermal insulation, and muscle activity. Heat is preserved by peripheral vasoconstriction and dissipated by peripheral vasodilation Thermal insulation is provided by white subcutaneous fat, which generally makes up 11% to 17% of a full-term infant's weight. Examples of muscle activity include increased activity and assumption of a tightly flexed position that limits the amount of exposed body surface.

Though researchers believe an infant may have some degree of shivering ability, the extent to which this shivering results in heat production is believed to be minimal.

Infants must also be protected against and assessed for hyperthermia. A cold-stressed infant must be rewarmed gradually. Though a newborn has six times the number of sweat glands of an adult, their function is limited until around the fourth week of life. When overheated, the newborn responds with peripheral vasodilation, evaporation of insensible water loss, and increased oxygen consumption and metabolic rate.

INITIAL ASSESSMENT

Apgar

The Apgar score is a five-part scoring method developed by Dr. Virginia Apgar in 1952. Each of the five signs are assessed/scored at one and five minutes of life. When added together, the score ranges from 0 to 10. A score of 8 to 10 indicates the newborn is not in any apparent distress, while a score of five to seven indicates mild respiratory, metabolic, or neurologic depression. A score below 5 indicates more detailed resuscitative measures may be indicated. *(See Table 8-1.)*

Gestational Age

In the 1950s, the World Health Organization (WHO) defined a premature infant as one that weighed 2,500 grams or less. During the 1960s, however, infants were identified who, though they met the weight criteria set forth by WHO, were indeed term or post-term according to their length of gestation. In the late sixties, Battaglia and Lubchenco developed a method by which infants are classified according to both their gestational age and birth weight (Colorado Intrauterine Growth Chart). The length of gestation is subdivided into three categories; less than 38 weeks

(pre-term); from the beginning of the 38th week to the end of the 41st week (term); and from the beginning of the 42nd week and beyond (pre-term). After plotting the infant's length of gestation on the horizontal (X) axis, the infant's weight in grams is plotted on the vertical (Y) axis. Where these two points intersect provides the examiner with a good understanding of the infant's gestational age and actual/potential needs. An infant is classified as small for gestational age (SGA) when its birth weight falls below the 10th percentile expected for that length of gestation. If the infant's birth weight is higher than the 90th percentile, a classification of large for gestational age (LGA) is made. If the infant's birth weight falls between the 10th to 90th percentile expected for that gestational age, the infant is considered appropriate for gestational age (AGA). An additional classification, very low birth weight (VLBW) was added in the 1980s. A VLBW infant weighs between 500 and 1499 grams.

There are several gestational age assessment tools available to assess the infant's growth and maturation based on external physical features and neurologic maturity *(see table 8-2)*. The most commonly used is the Ballard tool, which was last revised in 1988 to allow for assessment of newborns of 20 to 44 weeks gestation.

According to the Ballard tool, the criteria used to evaluate neuromuscular maturity are posture, square window, arm recoil, popliteal angle, scarf sign and heel to ear *(see table 8-2)*. The criteria used to evaluate physical maturity are skin, lanugo, plantar surface, breast, eye/ear, and genitalia. After each criterion is scored according to a predetermined description, the total score is determined and placed in the maturity rating box to determine the neonate's "age by exam" *(see table 8-2)*. The gestational "age by exam" may differ from the "age by dates" calculated by using Nagele's rule. Providing care based on the infant's "age by exam" will be individualized and comprehensive.

				TABLE 8-1			

TABLE 8-1
The Apgar Scoring System

Sign	0	1	2
Heart rate	Absent	Below 100	Above 100
Respiratory effort	Absent	Slow, irregular	Good, crying
Muscle tone	Flaccid	Some flexion	Active motion
Reflex irritability	No response	Crying	Vigorous crying
Color	Blue/pale	Pink body, blue extremities	Pink baby

NEUROMUSCULAR MATURITY

With the neonate in a supine position, posture is scored using the following criteria:

0 - elbows and knees are not flexed; 90-degree angle at ankle

1 - slight flexion of wrists, hips, and knees; 90-degree angle at ankle

2 - greater than 90-degree flexion of elbows, hips and knees; 90-degree angle at ankle

3 - 90-degree flexion of elbow, hips, knees, and ankles

4 - 45-degree flexion of elbow, hips, and knees; less than 90-degree angle at ankle

While flexing the neonate's wrist down onto the ventral aspect of the forearm, the square window sign is scored using the following criteria:

-1- the angle between the hand and forearm is >90-degrees

0 - the angle between the hand and forearm is 90-degrees

1 - the angle between the hand and forearm is 60-degrees

2 - the angle between the hand and forearm is 45-degrees

3 - the angle between the hand and forearm is 30-degrees

4 - the angle between the hand and forearm is 0-degrees

After placing the neonate in a supine position, first flex the forearms for five seconds, then pull the arms out and release. The arm recoil is scored using the following criteria:

0 - the elbows extend at a 180-degree angle

1 - the elbows flex at a 140 to 180-degree angle

2 - the elbows flex at a 110 to 140-degree angle

3 - the elbows flex at a 90 to 110-degree angle

4 - the elbows flex at less than a 90-degree angle

With the neonate in a supine position and pelvis flat, flex the knees upon the abdomen and extend the lower leg toward the neonate's head. The popliteal angle is scored using the following criteria:

-1- the legs are straight, pointing toward the head at a 180-degree angle

0 - the knees are flexed at a 160-degree angle

1 - the knees are flexed at a 140-degree angle

2 - the knees are flexed at a 120-degree angle

3 - the knees are flexed at a 100-degree angle

4 - the knees are flexed at a 90-degree angle

5 - the knees are flexed at less than a 90-degree angle

With the neonate in a supine position and head midline, one hand is pulled over the chest toward the opposite shoulder. The scarf sign is scored using the following criteria:

-1- the elbow passes the opposite axillary line

0 - the elbow slightly passes the opposite axillary line

1 - the elbow reaches the opposite axillary line

2 - the elbow reaches the midline of the trunk

3 - the elbow reaches the near axillary line

4 - the elbow does not cross over the near axillary line

With the neonate in a supine position, the legs are extended toward the head without forcing them. The heel-to-ear sign is scored using the following criteria:

-1- the legs reach the head, the knees are extended at a 180-degree angle

0 - the knees are flexed at a 160-degree angle

1 - the knees are flexed at a 145-degree angle

2 - the knees are flexed at a 110-degree angle

3 - the knees are flexed at a 90-degree angle

4 - the knees are flexed at less than a 90-degree angle

Physical Maturity

The skin is scored using the following criteria:

-1- transparent, sticky, and friable

0 - thin, numerous veins visible, gelatinous, red, translucent,

1 - smooth, pink, visible veins

2 - few vessels visible, superficial peeling or rash

3 - rare vessels visible, cracking, pale areas

4 - no vessels visible, deep cracking, parchment-like

5 - leathery, cracked, wrinkled, pale

Lanugo is scored using the following criteria:

-1- none

0 - sparse

1 - abundant over entire body

2 - thinning

3 - bald areas present

4 - mostly bald

The plantar surface is scored using the following criteria:

-2- heel-to-toe distance is ≤40 mm

-1- heel-to-toe distance is between 40-50 mm

0 - heel-to-toe distance is ≥50 mm; no creases present

1 - faint red marks over anterior half of sole

2 - anterior transverse mark present

3 - creases present over anterior two-thirds of sole

4 - creases over entire sole

The breast is scored using the following criteria:

-1- imperceptible

0 - barely perceptible

1 - areola flat, no bud present

2 - areola stippled; bud 1 to 2 mm

3 - areola raised; bud 3 to 4 mm

4 - full areola; bud 5 to 10 mm

The eyes and ears are scored using the following criteria:

-2- eyelids are tightly fused

-1- eyelids are loosely fused

0 - eyelids are open; pinna flat, remains folded

1 - pinna slightly curved; soft, slow recoil

2 - pinna well curved; soft but ready to recoil

3 - pinna formed and firm; instant recoil

4 - thick cartilage; ear stiff and remains erect from head

The male genitalia are scored using the following criteria:

-1- flat scrotum, no rugae visible

0 - empty scrotum, faint rugae visible

1 - testes in inguinal canal; rare rugae visible

2 - testes descending; few rugae visible

3 - testes descended; good rugae visible

4 - testes pendulous; deep rugae visible

The female genitalia are scored using the following criteria:

-1- prominent clitoris; labia flat

0 - clitoris prominent; labia minora small

1 - clitoris prominent; labia minora enlarging

2 - labia majora and minora equally prominent

3 - labia majora large; labia minora small

4 - labia majora covers clitoris and labia minora

ANOMALIES

Cardiac System

While congenital cardiac anomalies can occur during any stage of embryonic development, cardiac structures are most susceptible to defects from the third to ninth weeks of gestation. Though the majority of causes are unknown, the effect of genetic and environmental factors are being investigated. Approximately 30% of all deaths from anomalies result from those of a cardiac nature. Congenital cardiac anomalies are divided into cyanotic and acyanotic anomalies. Examples of cyanotic anomalies are tetralogy of Fallot, truncus arteriosus, complete transposition of the great vessels, tricuspid atresia, and anomalous venous return. In these defects, very high pressure in the right side of the heart allows right-to-left shunting of unoxygenated blood. Arterial blood oxygen becomes desaturated as the unoxygenated blood mixes with the oxygenated blood, resulting in decreased peripheral perfusion and cyanosis. Examples of acyanotic anomalies are patent ductus ateriosus, pulmonary stenosis, coarctation of the aorta, ventricular septal defects, and atrial septal defects. In these defects, increased pulmonary blood flow to the left ventricle can result in congestive heart failure and pulmonary edema.

Respiratory System

A diaphragmatic hernia, the most common respiratory tract anomaly, results from a congenital defect in the diaphragm. As a result, the abdominal contents herniate into the thoracic cavity, causing displacement of the heart and lung tissue. Bowel sounds may be heard over the chest wall and the anterior of the abdomen is scaphoid (sunken). Immediate surgical intervention is necessary. If the defect is large, severe herniation during the prenatal period results in incomplete lung tissue development, a condition that may be incompatible with extrauterine existence.

Unilateral or bilateral blockage of the posterior nares is known as choanal atresia. Since newborns are obligatory nose breathers, signs of respiratory distress are evident immediately after birth. Surgical intervention is necessary and the prognosis is excellent if there are no accompanying anomalies.

Gastrointestinal System

Tracheoesophageal malformations occur when the trachea and esophagus do not separate completely during the first trimester of pregnancy. Examples of these anomalies include tracheoesophageal fistula, esophageal atresia, and absence of the esophagus. The most frequently occurring anomaly is when the esophagus ends in a blind pouch (atresia), with a fistula connecting it to the trachea. When fed, the blind pouch fills up, fluid enters the trachea through the fistula, and the newborn suffers acute respiratory distress and cyanosis. Surgical intervention is required and the prognosis is excellent if the defect is not associated with other major anomalies.

An omphalocele is the protrusion of the abdominal contents through a defect in the abdomi-

TABLE 8-2
Newborn Maturity Rating & Classification

ESTIMATION OF GESTATIONAL AGE BY MATURITY RATING
Symbols: X - 1st Exam   O - 2nd Exam

NEUROMUSCULAR MATURITY

	−1	0	1	2	3	4	5
Posture							
Square Window (wrist)	>90°	90°	60°	45°	30°	0°	
Arm Recoil		180°	140°–180°	110°–140°	90°–110°	<90°	
Popliteal Angle	180°	160°	140°	120°	100°	90°	<90°
Scarf Sign							
Heel to Ear							

Gestation by Dates _____ wks

_____

Birth Date _____ Hour _____ am/pm

APGAR _____ 1 min _____ 5 min

MATURITY RATING

score	weeks
−10	20
−5	22
0	24
5	26
10	28
15	30
20	32
25	34
30	36
35	38
40	40
45	42
50	44

PHYSICAL MATURITY

Skin	sticky friable transparent	gelatinous red, translucent	smooth pink, visible veins	superficial peeling &/or rash, few veins	cracking pale areas rare veins	parchment deep cracking no vessels	leathery cracked wrinkled
Lanugo	none	sparse	abundant	thinning	bald areas	mostly bald	
Plantar Surface	heel-toe 40–50mm:–1 <40mm:–2	>50mm no crease	faint red marks	anterior transverse crease only	creases ant. 2/3	creases over entire sole	
Breast	imperceptible	barely perceptible	flat areola no bud	stippled areola 1–2mm bud	raised areola 3–4mm bud	full areola 5–10mm bud	
Eye/Ear	lids fused loosely:–1 tightly:–2	lids open pinna flat stays folded	sl. curved pinna; soft; slow recoil	well curved pinna; soft but ready recoil	formed & firm instant recoil	thick cartilage ear stiff	
Genitals male	scrotum flat, smooth	scrotum empty faint rugae	testes in upper canal rare rugae	testes descending few rugae	testes down good rugae	testes pendulous deep rugae	
Genitals female	clitoris prominent labia flat	prominent clitoris small labia minora	prominent clitoris enlarging minora	majora & minora equally prominent	majora large minora small	majora cover clitoris & minora	

SCORING SECTION

	1st Exam = X	2nd Exam = 0
Estimating Gest Age by Maturity Rating	_____Weeks	_____Weeks
Time of Exam	Date _____ Hour_____ am/pm	Date _____ Hour_____ am/pm
Age at Exam	_____ Hours	_____ Hours
Signature of Examiner	_____ M.D.	_____ M.D.

Source: Ballard, J. L., Khoury, J. C., Wedig, K., Wang, L., Eilers-Walsman, B. L. & Lipp, R. New Ballard Score, expanded to include extremely premature infants. *J Pediatr.* 1991;119:417–423.

nal wall at the umbilicus. The protruding bowel is covered by a thick membrane composed of amnion and peritoneum. Several surgeries may be needed to reduce the bowel if the defect is large. Prognosis is guarded if the defect is associated with other congenital anomalies or is very large and includes all major abdominal organs.

Gastroschisis refers to incomplete abdominal wall closure that does not involve the umbilical cord insertion site. Generally, the small intestine and part of the large intestine protrude and no membranous sac covers the protrusion.

Intestinal obstruction that results from obstruction of the terminal ileum by viscous meconium is known as meconium ileus. The colon atrophies and narrows beyond the site of obstruction. In the majority of cases, it is associated with cystic fibrosis, a genetic disease resulting from a pancreatic enzyme deficiency.

Central Nervous System

The majority of central nervous system anomalies are readily apparent. A meningomyelocele (or myelomeningocele) is a cystic protrusion of the meninges, cerebrospinal fluid, and spinal cord through a defect in the posterior wall of the vertebral column. There will be no motor or sensory function below the level of the defect and prognosis depends on the degree of involvement and level of the defect.

An encephalocele is a protrusion of the meninges and portion of brain tissue through the cranium, generally in the occipital area. As with a meningomyelocele, an encephalocele results from the failure of the neural tube to close during embryonic development. This anomaly may also be accompanied by hydrocephalus and paralysis.

Hydrocephalus is an abnormal accumulation of cerebrospinal fluid in the ventricles of the brain. This condition is frequently associated with myelomeningocele due to blockage in the flow of cerebrospinal fluid. The suture lines are separated,

fontanelles bulge and feel tense and the infant has a high-pitched cry.

Anencephaly refers to the absence of part of the cranial vault and underlying brain tissue and is incompatible with life.

RESUSCITATION

(Guidelines for Neonatal Advanced Life Support by the American Heart Association and American Academy of Pediatrics, 1994)

Within the first few minutes following delivery, the newborn undergoes many changes as he or she adapts to extrauterine existence *(see figures 8-4 and 8-5)*. Neonates are more likely to require resuscitative measures at this time than at any other time in their lives. Prompt, adequate resuscitation will directly affect the newborn's quality of life. At each delivery, properly trained health care professionals must be prepared to resuscitate the infant, if needed. Every delivery room should be equipped with the following:

- A radiant warmer for the newborn; sterile blankets; masks, gloves and protective eyewear (where indicated) for the attendant; tape; tongue blades.

- An oxygen source; newborn-sized ambu bag; an assortment of face masks suitable both for fullterm and post-term infants.

- Manual and wall suction that can be adjusted to low force; an assortment of soft-suction catheters in various pediatric sizes; suction bulbs.

- A newborn laryngoscope with an assortment of blades, including premature sizes; uncuffed endotracheal tubes in a variety of sizes from 2.0 to 4.5.

- An emergency drug box with pediatric concentrations of medications needed for full resuscita-

FIGURE 8-4
Resuscitation Flow Diagram

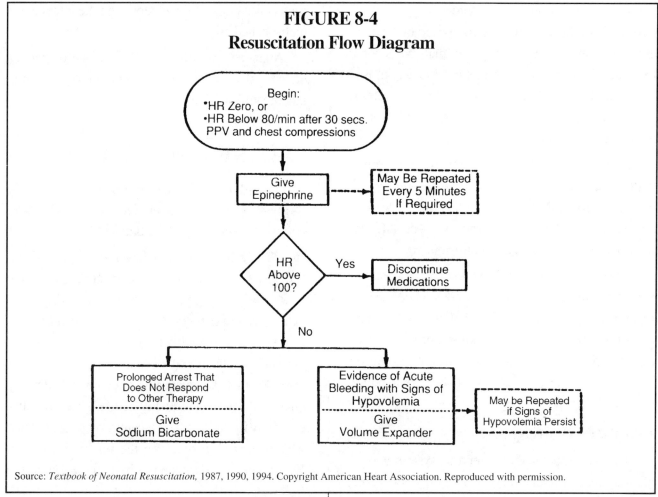

Source: *Textbook of Neonatal Resuscitation,* 1987, 1990, 1994. Copyright American Heart Association. Reproduced with permission.

tion of a newborn, including but not limited to atropine, epinephrine, and sodium bicarbonate. Syringes and labels should also be available.

- An umbilical vessel catheterization tray; intravenous fluids; intravenous catheters including butterfly needle sets; over-the-needle flexible catheters.

- An electrocardiogram monitor; leads; newborn-sized electrodes.

Approximately 80% of newborns will respond to the initial steps of neonatal resuscitation covered below.

1. Position the infant under a preheated radiant warmer.

2. Dry the infant thoroughly from head to toe with a prewarmed blanket or towel to prevent heat loss. (Important: If the amniotic fluid contained meconium, the trachea should be suc-

tioned immediately after the infant is placed on the warmer bed. This infant should not be dried yet since doing so may provide tactile stimulation that could induce aspiration of meconium before it can be suctioned.) Universal Precautions should be used when handling the newborn initial bath (Refer to the Appendix for the CDC Guidelines.)

3. Remove the wet linen from contact with the infant.

4. Position the newborn supine or supported on its side. Maintain the infant's head in a neutral position by placing a 3/4"–1" rolled blanket under the shoulders.

5. Suction the mouth first, then the nose. Suctioning the nose first may trigger a gasp reflex that could cause material (e.g. meconium) to be aspirated into the lungs. (A DeLee

FIGURE 8-5
Resuscitation in the Delivery Room

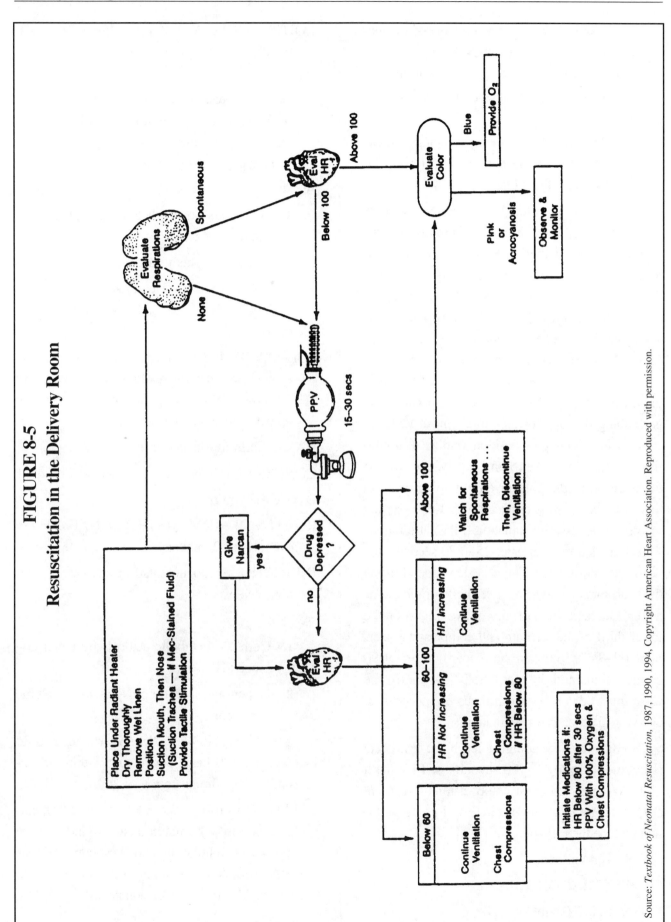

Source: *Textbook of Neonatal Resuscitation*, 1987, 1990, 1994, Copyright American Heart Association. Reproduced with permission.

suction trap is no longer recommended for suctioning.) Suctioning should be limited to 3 to 5 seconds at a time. The heart rate should be monitored during the suctioning to detect possible bradycardia.

6. Provide tactile stimulation by slapping or flicking the soles of the feet or by rubbing the infant's back a few times.

The next steps after the preceding measures will depend upon the infant's respirations, heart rate, and color. If there are spontaneous respirations, the nurse goes on to evaluate the heart rate. If the heart rate is above 100 beats per minute, the color is then evaluated. If the infant is pink or has acrocyanosis (peripheral cyanosis), the infant needs only to be observed and monitored. If the infant has central cyanosis, free flow oxygen at 5L/min is provided either by face mask (held firmly) or oxygen tubing directed towards mouth/nose with the hands held in a cupping position. Further resuscitative measures are taken immediately, however, if there are no respirations or only gasping ones. In this case, the infant is provided with 100% oxygen via positive-pressure ventilation (PPV) at a rate of 40–60 times a minute. After 15 to 30 seconds, the heart rate is evaluated. The next step depends upon the heart rate *(see table 8-3)*. If chest compressions are indicated, position the tips of two fingers on the lower third of the sternum and compress the sternum 1/2–3/4″. To obtain the proper number of 90 compressions and 30 ventilations (3:1 ratio), the chest must be compressed 3 times in 1.5 seconds, allowing .5 seconds for ventilation.

Medications are administered if the heart rate is below 80 following 30 seconds of PPV with 100% oxygen and chest compressions *(see table 8-4)*. Medications administered during resuscitation include the following:

NAME: **Epinephrine**

CONCENTRATION: 1:10,000

DOSAGE: 0.1–0.3 ml/kg

ROUTES OF ADMINISTRATION: IV or ET, rapidly

INDICATIONS: When the heart rate remains below 80 beats per minute despite a minimum of 30 seconds of adequate ventilation with 100% oxygen and chest compressions OR when the heart rate is zero.

ACTION:

1. Increases strength and rate of cardiac contractions

2. Causes peripheral vasoconstriction

ANTICIPATED SIGNS: Heart rate should increase to >100 within 30 seconds following administration.

FOLLOW-UP: If the heart rate remains below 100, epinephrine may be readministered every five minutes. Volume expanders and/or sodium bicarbonate should be considered.

NAME: **Sodium bicarbonate**

CONCENTRATION: 4.2% solution = 0.5 mEq/ml

DOSAGE: 2 mEq/kg

ROUTES OF ADMINISTRATION: IV slowly over at least 2 minutes

INDICATIONS: Documented or suspected metabolic acidosis

ACTION:

1. Corrects metabolic acidosis by increasing blood pH

2. Hypertonic solution provides some volume expansion

ANTICIPATED SIGNS: Heart rate should increase to ≥100 beats per minute within 30 seconds following administration.

FOLLOW-UP: If the heart rate remains ≤100, epinephrine may be readministered and volume expanders, ventilation, and chest compressions continued. Administration of dopamine should be considered if hypotension persists.

IMPORTANT POINTS:

1. The administration of sodium bicarbonate must be accompanied by effective ventilation.

2. Careful attention must be paid to the concentration and rate of delivery of sodium bicarbonate in order to avoid intraventricular hemorrhage.

3. While useful in a prolonged resuscitation, the use of sodium bicarbonate is discouraged in cases of bradycardia or brief arrests.

NAME: **Volume expanders** (i.e. Ringer's lactate, whole blood, normal saline, 5% albumin-saline)

DOSAGE: 10 ml/kg

ROUTES OF ADMINISTRATION: IV over 5–10 minutes

INDICATIONS: Signs of hypovolemia

a. Falling blood pressure

b. Weak pulse despite a good heart rate

c. Poor response to resuscitation

d. Pallor despite oxygenation

ACTIONS:

1. Vascular volume increased

2. Decreased metabolic acidosis due to increased tissue perfusion

ANTICIPATED SIGNS: Stronger pulse, increased blood pressure, and improved pallor.

FOLLOW-UP: If signs of hypovolemia continue, administration may be repeated. If there is little or no improvement, sodium bicarbonate for metabolic acidosis should be considered. The use of dopamine should be considered if the blood pressure persistently drops.

NAME: **Naloxone hydrochloride (Narcan)**

CONCENTRATION: 0.4 mg/ml or 1.0 mg/ml

DOSAGE: 0.25 ml/kg (0.4 mg/ml concentration)

0.1 ml/kg (1.0 mg/ml concentration)

ROUTES OF ADMINISTRATION: ET and IV are preferred routes, though IM and SQ are acceptable despite delayed onset of action.

INDICATIONS:

1. Signs of respiratory depression in the newborn.

2. Mother received narcotic within the last 4 hours.

ACTION: Narcotic antagonist

ANTICIPATED SIGNS: Spontaneous respirations

FOLLOW-UP: Closely monitor respirations and heart rate. Naloxone may need to be readministered if respiratory depression recurs.

TABLE 8-3		
If after 15–30 seconds of 100% oxygen via PPV, the heart rate is:		
Below 60	**60–100**	**Above 100**
Continue ventilation	HR NOT INCREASING Continue ventilation	Watch for spontaneous respirations, then discontinue ventilation
Initiate chest compressions	Initiate chest compressions if HR is below 80 and not increasing	Provide free flow oxygen as needed
	HR INCREASING Continue ventilation	

TABLE 8-4
Medication for Neonatal Resuscitation

Medication	Concentration to Administer	Preparation	Dosage/Route*	Total Dose/Infant			Rate/Precautions
				Weight	**Total mL**		
Epinephrine	1:10 000	1 mL	0.1-0.3 mL/kg IV or ET	1 kg 2 kg 3 kg 4 kg	0.1-0.3 mL 0.2-0.6 mL 0.3-0.9 mL 0.4-1.2 mL		Give rapidly May dilute with normal saline to 1-2 mL if giving ET
				Weight	**Total mL**		
Volume Expanders	Whole blood 5% Albumin-saline Normal saline Ringer's lactate	40 mL	10 mL/kg IV	1 kg 2 kg 3 kg 4 kg	10 mL 20 mL 30 mL 40 mL		Give over 5-10 minutes
				Weight	**Total Dose**	**Total mL**	
Sodium Bicarbonate	0.5 mEq/mL (4.2% solution)	20 mL or two 10-mL prefilled syringes	2 mEq/kg IV	1 kg 2 kg 3 kg 4 kg	2 mEq 4 mEq 6 mEq 8 mEq	4 mL 8 mL 12 mL 16 mL	Give *slowly*, over at least 2 minutes Give only if infant is being effectively ventilated
				Weight	**Total Dose**	**Total mL**	
Naloxone Hydrochloride	0.4 mg/mL	1 mL	0.1 mg/kg (0.25 mL/kg) IV, ET IM, SQ	1 kg 2 kg 3 kg 4 kg	0.1 mg 0.2 mg 0.3 mg 0.4 mg	0.25 mL 0.50 mL 0.75 mL 1.00 mL	Give rapidly IV, ET preferred IM, SQ acceptable
	1.0 mg/mL	1 mL	0.1 mL/kg (0.1 mL/kg) IV, ET IM, SQ	1 kg 2 kg 3 kg 4 kg	0.1 mg 0.2 mg 0.3 mg 0.4 mg	0.1 mL 0.2 mL 0.3 mL 0.4 mL	
				Weight	**Total µg/min**		
Dopamine	$6 \times \dfrac{\text{Weight (kg)} \times \text{Desired dose (µg/kg/min)}}{\text{Desired fluid (mL/h)}} = \dfrac{\text{mg of dopamine}}{\text{per 100 mL of solution}}$		Begin at 5 µg/kg/min (may increase to 20 µg/kg/min if necessary) IV	1 kg 2 kg 3 kg 4 kg	5-20 µg/min 10-40 µg/min 15-60 µg/min 20-80 µg/min		Give as a continuous infusion using an infusion pump Monitor heart rate and blood pressure closely Seek consultation

*IM, intramuscular; ET, endotracheal; IV, intravenous; SQ, subcutaneous

From *Textbook of Neonatal Resuscitation*, 1987, 1990, 1994 American Heart Association

IMPORTANT POINTS:

1. Naloxone acts for one to four hours. Because the action of the narcotic may exceed this time frame, repeated administration of naloxone may be necessary.

2. Administering naloxone to the infant of a narcotic-addicted mother may result in severe seizures.

Research and experience continually changes standards of neonatal resuscitation; thus the resuscitation of the newborn is best left to those trained and knowledgeable in the procedure. However, every nurse routinely involved in the delivery or care of newborns should have an understanding and knowledge of the techniques of newborn resuscitation. Remember that when resuscitation begins in the delivery room, it frequently takes place in front of the frightened new mother. Whenever possible, a nurse should be assigned simply to stay at her side and reassure her (and her partner, if present) that everything possible is being done for her infant and that the pediatrician or nurse will speak with her as soon as possible about the infant's condition.

GENERAL PHYSICAL ASSESSMENT

Vital Signs

Normal vital signs for the newborn.

Temperature: Axilla 36.5°–37.0°C (97.7°–98.6°F); rectal 36.6°–37.2°C (97.8°–99°F)

Pulse: 120–160

Respiration: 30–0

Blood pressure: Systolic blood pressure in the term infant ranges from 63–70 mm/Hg while the diastolic pressure ranges from 40–50 mm/Hg.

Vital Statistics

Birth weight: 2950–3515g (6.5–7.75 lbs.)

Length: 45–52.3 cm (18″–20.5″); the infant grows 10 cm (4″) within the first 3 months of life

Head circumference: 33–35 cm (13″–14″). The head circumference is generally 2 cm larger than the chest circumference and increases 2″ within the first 4 months of life.

Chest circumference: 31–33 cm (12″–13″)

Skin

The infant's skin color can provide many insights into its condition. Pale skin results from decreased hemoglobin or cutaneous vasoconstriction. Plethora indicates the skin has a ruddy, purplish hue because of increased hemoglobin levels. Cyanosis results from increased amounts of unsaturated hemoglobin.

Other skin findings include the following:

Vernix caseosa, a greasy substance with a cheese-like consistency is made up of epithelial cells and secretions from sebaceous glands. It first appears early in the third trimester and begins to diminish after 40 weeks gestation. Its purpose is to protect the skin from the drying effect of amniotic fluid.

Lanugo is a fine, downy hair that covers the fetus's body by 17 weeks gestation, peaks by 30 weeks, then begins to disappear first from the face, then trunk, and finally the extremities.

Acrocyanosis, the normal cyanosis of the hands and feet within the first 24 hours of life, is due to venous stasis of the extremities.

Milia, small, white, clogged sebaceous glands located on the nose, forehead, cheeks, and chin, disappear within the first few weeks of life.

Mongolian spots are areas of blue pigmentation on the back, sacral area or buttocks. Primarily seen in blacks, Asians and Native Americans, these spots usually disappear during the first few years of life.

The most common and variable of the benign transient lesions of the newborn is **erythema toxicum.** The lesions, irregularly shaped, small reddened areas with pale centers, are usually located on the trunk and diaper area. The lesions usually appear about the second day of life, but new ones may appear over the first week.

Head

Fontanels: The anterior fontanel is located at the juncture of the coronal, frontal, and sagittal sutures. Diamond-shaped and measuring 3 to 4 cm long by 2 to 3 cm wide, the anterior fontanelle gradually closes during the first 18 months of life. Closure of the anterior fontanel at birth is associated with inadequate brain development. The triangular-shaped posterior fontanel is located at the juncture of the sagittal and lambdoidal sutures. Measuring $1 \times 1 \times 1$ cm, it usually closes within the first three months of life, though molding of the newborn's head may cause it to be closed at birth. The fontanels, assessed while the infant is quiet or sleeping, should feel soft and flat to the touch. A sunken or depressed feeling may indicate dehydration, while bulging may indicate increased intracranial pressure.

Cephalhematoma, a collection of blood between a skull bone and the periosteum, does not cross suture lines. Resulting from pressures experienced during labor or trauma from forceps, the localized scalp swelling may last up to 8 weeks. The infant with a cephalhematoma is at increased risk of hyperbilirubinemia resulting from the breakdown of red blood cells within the collection. Caput succedaneum, localized swelling over the presenting part, does cross suture lines and usually disappears within 1 week.

Eyes

A newborn's eyes are generally blue or gray due to scleral thinness. The permanent eye color is established by 12 months of life. Tearless crying results from immature lacrimal glands and may last up to 3 months. Subconjunctival hemorrhages may result from vascular tension changes during birth. Transient strabismus is due to poor muscle control.

Mouth

The newborn's mouth should be symmetrical and an appropriate size for the face. If the mouth droops unilaterally, it could be due to damage to the seventh cranial (facial) nerve resulting from birth trauma. Downturning of both corners ("fish mouth") is frequently associated with fetal alcohol syndrome. An extremely wide mouth (macrostomia) or large tongue (macroglossia) is indicative of a metabolic disorder such as hypothyroidism. An unusually small mouth (microstomia) is frequently associated with a congenital syndrome. Deviation of the tongue to one side is seen in neurological defects such as cranial nerve palsy. The palate should be inspected for a high arch and cleft of the hard or soft palate. Unilateral or bilateral lip clefts may be present in conjunction with cleft palate or by themselves. By looking at the infant's profile, a small chin (micrognathia) can be observed. Micrognathia is frequently associated with Pierre Robin's syndrome. Epstein's pearls are protein deposits found on the gums and/or hard palate. The mouth should be inspected for a precocious or natal tooth, which should be removed if loose to prevent aspiration should it fall out.

Nose

Nares must be checked for patency since infants are obligatory nose breathers. This can be done using one of two methods: While closing off one nostril with the examiner's finger, evaluate the infant's ability to breath through the remaining nostril. Patency can also be evaluated by passing a catheter down each nostril. The infant should be assessed for nasal flaring, a sign of respiratory distress.

Ears

The top of the ear should be above or parallel to an imaginary line from inner to outer canthus of the eye. Low-set ears may indicate chromosomal abnormalities (e.g. trisomies 13 and 18, bilateral renal agenesis, and/or mental retardation).

Neck

A newborn's neck is short and weak with deep skin folds and full range of motion. Tilting of the head to one side and nuchal rigidity may indicate damage to the sternocleidomastoid muscle (torticollis). This injury occurs when there is contraction of the neck muscle due to a traumatic hematoma acquired in utero or during delivery. Abnormal skin folds or webbing of the neck is indicative of Turner's syndrome, a sex chromosome abnormality.

Extremities

The hands and feet should be assessed for the number of digits on each. Polydactyly means there are more than five digits on each extremity; syndactyly is the fusion of two or more digits. Though these findings may be isolated, they are also associated with congenital syndromes such as trisomy 13 (polydactyly) and Apert's syndrome (syndactyly).

Clavicles

The most common birth injury is a fractured clavicle, primarily the result of a difficult delivery. Signs of a fractured clavicle include crepitus (crackling or grinding sound on movement), asymmetrical movement or Moro reflex, and excessive crying when the affected extremity is moved.

Breast Tissue

There may be breast engorgement or a milky discharge from the nipple due to the withdrawal of maternal estrogen. The newborn may have supernumerary or accessory "nipples" located below and medial to the true nipples. To differentiate these accessory "nipples" from a nevus (mole) the tissue adjacent to the "nipple" is pulled laterally. An accessory "nipple" will dimple while a nevus will not.

Abdomen

The abdomen, which appears large in relation to the pelvis, is cylindrical in shape with some protrusion. Bowel sounds can be auscultated every 10–15 seconds. A scaphoid (sunken) appearance, is indicative of a diaphragmatic hernia, a surgical emergency.

Respiratory System

The newborn must be observed for signs of respiratory distress. These include tachypnea (respiratory rate 60/min), nasal flaring, grunting, retractions (substernal or intercostal), and cyanosis. Breath sounds should be assessed for rales and rhonchi. Rales are crackling sounds heard upon inspiration. The sound results from air entering bronchioles/alveoli that contain serous secretions. Rhonchi are continuous rumbling sounds that are more evident during expiration.

Umbilical Cord

The umbilical cord is whitish and gelatinous with two arteries and one vein. A single artery may indicate a congenital, cardiac, or renal disorder.

Genitalia

The majority of term males will have one to two testes descended into the scrotum at delivery. Epispadias exists when the urinary meatus is located on the dorsal surface of the penis. Hypospadias exists when the urinary meatus is on the ventral surface of the penis. A hydrocele, a collection of fluid in the testes, is a common, generally benign finding that resolves spontaneously. The foreskin of the uncircumcised male remains tight for two to three months. The female may have clear or bloody vaginal discharge due to the influence of maternal hormones. In the full-term female, the labia majora generally completely covers the labia minora and clitoris.

Spine

The back should be assessed for scoliosis, lateral curvature of the spine. Neural tube defects are midline abnormalities of the spine caused by failure of the neural tube to close properly during the fourth week of development.

Anus

Anal patency is checked by taking the initial temperature rectally. Thereafter, axillary temperatures are recommended in order to avoid trauma to mucous membranes of the rectum.

Hips

Signs of congenital dislocation of the hips are:

- Uneven leg lengths: Upward displacement of the head of the femur out of the acetabulum would make the dislocated side to be shorter.

- Asymmetrical gluteal folds.

- Positive Ortaloni's sign: With the infant on its back, flex the knees up against the abdomen and abduct the legs. Feeling or hearing a hip click or the inability to achieve at least a 65-degree abduction angle indicates a dislocated hip.

NEUROLOGICAL ASSESSMENT

In addition to the neurological components of a gestational age assessment tool, the nurse should also assess the infant's cry and reflexes. A full term infant's cry will be loud and strong while a high-pitched cry may indicate increased intracranial pressure or drug-withdrawal.

Moro reflex. When the neonate is lifted above the crib and then suddenly lowered, there is a symmetric extension then abduction of the arms;

the index finger and thumb form a "C" shape. This reflex remains for approximately four months. An asymmetrical response may result from birth injuries such as brachial plexus palsy or a fractured clavicle.

Startle reflex. In response to a loud noise or sudden motion, the newborn abducts its arms with flexion of the elbows; the hands remain clenched. The startle reflex diminishes by four months. Complete and consistent absence of response to loud noises may indicate deafness. An infant's response may be absent or diminished during deep sleep.

Rooting reflex. Stroking the infant's cheek will cause him to turn his head in the direction of the stroke. The rooting reflex disappears within six to seven months. No response may occur in premature infants or those with neurological involvement.

Stepping reflex. Holding the infant upright with the feet touching a flat surface results in dancing or stepping movements. This reflex is most prominent immediately after birth and lasts approximately 4–5 months.

Palmar reflex. The infant will grasp any object when the palms of the hands are touched. While this reflex decreases by three to four months, it is replaced by a voluntary movement by 8 months of age. Asymmetry of response indicates neurological damage.

Tonic neck reflex (fencing position). While supine, the infant will extend the arm and leg of the side to which he is facing while the opposite extremities are flexed. This reflex remains until three to four months; if it is absent after one month of age or is persistently asymmetric, a cerebral lesion may be present.

Babinski reflex. Stroking upward on the lateral aspect of the sole and then across the ball of the foot makes the toes hyper extend (fan upward). While a positive Babinski is an abnormal finding in an adult, it is normal in a child up to one year of age. The lack of a Babinski reflex in a full-term infant indicates a spinal cord defect.

Trunk incurvation. Stroking alongside the infant's spine while in a prone position causes the trunk to turn toward the stimulated side. If not initially seen in the first few days, it should appear by the end of the first week of life and then disappear by four weeks. A lack of response indicates neurological damage.

Observation During Stabilization Period

The first several hours following delivery are characterized by a predictable and identifiable series of behavioral and physiological findings. Infants go through three distinct periods that have been identified as the initial period of reactivity, the period of relative inactivity, and the second period of reactivity. Infant behaviors and responses during these periods can be affected by maternal medications, anesthesia, stress, and labor duration.

The initial period of reactivity last approximately 15–30 minutes following delivery. During this time, neonatal adaptations are regulated mainly by the sympathetic nervous system. Respirations are irregular, peaking at 60–90/minute. There may be transient rales, grunting, nasal flaring, retractions, and periodic breathing, but they should subside quickly. Tachycardia, with a mean peak of 180/minute at three minutes of life, and some lia-

bility of the heart rate are to be expected. Acrocyanosis and brief period of cyanosis are also normal. The infant is subject to heat loss if preventive measures are not taken. The infant is alert, exploratory, and intensely active. This is an excellent time to initiate parental-infant bonding.

The period of relative inactivity lasts from 30 minutes to two hours. The respiratory rate decreases and is characterized by periods of rapid respiration with dyspnea, shallow synchronous breathing, and by barreling of the cheek, which disappears when the infant cries or is handled. The heart rate decreases to approximately 120–140/minute. There is color improvement with flushing upon crying. The body temperature is low. The infant is in a sleepy or drowsy state. Spontaneous jerks and twitches are common. Attempts to initiate feeding during this period may be difficult because the infant is sleepy.

The second period of reactivity lasts approximately two to six hours. During this period, there are exaggerated responses to internal and external stimuli. There are brief periods of rapid respiration, which are related to stimuli and activity. There are also episodes of periodic breathing (irregular respiration with short periods of cessation). The heart rate is labile, with wide swings from bradycardia to tachycardia related to activity and external stimuli. There are abrupt color changes and variable activity levels.

EXAM QUESTIONS

CHAPTER 8
Questions 49–60

49. The cardinal movement of labor which occurs when the fetal chin rests against the chest is called

    a. expulsion.

    b. descent.

    c. internal rotation.

    d. flexion.

50. Which of the following must be completed prior to transferring a newborn from the delivery room to the nursery?

    a. administration of aquamephyton

    b. placement of identification bands

    c. weighing

    d. complete set of vital signs

51. Following rupture of membranes, the nurse's *initial* action should be which of the following?

    a. change the patient's underpad

    b. notify the physician

    c. monitor fetal heart rate

    d. monitor the frequency and duration of contractions

52. One of the most important nursing interventions to assist the neonate in adapting to extrauterine life is to

    a. maintain a stable body temperature for the neonate.

    b. initiate breastfeeding immediately.

    c. perform a heelstick to assess for hypoglycemia.

    d. transfer the baby to the nursery as soon as possible.

53. An Apgar score of five to seven at one minute of life indicates the neonate has

    a. no apparent distress.

    b. good cardiorespiratory rate, vigorous cry, and pink skin color.

    c. mild respiratory, metabolic, or neurologic depression.

    d. severe depression requiring resuscitation.

54. The appropriate rate for positive pressure ventilation is_____times per minute.

    a. 65–75

    b. 40–60

    c. 25–35

    d. 15–25

55. During neonatal resuscitation, chest compressions are to be initiated when the heart rate is below

    a. 120 bpm.

    b. 80 bpm and not increasing.

    c. 80 bpm and increasing.

    d. 100 bpm.

56. Placing an infant on an unpadded scale for weighing can lead to loss of body heat via

    a. evaporation.

    b. conduction.

    c. convection.

    d. radiation.

57. The most common benign transient lesion in the newborn is called

    a. lanugo.

    b. mongolian spot.

    c. milia.

    d. erythema toxicum.

58. A condition in the newborn in which a collection of blood develops between a skull bone and the periosteum without crossing suture lines is called

    a. caput succedaneum.

    b. intraventricular hemorrhage.

    c. bulging fontanelles.

    d. cephalhematoma.

59. A sign of respiratory distress in the newborn is

    a. a heart rate of 120 beats per minute.

    b. grunting.

    c. acrocyanotic skin color.

    d. respirations greater than 30/minute.

60. The initial period of reactivity for the newborn lasts for about

    a. 5–10 minutes.

    b. 1 hour.

    c. 15–30 minutes.

    d. 2 hours.

CHAPTER 9

THE POSTPARTUM PERIOD

CHAPTER OBJECTIVE

After studying this chapter, the reader will be able to identify physiological and psychological changes that normally occur following childbirth and select effective nursing assessment and intervention strategies for postpartum patients.

LEARNING OBJECTIVES

After studying this chapter, the student will be able to

1. Identify normal physiological and psychological changes that occur in women immediately following childbirth.

2. Select critical parameters of physiological and psychological adjustments that should be assessed for all postpartum patients.

3. Recognize common postpartum complications and select effective nursing intervention strategies for each one.

4. Indicate elements of postpartum nursing care.

5. Choose appropriate strategies for helping postpartum patients cope with grief and loss.

INTRODUCTION

This chapter focuses on the postpartum period, which is for the purposes of this chapter defined as the first six weeks after childbirth. First, the physiological and psychological changes the new mother undergoes are described. A section on postpartum complications follows nursing assessment of the postpartum patient is then reviewed. The chapter finishes with a discussion of nursing strategies for care of the postpartum patient. Post-anesthesia care, pain management, intervention in abnormal psychological responses, nutritional concerns, and parent education needs are all addressed. The chapter also includes a brief discussion of strategies for supporting grieving families who have lost their infant or whose infant is born ill.

CHANGES IN THE POSTPARTUM PERIOD

The postpartum period is the time frame from childbirth to stabilization of the mother's body in a nonpregnant state, generally considered to be about six weeks. Some professionals identify the first two hours of this period as the fourth stage of labor. During this period there are rapid changes as the mother's body systems stabilize and attempt to achieve equilibrium after the birth. Later, the postpartum period is a time that requires not only emotional adaptation, but also a time when the female body undergoes amazing changes. The following is a review of those changes.

Breasts. Throughout the pregnancy, the breasts have been preparing to nourish the offspring. Enlarged and with darkened areolae, the breasts begin to secrete colostrum shortly after delivery. This thin yellow fluid is the precursor to breast milk. Emptying the breasts stimulates the production of additional milk through a complex set of neurohormonal events mediated by the hormone prolactin. If the mother is not breastfeeding, failure to empty the breasts will suppress lactation and milk production will cease. (Chapter 10 covers lactation and breastfeeding in greater detail.) Engorgement of the breasts after childbirth is not uncommon, and it usually subsides in one or two days.

Genital and reproductive organs. The reproductive organs never quite return to the size and condition of never-pregnant organs. The uterus, cervix, and vagina, which are no longer as resilient as never-pregnant organs, undergo significant changes after childbirth. Some of these, such as weakening of the supporting structures, can be frustrating or even devastating, especially in the woman who has borne several children. The following is a review of the gynecologic changes that occur postpartum:

Uterus: During the postpartum period, the uterus contracts and shrinks back down into the pelvis in a process known as involution *(see figure 9-1)*. This versatile organ is transformed from a womb weighing about two pounds to a mere 1-1/2- to 2-ounce structure when involution is complete (Reeder & Martin, 1987). The process takes about six weeks. After delivery, the lining of the uterus, or endometrium, is shed in preparation for regeneration and restoration. The area where the placenta was attached takes the longest time to heal. A discharge known as lochia results as this wound on the surface of the inner uterus heals. Initially, the lochia will be red (lochia rubra), then serosanguineous or brown (lochia serosa), and finally pale or brown (lochia alba). A foul odor to lochia is inconsistent with a normal recovery and should be reported to the obstetrician or nurse midwife.

Cervix: The cervix, generally lacerated and traumatized during delivery, seldom regains a nulliparous appearance. Instead, depending on the degree of birth trauma, the os, or opening, remains open a bit.

Vagina: The vagina also seldom returns to its previous condition. Swelling, engorgement, and edema are common in the first few weeks after childbirth. Thereafter, tone begins to return. Dryness may cause discomfort and impede intercourse until ovulation resumes and the resulting hormonal action enhances natural lubrication and elasticity.

Cardiovascular. After rising in anticipation of childbirth, the blood volume begins to drop after delivery, stabilizing between 10 to 14 days later. About 500 ml is normally lost during a routine vaginal delivery and about 1,000 ml during a Cesarean section. The blood volume is also reduced by diuresis following childbirth. The blood pressure generally remains stable during this transition, although there is sometimes a decrease in the heart rate.

Intestinal. Digestion, gastrointestinal motility, and intestinal function usually climb to previous levels of functioning in a matter of days to a week or two. Constipation is a common complaint of the postpartum patient, probably due to perineal pain, decreased activity, lack of oral intake, and narcotics administered during labor. Weight loss after delivery is dramatic initially, then levels off *(see table 9-1)*.

Urinary system. As mentioned above, diuresis follows delivery, yet some new mothers find it difficult to void in the first hours after childbirth. Birth trauma can damage the urethra, the outlet from the bladder to the outside of the body; edema of the vulva and perineum can making voiding painful or difficult. Retention of urine is a common concern, and a distended bladder can interfere with involution of the uterus. After a Cesarean section, many patients will have an indwelling catheter in place. If conservative measures to help the patient void spontaneously fail, catheterization may be indicated.

Abdomen: The abdominal musculature, stretched by the expanding uterus during pregnancy, is flabby and loose in the postpartum period, a fact many women find quite distressing. Exercise and the natural weight loss that follows delivery will help return the abdomen to a pre-pregnant state, although many women never achieve the muscle tone and firmness they had before pregnancy.

Menstrual cycle: Women who elect to breastfeed their infants may find ovulation and menstruation suppressed for the duration of lactation. Women who do not breastfeed will generally begin to menstruate again in about six to ten weeks (Pelletteri, 1995).

POSTPARTUM COMPLICATIONS

The first hours after childbirth are usually consumed with the mother's exploring her newborn and rejoicing with her family in the excitement of the birth. It's also a time for her body to begin its journey back to the nonpregnant

---

TABLE 9-1

Sources and Amount of Weight Loss During the Postpartum Period

Fetus, placenta, amniotic fluid, and blood loss
12–13 lbs./5.5–6.0 kg.

Perspiration, diuresis in first postpartum week
5–8 lbs./2.5–4.0 kg.

Uterine involution and lochia
2–3 lbs./1 kg.

Total weight loss
19–24 lbs./9–10 kg.

Source: *Maternity Nursing,* 16th Ed., Reeder, S. J. & Martin, L. L., 1987, JB Lippincott, Philadelphia, PA.

---

state. This opens the door for a host of potential complications.

Postpartum hemorrhage. Postpartum hemorrhage (PPH) is defined as blood loss greater than 500 ml and classified as *early* if it develops in the first 24 hours after childbirth, and *late* if develops after this time. Causes of PPH include uterine atony (90%), genital tract lacerations (6%), and retained placental fragments (4%) (Rivlin, Morrison, & Bates, 1982). Normally the uterus begins to contract and shrink after childbirth. This is aided by breast-feeding, which causes the uterus to contract, gentle massage of the fundus of the uterus, and in some cases by the administrating of oxytocin, a powerful uterine stimulant that helps the uterus contract. If involution doesn't proceed normally, subinvolution is said to have occurred and hemorrhage may result. Blood loss can be swift and significant, so prevention plays an important role in this serious complication. The mother who doesn't breastfeed is more likely to suffer this complication, as are those women with infections, hormonal imbalances, hypertension, and clotting disorders. Treatment includes massaging the fundus to speed involution and administrating oxytocin. Intravenous fluids to support maternal circulation may be required. In rare cases, surgical intervention and even an emergency hysterectomy may become necessary.

Infection. Maternal infections decreased dramatically when aseptic techniques and strict handwashing protocols were instituted for professionals. Nevertheless, maternal infections continue to be a concern. Again, prevention is the key. Since most women deliver their infants in a hospital, the infection is generally transmitted by their healthcare provider or by instruments used in their care. Staphylococci, streptococci, and coliforms are some of the more common microbes that infect postpartum women. Several areas are especially susceptible to infection in the postpartum period:

Urinary tract infection: Urinary tract infections occur in about 5% of all postpartum patients and in 15% of women who were catheterized before delivery (Reeder & Martin, 1987). Prevention includes strict handwashing and aseptic techniques by the healthcare provider, especially when examining or catheterizing the patient. Evaluating the vital signs for changes such as increased temperature and heart rate will also help detect urinary tract infections. The infection may be confined to the bladder, or it may ascend to the kidneys. Treatment involves antibiotics and fluids.

Endometritis: When the lining of the uterus becomes infected, the patient is suffering from endometritis. Alternatively, the infection may involve other structures in the reproductive system. Symptoms include fever, chills, malaise, abdominal pain, and foul-smelling lochia. Treatment includes fluids, analgesics, and antibiotics.

Wounds: Infection is the primary concern with genital tract lacerations, an episiotomy, or a Cesarean section wound. Keeping the area clean and dry will promote healing. Some physicians and nurse midwives will prescribe ice packs, sitz baths, or heat lamps to promote the healing of an episiotomy. Treatment of a wound infection usually requires antibiotics but may necessitate a return to surgery to drain and repair an abscess if the infection is severe.

Thrombophlebitis. Thrombophlebitis is an inflammation of the inner wall of a vein coupled with clot formation. Sometimes this condition does not become evident until one to two weeks after giving birth. The patient frequently appears quite ill, complaining of fever and malaise. Her leg may appear swollen or discolored. This complication must be reported immediately to the obstetrician or nurse midwife. Treatment of thrombophlebitis usually consists of subcutaneous heparin and rest. Women are at increased risk for thrombophlebites during pregnancy and soon after delivery as the result of hypercoagulability, blood stasis in the lower extremities due to uterine pressure and vessel damage.

Pneumonia. Because the mother is less inclined to cough/deep breathe and ambulate with an abdominal incision, pneumonia is more common after Cesarean delivery. It can usually be prevented by the turn, cough, deep breathe regimen and early ambulation. When pneumonia does develop, treatment is usually with fluids, rest, and antibiotics.

Dehydration. Sweat and blood or fluid loss during labor and delivery can leave the mother dehydrated in the immediate postpartum period. Adequate hydration is essential to a normal postpartum recovery. If the patient has an intravenous catheter in place, it can be used for hydration as ordered by the physician or nurse midwife. If not, and she is stable, fluids may be offered by mouth.

Hematomas. Tissue damage by definition includes disruption of blood vessels. Even after the outermost layers of the wound are repaired and closed, blood may continue to leak beneath the surface, causing a blood-filled enlargement called a hematoma. Hematomas can develop postpartum in the vulva, vagina, and also around a Cesarean section incision or the episiotomy. Hematomas appear as an area of purplish discoloration and obvious swelling which is very tender to the touch. Good surgical technique and hemostasis generally will prevent this complication. If a hematoma does develop, early detection is crucial to successful management. The nurse should be aware that unilateral vulvar edema can signal an ominous but rare and sometimes fatal postpartum complication. Treatment may require a return to surgery to explore the wound and stop any bleeding.

Postpartum depression. The postpartum period is a time of tumultuous hormone changes accompanied by incredible alterations in maternal physiology. The new mother now finds herself responsible for another human being, and her life is never the same as it was before she had a child. It's no wonder, then, that the new mother feels overwhelmed, anxious, tearful, hopeful, depressed, and excited during this turning point in her life. Once again, the nurse is the one who will need to guide the mother through these challenging times. The majority of women will admit to some degree of depression or blue mood after they give birth that lasts a few days to a week or two. Given the physiological changes in the body and the life style changes that accompany the birth of an infant, this is not surprising. Time generally reverses this depression and no intervention is necessary. However, around 1 to 2% of women will experience a serious postpartum depression (Rivlin, Reeder). Rivlin, Morrison and Bates (1982) identified three elements that play a role in

postpartum depression: the physiological changes of pregnancy; an underlying psychiatric disorder; and negative social factors. It is likely that the hormonal changes occurring during pregnancy and the postpartum period have significant influences on mood. Also, bringing a child into the world is quite overwhelming to many women. Regardless of the cause, it is frequently the nurse who will suspect and identify postpartum depression. Signs include crying, irritability, insomnia, and anorexia. The patient often expresses anger, frustration, or feelings of hopelessness and sadness. While the common "baby blues" usually resolves spontaneously, the patient with a severe postpartum depression will generally require psychiatric treatment. Without treatment, some women have been known to harm themselves and their babies, so early identification and intervention may be essential to averting a tragedy.

Failure to bond. Bonding is the process through which the parents and infant become psychologically and emotionally attached to each other. Every woman fantasizes and dreams about her baby as she carries it through pregnancy; then childbirth brings her face to face with the infant. If the baby meets the mother's expectations or fulfills her dreams, she is more likely to bond with the child than if the infant is not what she expected. Bonding with the infant is critical during the first early days after delivery, and the nurse can play a crucial role in seeing that bonding is established during this period. Bonding can be disrupted by many factors; early identification of a troubled relationship can help avert future disasters.

NURSING ASSESSMENT OF THE POSTPARTUM PATIENT

Immediately after the birth of an infant, the mother and her partner or support person are typically consumed with exploring the infant and celebrating the birth. In the healthy postpartum patient without complications, nursing care can be unobtrusive to allow the new mother to bask in the glory of her femininity and the joyous occasion. But this idyllic scene can be splintered in just moments by a postpartum complication. Indeed, the safe birth of the infant does not mean that professional care is no longer indicated; the potential for serious or fatal maternal complications still exists. That is why a conscientious and astute nursing assessment of the postpartum patient is essential to a positive outcome for both mother and child. The following is a presentation of the basic nursing assessment of the normal postpartum patient. This is in addition to the usual nursing assessment performed for every patient. It is not intended to be an exhaustive or complete review, because that is beyond the purpose and scope of this text. Nursing strategies for the care of the postpartum patient are covered after this section.

Nursing assessment of the postpartum patient can be remembered by the using the mnemonic "BUBBLE" for *breasts, uterus, bowels, bladder, lochia, episiotomy, and extremities.* Remember to inform the obstetrician or nurse midwife of any abnormalities you detect or suspect.

Breasts. Nursing assessment of the breasts involves evaluating their color, temperature, and consistency or elasticity. The breasts may be palpated for tenderness and visually inspected for any variations in symmetry or obvious malformations. As mentioned earlier, engorgement and congestion of the breasts is relatively common following childbirth, and the patient with this condition will understand-

ably be reluctant to have the breasts examined. Breastfeeding generally relieves some of the pain, but the woman who elects not to breast-feed may experience some discomfort for one to two days. Documentation should include patient comments or complaints about the breasts and the appearance of the breasts.

Uterus. In the immediate postpartum period, evaluation of the uterus occupies a key role in the nursing assessment, because it is a primary source of postpartum complications such as hemorrhage. Contraction of the uterus is essential to involution and control of hemorrhage. The uppermost part of the uterus is the fundus; it can be palpated after childbirth. Fundal height and uterine tone should be assessed at regular intervals during the first few postpartum days *(see figure 9-1)*. The height of the fundus in relation to the umbilicus is what is usually recorded in the nursing notes. In the first two hours after childbirth, experienced obstetric nurses will check the fundus, massage if necessary, and evaluate the amount and quality of the discharge from the uterus. The consistency of the uterine muscle guides the nurse in performing massage; a boggy uterus indicates massage may be necessary. Documentation should include the patient's comments or complaints, consistency of the uterus, fundal height, and amount/type of discharge.

Bowels. As discussed earlier, gastrointestinal motility is often impaired in the postpartum patient due to a number of factors. Nursing assessment of the gastrointestinal system includes inspection, palpation, and auscultation of the abdomen. The nurse should also elicit information from the patient about the presence or absence of such symptoms as pain, nausea, flatus, or bowel movement.

Bladder. Birth trauma can make voiding difficult, if not impossible, in the immediate postpartum period. Nursing assessment includes inspection and palpation of the abdomen to determine if the bladder is distended, location of the fundus, plus noting patient complaints of discomfort. Examining the color, amount, and clarity of any urine is also essential. Documentation should include recording objective observations and the patient's comments or complaints.

Lochia. Inspection of the lochia, the discharge from the uterus following childbirth, is an integral aspect of the nursing assessment of the postpartum patient. Beginning as a red, bloody flow, the lochia fades to brown and finally to a pale brown as recovery progresses. While the lochia may possess a scent much like menstrual flow, the lochia should never have a foul smell. Documentation should include the amount, color, odor, and consistency of the lochia. The amount of lochia is best assessed and described for the nursing record by noting the color and consistency, and then recording how much of the pad is saturated and how frequently the pads must be changed.

To more accurately estimate blood loss the nurse can use the following methods:

- Calculate the amount of blood that is necessary to saturate the peripads used in the particular institution; given this determination, one can estimate the amount of the peripad saturated.

- Weigh all items saturated with blood and blood clots; generally, 1cc of blood equals 1 gram in weight.

- Draw a hemoglobin and/or hematocrit. The loss of 500cc of blood decreases hemoglobin by 1 to 1.5mg/dl and the hematocrit decreases by 3% to 4% (Luegenbiehl, D., et al., 1990).

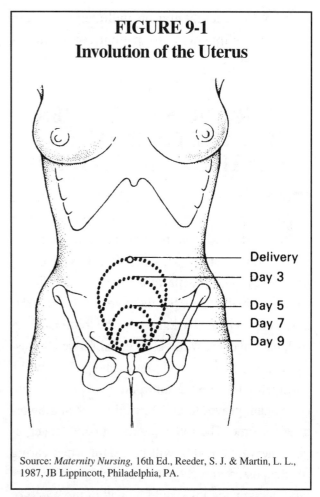

**FIGURE 9-1
Involution of the Uterus**

Delivery
Day 3
Day 5
Day 7
Day 9

Source: *Maternity Nursing,* 16th Ed., Reeder, S. J. & Martin, L. L., 1987, JB Lippincott, Philadelphia, PA.

Episiotomy. Inspection and assessment of the perineum and episiotomy (if present) will require protecting the patient's privacy and providing adequate lighting. Some swelling and edema of the vulva and perineum are common in the first days after childbirth. Any undue swelling, discoloration, separation, or discharge other than lochia should be noted, along with patient complaints of pain or discomfort. Documentation should include the condition of the perineal area and any patient complaints or comments.

Extremities. Assessment includes inspection of the legs and soliciting patient complaints of pain or discomfort in the calf area. With the patient supine, her leg is held straight and her foot flexed back *(see figure 9-2)*. If this maneuver produces pain in the calf, thrombophlebitis should be suspected. The extremities should not be massaged if thrombophlebitis is suspected. Documentation includes recording your findings and any patient comments or complaints.

NURSING STRATEGIES FOR THE CARE OF THE POSTPARTUM PATIENT

The overall nursing goal in caring for the postpartum patient is to ensure that mother and child have the best possible outcome; nursing interventions are directed at this goal *(see table 9-2)*. The postpartum period ordinarily is calm and predictable, but the potential for disaster always lurks in the background. Childbirth is a normal, natural event with the potential for deadly disaster, so the nurse must be ever-vigilant when caring for the postpartum patient. Nursing care once again proves to be a critical factor in a favorable outcome. The following are nursing strategies and interventions that will be useful when caring for the postpartum patient. In clinical practice, specific nursing actions should be within the scope of the institution's practice guidelines and the state Nurse Practice Act, commensurate with the nurses skills and training, and appropriate to the clinical situation at hand.

The Postpartum Period

Maternity patients require the most intensive nursing care in the first hours after delivery; this need gradually diminishes as the mother recovers and begins to resume self-care. Some women leave the hospital or birthing center in a matter of hours, others will stay for days, especially if they have had a Cesarean section. Nursing strategies for this patient not only include all those actions appropriate for any hospitalized patient but also the special care necessary when there is another person, namely the infant, involved.

- Since time is generally a critical factor in the outcome, notify the obstetrician or nurse-mid-wife immediately when any serious postpartum complications occur. When in doubt, let them decide whether the patient is experiencing a complication that requires intervention.

- Explain to the patient what is being done and why. Remember that what is a common, everyday activity to the nurse is not common or everyday to a new mother. Explanations should help reduce the mother's anxiety and enhance her recovery.

- Recover the woman who has had a Cesarean section as any patient who has had major surgery: Monitor vital signs every 15 minutes $\times$ 4; then every 30 minutes $\times$ 2; then every 4 hours $\times$ 24 hours. Never leave the patient unattended and have suction and oxygen available at the bedside. Maintain a patent IV and be aware of any changes in the patient's condition that might indicate an impending complication. Prompt intervention in any complication will help enhance the probability of a good outcome.

- Monitor the patient who had a normal spontaneous vaginal delivery (without general or regional anesthesia) as indicated by her condition, or at least every 15 minutes for the first 2 hours post-op or until her vital signs are stable. Careful monitoring will help detect trends or changes in the vital signs that may indicate a complication is on the horizon.

- Prepare for the onset of shock and cardiovascular collapse in any postpartum patient who complains of severe abdominal pain and who has excessive vaginal bleeding, tachycardia, or whose blood pressure dropped. A serious PPH may have developed. Medical management of this patient may consist of fluid and oxytocin administration, blood transfusion, and oxygen administration. Emergency surgical intervention, including uterine curettage or hysterectomy, may be necessary.

- Don't let the postpartum patient experiencing a serious complication (such as PPH) eat or drink until she has been evaluated by the doctor or nurse midwife. Should general anesthesia become necessary, anything in her stomach could be aspirated into the lungs, where it would cause a potentially fatal pneumonia.

- Investigate all complaints of a change in the patient's comfort level, since these changes may indicate a postpartum complication.

- Administer analgesics as ordered to the postpartum patient, because pain from the episiotomy or contractions of the uterus may make her uncomfortable. Uncontrolled pain can lead to a sympathetic response, with elevations in blood pressure and heart rate. Sometimes a change in position, extra pillows, and warm blankets are all that is necessary to promote comfort. Remember that medications administered to the mother should be expected to cross to the infant in the breast milk unless proven otherwise; advise the obstetrician or nurse midwife that the patient is breastfeeding.

- Monitor closely any intravenous infusion that contains oxytocin, because rapid administration of this agent can cause uterine rupture from tonic contractions.

- Know the location of the emergency drug cart, cardiac defibrillator, resuscitation equipment, and fire extinguisher before accepting a patient care assignment on the maternity ward. Know the unit's procedure for summoning a resuscitation team. Memorize emergency numbers such as those used to call the resuscitation team and the anesthesia team so they won't have to be searched for in the event of an emergency.

- Check the odor, amount, and consistency of the lochia; document findings. Atypical changes in the lochia may herald the onset of a postpartum complication. Implement a peripad count when the amount of lochia appears increased.

TABLE 9-2
Goals of Postpartum Nursing Care

- Promote normal involution

- Prevent or minimize complications

- Promote comfort and healing

- Assist in restoration of normal body functions

- Increase client understanding of physiological and emotional changes

- Support self-care

- Promote family adaptation and integration of the infant

- Support parenting abilities and parent-infant relationships

Source: *Maternity Nursing,* 16th Ed., Reeder, S. J. & Martin, L. L., 1987, JB. Lippincott Philadelphia, PA.

- Respect the patient's dignity by providing privacy when examining her, and note that adequate light and exposure are essential to an accurate assessment of the external genitalia.

- Teach the new mother proper perineal hygiene and follow the doctor or nurse midwife's instructions for care of the episiotomy. This will promote healing and reduce the incidence of infection.

- Use the postpartum period to remind the new mother of the importance of performing a monthly self-breast exam (SBE) and of talking with her doctor or nurse practitioner about regular mammograms. One in nine women will develop breast cancer, and this is an excellent opportunity for the nurse to teach the patient about SBE and cancer detection.

- Teach the new mother how to care for her breasts, since prevention of mastitis is easy but treatment can be difficult.

- Remind the new mother that she should use perineal pads rather than tampons until advised

FIGURE 9-2

Method to Identify Presence of Thrombosis in the Calf (Homan's Sign)

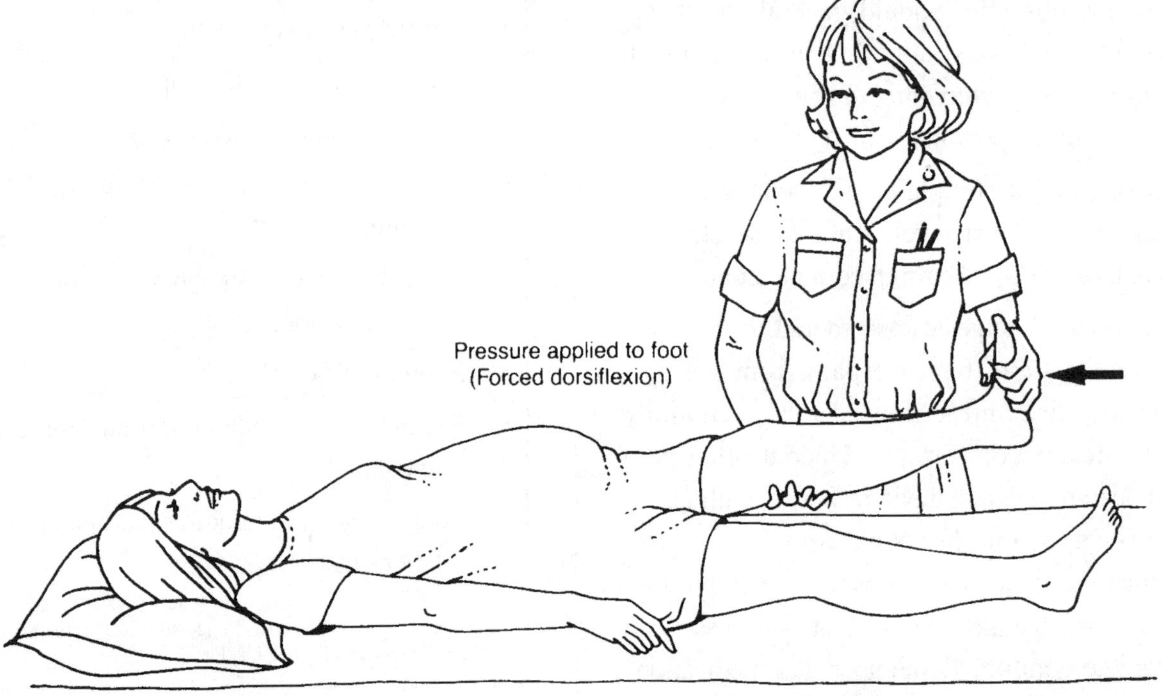

Pressure applied to foot
(Forced dorsiflexion)

Pain experienced behind calf
or in calf when thrombosis is present

Source: *Maternity Nursing,* 16the Ed., Reeder, S. J. & Martin, L. L., 1987, JB Lippincott, Philadelphia, PA.

otherwise by her doctor or nurse practitioner, because tampons have the potential to introduce or hold organisms in the genital tract.

- Check with the obstetrician or nurse midwife about application of ice or heat packs and a breast binder for the woman who complains of breast engorgement and who is not breastfeeding. Such measures may enhance her comfort.

- Ask the patient who appears to be suffering from postpartum depression if she can describe more about how she is feeling. In most cases of the "baby blues," simply allowing a woman to express her concerns and then showing support and empathy will provide significant relief. In other cases, it will offer additional information that can be used to determine if further intervention is necessary.

- Explain to the family of the patient with postpartum depression that their support and under-

standing can be instrumental in the patient's recovery.

- Explain to the new mother that she must call for assistance when getting out of bed or showering for the first time after delivery. She may experience some transient postural hypotension and the nurse's or attendant's presence will help prevent a fall with subsequent injury.

- Instruct the new mother in the importance of and rationale for frequent turning, coughing, and early ambulation to reduce the incidence of pneumonia and thrombophlebitis. Demonstrate effective coughing technique by holding a pillow across the abdomen (to minimize pain), leaning over it, and coughing. Have the patient demonstrate back the technique to validate her learning.

- Follow the physician's instructions when carrying for the patient with a surgical wound from

Cesarean section, since this will help prevent infection and promote healing.

- Whether or not the new mother elects to breastfeed, good nutrition forms the foundation of her body's recovery from childbearing. Since many physicians will not cover this topic or will only give nutrition a cursory review, it is up to the nurse to teach the patient about the role of nutrition in a lifetime of good health, not just during the postpartum period. This is also an excellent opportunity for the nurse to discuss the role of nutrition in the baby's life. Teach the new mother about the importance of a healthy diet as her body recovers from giving birth. Women who are breastfeeding must be especially conscientious about their dietary intake. Encourage the ingestion of fresh fruits and vegetables, and the reduction of salty or fatty foods from the diet. Ask the hospital's or local health clinic's dietician to give detailed guidance to the patient who has unusual nutritional needs or unique dietary preferences.

- Advise the new mother to check with her doctor or nurse midwife about a return to exercise and work. Many professionals advise an "as tolerated" plan that lets the mother set her own pace for returning to work and activity. In any case, it is essential that the new mother not wear herself out while her body attempts to recover from giving birth. Ask her to request and expect help from other family members and omit tasks that will not have serious, deleterious consequences should they remain undone.

- Teach the new mother about the value of exercise in promoting health, aiding in weight loss after pregnancy, creating energy, and warding off the "baby blues." Tell her to check with her doctor or nurse midwife before beginning any exercise program.

Breastfeeding

Women who elect to breastfeed may require extra attention and care from the nurse if they are new to the task. This may be a drain on the nurse's time, but the payoff is enormous and tremendously rewarding for all involved.

- Don't give a bottle to the baby of the mother who wishes to breastfeed without first offering her the opportunity to put the infant to the breast. Supplementing with a bottle can reduce the mother's chances of success with breastfeeding.

- Remind the new mother to wash her hands before nursing. It is not necessary to wash the breasts before each feeding since this practice may lead to drying of the nipples and cracking. Prevention of dry and cracked nipples is paramount in avoiding infection and development of mastitis.

- Offer encouragement to the breastfeeding mother because she may get discouraged easily, especially if this is the first infant she has nursed.

- Refer the patient to a breastfeeding support group (i.e., La Leche League) that promotes breastfeeding. Ideally, the decision to breastfeed is made during the pregnancy, and she can use that time to learn more about breastfeeding.

- Note that the mother who keeps her baby with her in her hospital room may have more success with breastfeeding, since she will become immediately aware of the infant's hunger and won't have to rely on someone to bring the infant to her.

Bonding

After birth, the mother must begin to explore her infant and make him or her a part of her life. Above all, the nurse must be sensitive to each woman's individual reactions and not impose feelings or standards on the patient.

- Check the institution's policy on the instillation of eye drops after birth. These drops, required by many states to prevent sexually transmitted diseases from afflicting the eyes of the newborn, can obscure the infant's vision. Some professionals believe that the drops should be avoided during the first critical minutes of bonding, when an infant and his or her parents lock eyes for the first time.

- Provide privacy and unobtrusive nursing care for the parents in the first few hours after delivery, when attachments to the infant may begin to form.

- Review *Table 9-3: Potential Adaptive and Maladaptive Mothering Behaviors* (Johnson, High Risk Parenting) to determine if the patient's mothering responses can be classified as adaptive or maladaptive. If a high-risk parenting situation is identified, ask the obstetrician or nurse midwife to make a referral to a social worker for evaluation.

Caring for the Woman Whose Baby is Extremely Ill or Dead

Infant death or illness. Every couple hopes to have a perfect, happy, healthy baby. Yet life is not perfect and sometimes a tragedy strikes. The baby may be premature, ill, malformed, or dead. In some cases, the parents have been made aware of this possibility during the pregnancy. In others, the painful twist of events comes as a stunning blow after the birth of the child. The causes of the pathology may be unknown or known, as in maternal alcohol abuse. This situation will turn the parents' world upside down, and leave them bewildered, hurt, and confused. A discussion of nursing intervention techniques in this situation would fill a whole textbook and is not possible here. Suffice it to say that this family will require professional assistance from a team of nurses, doctors, social workers, and others to develop coping skills and return them to their highest possible level of functioning after this tragedy.

- Offer the patient an opportunity to see or hold an infant who died before or during delivery, since this may help facilitate her grief process. Dress the baby in a shirt and diaper and swathe it in a soft blanket; allow the mother to expose the child's body gradually to her own level of comfort. Because some tranquilizers given to the mother during delivery can cause amnesia, it may be appropriate to photograph the baby in the event the mother wants to see it later or cannot recall having seen it earlier. This nursing strategy is also appropriate in the case of the birth of a severely malformed infant. If the fetal head is malformed, put a cap on the baby in addition to the shirt and diaper. A cap can be styled from a short length of stockinette (like that used for orthopedic casts) fastened at one end with a rubber band.

- Ask the doctor or nurse midwife to consider moving the mother who lost her child to a nonpostpartum floor. Many professionals feel being around women with healthy babies makes recovery more difficult and painful. Referral to a social worker or chaplain may be helpful. Many communities have a perinatal loss support group.

Discharge Planning

Leaving the hospital with a newborn baby in her arms is an exciting moment for the mother. But before she leaves, the nurse should be certain the patient possesses the skills necessary to care for the infant at home.

- Make transportation safety a part of discharge teaching. Teach the parents that an infant held in a passenger's lap is not safe in a collision, and in many states it is a violation of the law.

TABLE 9-3 *(1 of 3)*
Potential Adaptive and Maladaptive Mothering Behaviors

Time/Situation	Adaptive	Maladaptive
Delivery	Attempts to position head to see infant as soon as delivered and while infant is on warming table.	Does not position head to see baby. Stares at ceiling.
	When shown infant: Smiles. Keeps eyes on infant, looking at all parts exposed. Attempts en face position. Uses fingertip touch on face and extremities. Asks to hold baby. Partially opens blanket to see more of infant. Talks to baby. Asks questions about baby.	When shown infant: Frowns. Stares at baby without expression. Does not assume en face position. Turns head away. Does not touch baby. Does not ask to hold baby. Declines offer to hold. If infant placed in her arm, lies still, and does not touch or stroke face or extremities. May not look at infant. Does not talk to baby. Asks few or no questions.
	Makes positive statements about baby: "She is so cute." "He is so soft!"	Makes no comments or makes only negative statements: "She looks awful." "He's ugly."
	May cry out of joy or relief that infant is normal or of desired sex.	May cry, appearing unhappy or depressed.
	May smile and cry at the same time. To differentiate from crying out of dissapointment, must note facial expressions and verbal statements.	When asked why she is crying, states being disappointed in baby.
	Expresses satisfaction with or acceptance of sex of infant. "We really wanted a girl, but it is more important that he is healthy." "I can't believe, a boy at last!"	Expresses dissatisfaction with sex of baby. "Not another girl. I should have known better than to have tried again for a boy." "I don't even want to see him." May use profanity when told sex.
	Predominant affect—appears pleased and happy.	Predominant affect—appears sad, angry, or expressionless.
	Suddenly decides she wants to breast feed.	Suddenly decides against breast feeding.
First Week	Initially uses fingertips on head and extremities. Progresses to using fingers and palm on infant's trunk. Eventually draws infant toward her, holding infant against her body.	Uses fingertip touch, without progressing to using palm on trunk or drawing infant toward her body.
	Snuggles infant to neck and face.	Does not hold infant to neck or face.
	Makes spontaneous movements, kissing, stroking, rocking.	Makes few or no spontaneous movements with infant.
	Attempts to establish eye contact by moving infant, assuming en face position, or shielding infant's eyes from light.	Does not use en face position or attempt to establish eye-to-eye contact.
	Handles and holds baby at times other than when giving direct care.	Handles only as necessary to feed or change diapers.
	Talks to infant.	Does not talk to infant.
	Smiles at baby frequently—changes affect appropriately, such as when infant cries.	Rarely smiles at baby. *or* Smiles all the time without change in affect.
	Makes many specific observations of infant: "Her eyes look like they might turn brown." "One foot turns in just a bit."	Makes no observations. Makes few observations which are either general or negative.

TABLE 9-3 *(2 of 3)*
Potential Adaptive and Maladaptive Mothering Behaviors

Time/Situation	Adaptive	Maladaptive
First Week (cont)	Discusses infant's characteristics attempting to relate them to others in the family: "He has my ears, but his daddy's chin." "She really doesn't look like either of our baby pictures, she just looks like herself."	Does not discuss infant's characteristics in relation to characteristics of family members.
	With a positive affect and affectionate manner, uses animal characteristics to describe baby: "She is just like a cuddly little kitten." "His hair feels like down."	In a negative or hostile manner, uses animal characteristics to describe baby: "She looks awful, just like a drowned rat." "He looks just like an ape to me."
	Asks questions about caring for infant after discharge.	Asks no questions about care.
	By the time infant is discharged, has obtained basic supplies for caring for infant.	Has made no plans for obtaining basic supplies.
First Few Weeks	*If infant remains hospitalized after mother is discharged*	
	Calls every 1–2 days.	Calls less frequently than every other day, or not at all.
	Visits minimum of twice a week.	Visits less frequently than twice a week, or not at all.
	Visits minimum of 30 minutes.	Visits fewer than 30 minutes.
	Asks specific questions about infant's condition.	Asks few specific questions. Asks very few questions. Asks inappropriate questions.
	Spends most of visit looking at and handling infant.	Spends most of visit observing unit activities and other infants (this may be normal behavior first 1 or 2 visits). Has little or no interaction with infant during visits.
	Becomes involved with care when encouraged and supported by staff.	When encouraged by staff to participate in care, refuses, terminates visit, or does only minimal care.
	Although visits are frequent and last longer than 30 minutes, makes statements about missing infant, e.g., expresses that she misses baby at home or that she wishes she could visit more often and stay longer.	Makes no statements about missing infant. *or* States she misses baby at home and wishes she could visit more often, but comments are not validated by frequent or lengthy visits.
	Expresses reluctance to terminate visit.	Leaves nursery with little hesitation.
	Waits until infant is asleep before leaving. Touches or talks to baby just before leaving. May stand outside window and look at baby before leaving unit.	Frequently asks nurse to complete feeding, or to change and settle infant.
First Months	Holds infant close to her body.	Does not hold infant securely against body.
	Supports infant's trunk and head in position of comfort.	Head and body of infant are not well supported.
	Muscles in arms and hands are relaxed and conform to curvature of infant's body.	Shoulder, arm, and hand muscles appear tense. Hands and fingers to not conform to infant's body.
	During feedings, holds infant in well-supported position against her body.	Holds infant away from body during feedings, or props infant or bottle.
	Positions during feedings so eye-to-eye contact can occur.	Position during feeding prevents eye-to-eye contact.

TABLE 9-3 *(3 of 3)*
Potential Adaptive and Maladaptive Mothering Behaviors

Time/ Situation	Adaptive	Maladaptive
First Months (cont)	Minimizes talking to infant while he is sucking.	Continues talking to infant during feeding, even though infant is distracted and stops sucking.
	Refers to infant using given or affectionate name.	Refers to infant in impersonal way, e.g., "the baby," "she," or "it."
	Plays with infant at times unrelated to direct care.	Handles infant mainly during caretaking activities.
	When infant is in infaseat, playpen, etc. frequently interacts with him.	Leaves infant for long periods in infaseat, playpen, or crib interacting only after baby becomes fussy.
	Places infant, when awake, in an area where he can observe and interact with others.	Leaves infant, when awake, alone for long periods of time in bedroom or isolated area.
	Occasionally leaves infant with someone else.	Frequently leaves baby with someone else. *or* Refuses to leave baby with someone else.
	Uses discretion in selecting babysitter and provides her with instructions on baby's routines, likes, and dislikes.	Does not use good judgment in selecting babysitter. Provides inadequate or no instructions for care.
	Provides infant with routine well-baby care.	Fails to provide infant with well-baby care, seeking medical assistance only after problems arise. *or* Keeps all appointments, and makes additional phone calls or additional visits to physician or emergency room for imagined or insignificant problems.
	Carries out medical plan for management of specific problems or conditions, e.g., thrush, anemia, or an ear infection.	Fails to or is inconsistent in carrying out medical plan for specific problems.
	Remains close to infant during physical exams, and attempts to soothe baby if he becomes distressed.	Remains seated at a distance from the exam table. Does not soothe infant during exam. Frequently arranges for someone else to take infant for medical appointments.
	Makes positive statements about mothering role.	Makes negative statements about mothering role.

Source: *High-Risk Parenting: Nursing Assessment and Strategies for the Family at Risk,* Hall Johnson, S., 1979.

Most states now dictate that an infant cannot leave the hospital unless secured in an appropriate infant car seat. Statistics prove such seats prevent infant injuries. A number of social service agencies will provide or help procure a seat for families who cannot afford one.

- Ensure that the new mother knows whom to call if she feels she is experiencing complications and knows how to take any medications she is taking home from the hospital. This information can help avert complications.

- Be aware of and advise the new mother of parenting classes offered in the community. Many hospitals, social organizations, and churches offer parenting classes at little or no cost. These can help her gain valuable parenting skills.

EXAM QUESTIONS

CHAPTER 9
Questions 61–75

61. The postpartum period generally is considered to end how long after delivery of the infant?

    a. 2 hours.

    b. 2 weeks.

    c. 6 weeks.

    d. 6 months.

62. Which of the following findings during the *immediate* postpartum period should be reported to the physician?

    a. Foul smelling lochia.

    b. Decreased heart rate.

    c. Constipation.

    d. Uterine cramping.

63. The discharge after childbirth is initially termed lochia rubra, which then becomes

    a. Lochia uterine.

    b. Lochia alba.

    c. Lochia sanguina.

    d. Lochia serosa.

64. After childbirth, the vaginal dryness that may cause discomfort and impede intercourse is generally due to

    a. poor maternal hygiene.

    b. insufficient uterine healing.

    c. lack of ovulation.

    d. postpartum depression.

65. About how much blood is generally lost during a routine vaginal delivery?

    a. 500 ml

    b. 1000 ml

    c. 200 ml

    d. 50 ml

66. When involution is complete, the uterus will weigh about

    a. 5 lbs.

    b. 2 oz.

    c. 12 oz.

    d. 1 lb.

67. Serosanguineous or brown discharge postpartum is called

    a. lochia rubra.

    b. lochia alba.

    c. lochia serosa.

    d. lochia candida.

68. About how much blood loss would the nurse expect in a patient undergoing a Cesarean section?

    a. 500 ml

    b. 2500 ml

    c. 250 ml

    d. 1000 ml

69. While examining a postpartum patient who delivered 12 hours ago, the nurse notices the patient's lochia is very heavy. What should be the nurse's *initial* action?

    a. Notify the physician.

    b. Check her vital signs.

    c. Ask how large the infant was.

    d. Palpate the fundus.

70. The average weight loss in the postpartum period is

    a. 4–10 lbs.

    b. 10–17 lbs.

    c. 19–24 lbs.

    d. 25–29 lbs.

71. In the woman who does not breastfeed, the menstrual cycle usually resumes in about

    a. 1–2 weeks.

    b. 2–4 weeks.

    c. 3–5 weeks.

    d. 6–10 weeks.

72. The primary cause of postpartum hemorrhage is

    a. retained placental fragments.

    b. uterine atony.

    c. genital tract lacerations.

    d. perineal hematomas.

73. Mastitis is most commonly caused by which of the following organisms?

    a. *E. Coli.*

    b. *Haemophilus.*

    c. Staphylococci.

    d. *Candida.*

74. A nursing action when caring for the postpartum patient who complains of pain in the leg is to

    a. massage the leg.

    b. call the physician immediately.

    c. ask her family to perform range of motion exercises.

    d. assess the leg for swelling or discoloration.

75. A positive Homan's sign may indicate

    a. endometritis.

    b. thrombophlebitis.

    c. mastitis.

    d. cervicitis.

CHAPTER 10

LACTATION

CHAPTER OBJECTIVE

After studying this chapter, the reader will be able to recognize the physiology of lactation, identify advantages and disadvantages of breastfeeding, and choose effective problem-solving techniques that benefit breastfeeding women.

LEARNING OBJECTIVES

After studying this chapter, the student will be able to

1. Identify the anatomic and physiological changes that occur during postpartum which are necessary for initiation and maintenance of lactation.

2. Select appropriate positioning and latch-on techniques that contribute to successful breastfeeding.

3. Choose nursing strategies for managing specific breastfeeding challenges.

4. Recognize the role of lactation educators and consultants in supporting breastfeeding families.

INTRODUCTION

This chapter focuses on lactation and breastfeeding of the newborn. Breast milk is the natural nourishment for newborns. Because nurses are often responsible for patient and parent education, all nurses should have an understanding of the value of breastfeeding and techniques for successful breastfeeding. Topics covered include the anatomy of the female breast and the physiology of lactation; the advantages and disadvantages of breastfeeding versus bottlefeeding; breastfeeding techniques; and problem solving with breastfeeding mothers. The chapter closes with a review of the resources available to breastfeeding mothers.

ANATOMY OF THE FEMALE BREAST AND PHYSIOLOGY OF LACTATION

Essential to providing nursing care to the pregnant patient is an understanding of the anatomy of the female breast and the physiology of lactation, both of which are reviewed below.

Anatomy of the Female Breast

The female breasts are secondary sex characteristics that develop during puberty and provide nourishment for the newborn should pregnancy occur. Also referred to as mammary glands, the breasts are composed of glandular tissue and fat cells (see figure 10-1). Connective tissue encloses each breast, which is covered with fatty tissue that gives the breast its size and shape.

Basic Components of the Breast

Lactiferous ducts: Each breast has about 20 lobes; each lobe contains a single lactiferous duct system. Breast milk is produced in the alveoli and then stored in widened areas of the lactiferous ducts until being released by the infant's suckling or by manual expression.

Nipple: The projectile tissue located at the tip of the breast. Each lactiferous duct ends at the nipple, where milk is expressed.

Areola: The dark area around the nipple. The areola typically darkens and enlarges during pregnancy.

Lactation

Lactation refers to the secretion of milk from the breasts. Lactation occurs as a result of a complex set of neurohormonal events orchestrated by the pituitary gland but also involving the hypothalamus, adrenal glands, and thyroid gland. The lactogenic hormone prolactin from the pituitary is a primary factor in the anatomical and physiological changes that occur with lactation, although a number of other hormones are also involved.

During pregnancy, prolactin stimulates the breasts to develop in preparation for lactation, but estrogen and progesterone suppress milk secretion. After delivery of the placenta, blood levels of estrogen and progesterone drop, leaving prolactin's effect dominant, and lactation occurs (Reeder & Martin, 1987). Continued lactation depends on continued stimulation. The breasts must be emptied to generate additional milk production. If the breasts are not emptied, milk production ceases within a few days. Breastfeeding mothers are often quite sensitive to their infant's needs and may find that milk secretion or the "let-down reflex" is stimulated by the sound of their infant's crying.

Secretions Produced Through the Physiology of Lactation

Colostrum: This antibody-rich yellow fluid is the initial secretion from the breasts postpartum. It may start to leak from the breasts during the latter stages of pregnancy. Colostrum serves to nourish the newborn and offers the baby valuable protection against infection.

Breast milk: On about the third postpartum day, the white breast milk appears. Once breastfeeding is established, the mother will produce about 200 ml to 300 ml of breast milk per day by the end of the first week, increasing up to as much as 900 ml a day as the infant grows

FIGURE 10-1

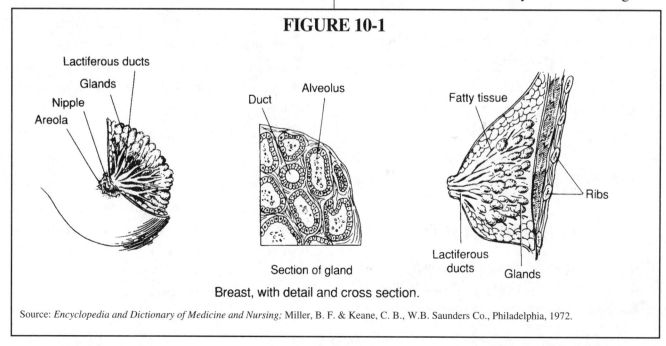

Breast, with detail and cross section.

Source: *Encyclopedia and Dictionary of Medicine and Nursing;* Miller, B. F. & Keane, C. B., W.B. Saunders Co., Philadelphia, 1972.

(Reeder & Martin, 1987). Breast milk is nature's most perfect food for infants. While artificial formulas can closely duplicate the nutritional content of breast milk, they do not contain the mother's antibodies, which can enhance and protect the infant's health.

Suppression of Lactation

Because emptying the breasts stimulates further milk production, lactation will be suppressed when the breasts are not emptied by suckling or manual expression. If the new mother elects not to breastfeed, or there has been a tragedy such as a stillbirth, lactation suppression can be accomplished by avoiding stimulation or suckling. The use of hormonal preparations are no longer recommended due to the possibility of adverse effects. Others recommend a tight bra or breast binder to suppress lactation. In any case, if the breasts are not emptied, milk production will cease.

Uterine Effects

The infant's suckling stimulates the release of oxytocin, a pituitary hormone that causes the uterus to contract. This helps reduce blood loss immediately postpartum and promotes involution. Many women note some cramping sensations when breastfeeding. Breastfeeding frequently suppresses ovulation and the return of menstruation, although it should not be considered a reliable method of birth control.

ADVANTAGES & DISADVANTAGES OF BREASTFEEDING VERSUS BOTTLEFEEDING

In Rudolph (1977), T. E. Cone discusses the first reports of artificial feedings of infants that were described in 1472, and the subsequent infant mortality, which was reported as high as 90%. Between 1890 and 1908, the process of pasteurization was developed and helped ensure that the milk supply was sanitary, thereby enhancing the survival of artificially fed infants.

Clearly, breast milk is nature's food for infants. Cow's milk is nature's food for calves. It seems logical that infants should be raised on breast milk rather than cow's milk, and most authorities agree. Unfortunately, the issue is not that simple. Currently in America, life styles and personal preferences generally are the most influential factors in the decision to breastfeed or bottlefeed infants. The advantages and disadvantages of each are briefly reviewed below.

Breastfeeding

As described previously, breast milk is a logical choice for infants, although it is not always the first choice of the mother because of the perceived disadvantages associated with it.

Advantages: Colostrum and breast milk contain anti-infective factors and antibodies, complement, lysozymes, lactoferrin, and interferon. Breast milk is also economical and readily available. Breastfeeding offers the mother an opportunity to touch and bond with her infant. Also, uterine contractions stimulated by breastfeeding hasten involution. Breastfeeding also helps promote development of the baby's facial muscles, teeth and jaw. Further, it reduces the incidence of allergies in the baby and decreases the incidence of maternal breast cancer.

Disadvantages: Because breastfeeding can be done only by the mother, it will be her responsibility to awaken in the night to feed the baby. She will also have to be available to nurse the infant at feeding times or express milk to be bottlefed later. Some infants, however, may be fussy when offered breast milk via an artificial nipple rather than the breast. Sore, cracked nipples can be uncomfortable both during and after breastfeeding. Milk may leak from the breasts in response to an infant's crying or other stimuli. Drugs, alcohol, and foods ingested by the nursing mother will in most cases be passed on to the infant. Because the composition of breast milk will reflect the mother's diet, she must be conscientious about her nutritional intake. Certain maternal illnesses, such as the Human Immunodeficiency Virus (HIV), can be passed to the infant via the breast milk.

Bottlefeeding

Artificial infant formulas, now made to closely mimic human milk, are the choice of many women, and are widely accepted as sufficient for the nutritional needs of infants. Dairy milk, canned milk, and diluted versions of infant formula do not provide adequate nutrition and are not considered acceptable for bottlefeeding.

Advantages: Commercially available infant formulas, correctly prepared in the home, are considered nutritionally adequate by many authorities. These preparations are convenient, easy to prepare, and can be administered by any caregiver, not just the mother. Artificial formulas are readily available, even in the case of illness or absence of the mother.

Disadvantages: The infant loses the opportunity to receive antibodies and anti-infective agents from the mother when infant formula is substituted for breast milk. The opportunity for skin to skin contact can be lost. The mother loses the physiological benefits of lactation, such as contraction of the uterus and suppression of menstruation. Improper preparation, diluting the formula, or substituting cow's milk for formula can lead to malnutrition and disease. Infant formulas must be purchased so they are not as economical as breast milk.

BREASTFEEDING TECHNIQUES

For many women, breastfeeding is a tremendously rewarding yet demanding task. It is easy for the new mother to become discouraged in the first few days postpartum, so every nurse should have an understanding of breastfeeding techniques in order to support a new mother's efforts. The nurse who is not skilled or comfortable with teaching breastfeeding techniques can refer the patient to a lactation consultant or organizations that support and promote breastfeeding, such as La Leche League, or put her in touch with a woman who has successfully breastfed her own infant.

Preparation for breastfeeding should begin during pregnancy with care of the breasts and nipples. The mother should avoid soap that may dry or crack the nipples. Some health care providers may recommend nipple creams or special brassieres to help prepare the breasts. In most instances, the mother is allowed to nurse her infant immediately after birth in the delivery room. Before breastfeeding, the mother should wash her hands thoroughly, since the hands are common sources of contaminants.

TECHNIQUES FOR BREASTFEEDING

Position

Experimenting with the best position will help the nursing mother determine what is most comfortable for her and her baby. The infant should not have to turn or search for the nipple. Mother and baby may sit or lie with their abdomens touching, or the mother may hold the baby like a football, with the feet toward her back, her arm supporting the baby's head and trunk, and the infant supine and facing her *(see figures 10-2, 10-3, and 10-4)*.

Sitting: Assuming a comfortable position in a chair, the mother lays the infant across her lap. She may want to support the baby on a pillow and place her own feet on a footrest so her arms won't fatigue as quickly. With the infant's head cradled in the crook of her elbow, the mother supports the baby's back and bottom with her arm and hand. The infant's abdomen touches the mother's abdomen. The mother's other hand is free to support the breast, guide the infant to the breast, or stroke the infant as he or she nurses.

Lying down: The mother and baby lie face to face, with the infant enfolded in the mother's arm for support. A pillow may be necessary for additional support for either the mother or the baby.

Latching On

Supporting the breast with the hand that is not supporting the infant allows the infant to latch on to the nipple and areola. The infant must grasp more than just the nipple to nurse successfully. The nipple should be brushed against the infant's lips to stimulate the rooting reflex. The infant should then draw the nipple and surrounding areola into his or her mouth and press it against the hard palate in order to suck. Care should be taken during nursing to support the breast so the infant's nostrils are not blocked during suckling. When the breast is withdrawn, the suction created should be gently broken to prevent irritating the nipples. Inserting a finger into the corner of the infant's mouth, between his or her gums, will break this suction.

Feeding Patterns

Every infant is unique and will feed in its own fashion, so it is important for the nurse and mother to be flexible and not rigid in feeding schedules and breastfeeding plans. Most authorities recommend feeding a newborn about every three hours

(or as demanded by the child), with about 10 minutes on each breast. Because the infant will nurse most vigorously from the first breast offered, the opposite breast should be the first breast offered at the next feeding. The infant can be given a chance to burp and remove swallowed air from the stomach when switching between breasts or whenever necessary.

Expressing Milk

When a mother cannot be available to breastfeed her infant, she can express the milk and store it to be bottlefed to the infant later. There are other reasons for expressing milk, such as a mother who is taking medication, ill, or having surgery. The breasts must be emptied to ensure continued milk supply, and in these cases the milk can be discarded and breastfeeding resumed when the mother's condition improves. Breast milk can be expressed by using a breast massaging technique, or a manual or electric breast pump may be used. The milk should be refrigerated or frozen for later use. If frozen, breast milk should not be thawed in a microwave oven, on the stove, or at room temperature, but only under lukewarm water or in the refrigerator. It should not be refrozen.

Weaning

Weaning from the breast begins when the mother is no longer able or willing to breastfeed, or as the infant grows and loses interest in the breast. Many women breastfeed their infants even past the first year, but each mother should check with her baby's healthcare provider about this important decision. In general, weaning should be a gradual rather than an abrupt process, with a bottle or cup substituted at intervals for the breast. A recommended method of weaning is for the woman to eliminate one particular feeding until her milk production adjusts (generally several days). After that she eliminates another feeding until the infant is totally weaned to the bottle or cup.

PROBLEM SOLVING WITH THE BREASTFEEDING MOTHER

Breastfeeding is a joyous and rewarding experience for most women. However, it requires adaptation on the part of the mother and her support system and can initially prove to be frustrating. The role of the nurse and other healthcare providers in supporting the breastfeeding mother is essential to her success with breastfeeding.

Common Challenges Presented by Breastfeeding

Flat or inverted nipples. Mothers with flat or inverted nipples can successfully breastfeed. In most cases, this patient should be identified during pregnancy and steps made to counter the concern. In some cases, the physician or nurse midwife will prescribe nipple stretching exercises or advise the patient to wear a special breast shield (Ross Laboratories, 1987). Use of the nipple shield should be used only as a last resort since the volume of milk produced is less and the infant could prefer having the nipple shield used at each feeding.

Cracked and sore nipples. Breastfeeding can result in sore nipples, but in general the nipples will become less tender as nursing progresses. Keeping the nipples clean and dry will significantly reduce the incidence of cracking. When possible, cracked nipples should be left exposed to air for a brief period each day to allow drying and healing. Breaking suction each time the breast is withdrawn rather than simply pulling the nipple from the infant's mouth will help relieve sore nipples. When nipple conditions interfere with breastfeeding, the mother should contact her healthcare practitioner for guidance.

Fussy babies. Even though it is perfectly natural, breastfeeding takes some getting used to. It is not uncommon for both mother and child to be somewhat irritable in the beginning. In general, a crying baby should be offered the breast and if it is refused, it may simply mean that the infant needs consoling or requires a diaper change. This is generally more of a problem with first-time mothers and during the first few days after childbirth, when the mother is most likely to be tired and feeling overwhelmed.

Sleepy babies. As a general rule, if the infant is sleeping, he or she isn't hungry and shouldn't be awakened for feeding. Unwrapping and stroking or talking before a feeding usually helps arouse the sleepy baby. But as a general rule, a baby who is sleeping soundly is not hungry. The mother can be reassured that the infant will let her know when he or she is hungry.

Breast engorgement. Breast engorgement is common in the first week after childbirth. Engorgement is easier to prevent than treat, and is often headed off by regular emptying of the breasts, massage, and application of intermittent heat or cold. Engorgement that does not subside in one to two days or that is accompanied by fever and excessive pain or discoloration of the breasts should be reported to the patient's healthcare practitioner.

Mastitis. This infection in the mammary gland generally appears 7 days to several weeks/months after delivery. Most commonly due to Staphylococcus aureus, the organism usually enters through a cracked or fissured nipple or is introduced from a nosocomial source. Symptoms of mastitis include chills, rapid rise in temperature, increased pulse and breathing rate, as well as localized tender, hardened breast tissue. Treatment depends upon the causative agent but usually begins with antibiotic therapy. Fluid intake should be increased,

FIGURE 10-2
4 Common Breastfeeding Positions

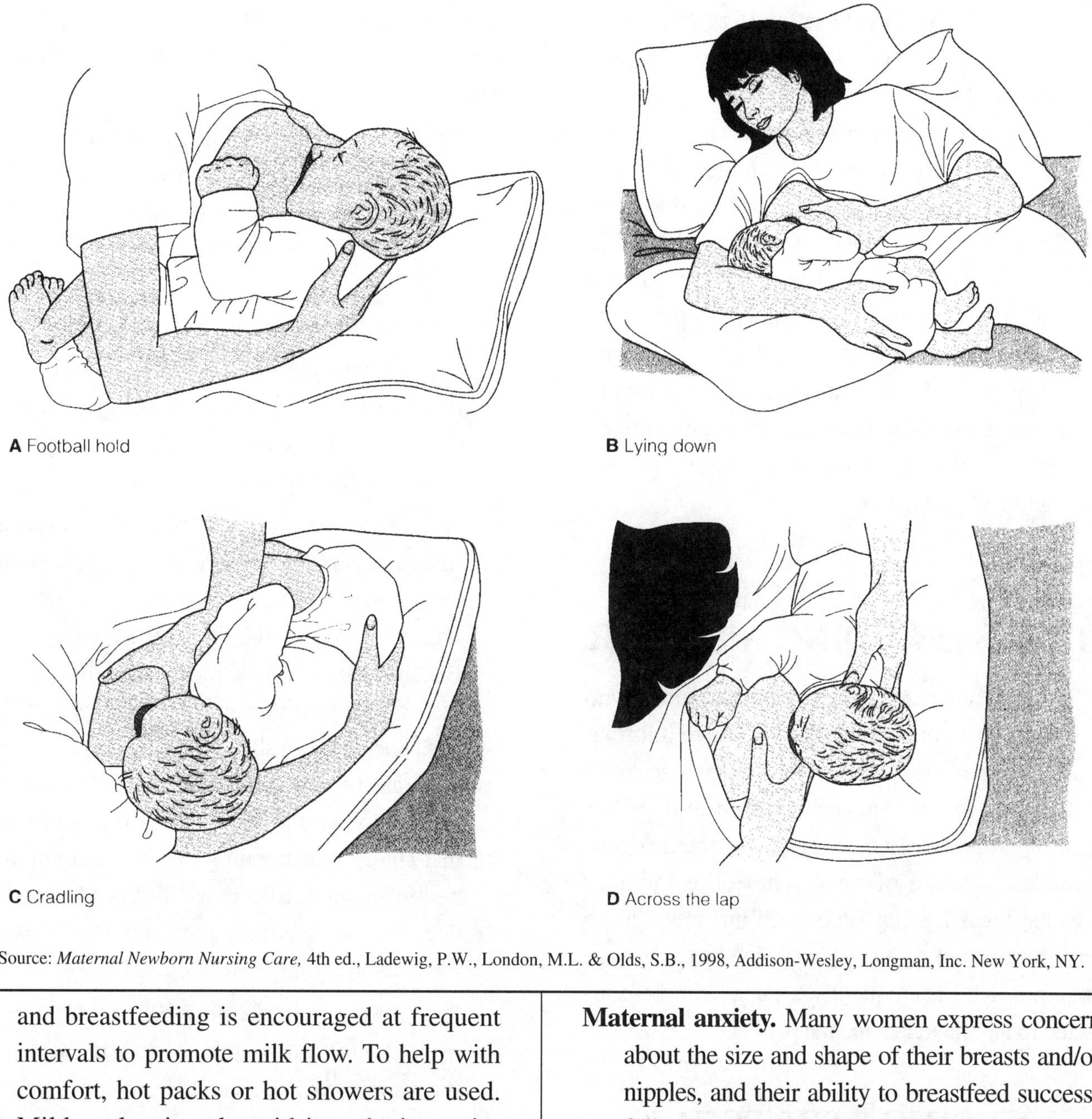

A Football hold

B Lying down

C Cradling

D Across the lap

Source: *Maternal Newborn Nursing Care,* 4th ed., Ladewig, P.W., London, M.L. & Olds, S.B., 1998, Addison-Wesley, Longman, Inc. New York, NY.

and breastfeeding is encouraged at frequent intervals to promote milk flow. To help with comfort, hot packs or hot showers are used. Mild analgesics also aid in reducing pain. Maternity nurses play a key role in preventing mastitis by early assessment of feeding techniques and by providing thorough patient education (especially hand washing prior to feeding) and ongoing support, especially following discharge home.

Maternal anxiety. Many women express concern about the size and shape of their breasts and/or nipples, and their ability to breastfeed successfully. The size of the breasts is irrelevant to successful breastfeeding. Maternal anxiety is best relieved by listening to and addressing the mother's concerns, assisting her when necessary, guiding her in proper techniques, and encouraging her not to give up too quickly.

Insufficient milk supply. Nature generally provides an adequate milk supply for the infant, although some mothers may worry that their supply is inadequate. The baby who nurses regularly, wets diapers, passes stools, and gains weight is probably getting enough milk. The breastfed baby may nurse for 15 to 20 minutes and then sleep for two to three hours. After the first 24 to 48 hours of life, the newborn should have six to eight wet diapers a day. The baby should also have normal skin turgor and moist mucus membranes. To determine adequate fluid intake, the infant can be weighed before and after each feeding. The diapers can also be weighed to calculate approximate output. If the parents are concerned about the baby's having adequate intake of breast milk, they can turn to their pediatrician, pediatric nurse practitioner, and/or lactation consultant for further assessment and evaluation.

RESOURCES FOR THE BREASTFEEDING MOTHER

There are resources available to women who wish to breastfeed but need more information or support. Nurses must lead the cause and discern the patient's concerns, then guide her to the appropriate resource. The nurse should determine in advance of need where the local or regional breastfeeding support groups meet in the area. La Leche League or a certified lactation consultation, who is frequently a nurse, can be contacted to aid the nurse and the patient.

NURSING STRATEGIES FOR THE CARE OF THE LACTATING PATIENT

Lactation is a normal event in which nurses play a critical role. A favorable outcome is, as always, often dependent on quality nursing care and prompt intervention. The following are nursing strategies that may prove useful when caring for a lactating woman. Any nursing actions taken should be within the scope of the institution's practice guidelines and the state Nurse Practice Act, commensurate with the nurse's skills and training, and appropriate to the clinical situation at hand.

- Dispel myths that breastfeeding results in sagging breasts or that women with small breasts will have insufficient milk supply. Addressing the patient's concerns about breastfeeding will help her make an informed decision about breastfeeding her infant.

- Support the patient's decision to breastfeed and help her through what may be difficult early days of breastfeeding by offering encouragement, reassurance, and guidance.

- Assume that a drug will pass into the breast milk unless proven otherwise. This means that, in general, whatever drugs the mother receives, expect the infant to receive also. Because this is often undesirable, the mother may be advised to pump her breasts and discard the milk if she is taking certain drugs such as tranquilizers. Tell the breastfeeding mother to inform her healthcare practitioners that she is breastfeeding before accepting any treatments or medications. Tell her to call her doctor if she has any questions about taking medications while breastfeeding.

- Remind the breastfeeding mother that breast milk should not be reheated or thawed in a microwave oven and should be stored in plastic, not glass containers, because some of the valuable nutrients in breast milk will cling to glass.

- Explain to the woman who experiences a multiple birth that twins and other multiple births can be breastfed. This mother will need to monitor her own diet even more carefully when breastfeeding more than one child to ensure that everyone gets adequate nutrition.

- Explain to the mother of a hospitalized post-term infant that she can express, freeze, and store breast milk for her infant. The nursery can use this milk when the infant is able to begin feedings. Later, when the infant is strong enough, the mother can begin breastfeeding. This not only benefits the infant but also helps the mother feel involved in the care of her child.

- Monitor closely the mother's progress with breastfeeding so intervention strategies can be planned should she become discouraged or face challenges during the process.

- Teach the new mother how to care for her breasts, since preventing mastitis and engorgement is easier than treating these conditions.

- Teach the new mother the steps to proper hygiene and care of her breasts following childbirth. This will promote healing and reduce the incidence of infection.

- Investigate local and regional resources for breastfeeding mothers before the need arises so the mother can be promptly referred to the appropriate support group.

- Guide the woman who is faced with choosing between breast and bottlefeeding to the decision that is most appropriate for her. The informed woman who makes a decision to bottlefeed must never be scorned or made to feel like a failure after she makes an informed decision that she feels is best for her and her baby.

- Encourage family members to support the mother's decision to breastfeed. This will help lessen the pressure on the new mother and enhance the success of breastfeeding.

- Remind the woman that many new mothers continue to breastfeed after returning to work. Most women manage this by expressing milk that will be fed to the infant later by the caregiver. A few women are fortunate enough to be in an employment setting where the infant can be brought to them, or they can return to the infant for feedings.

- Advise mothers that cow's milk from the dairy case, canned milk, and improperly diluted infant formulas will not provide adequate nutrition for their infants and are not acceptable. Adequate nutrition is essential to normal growth and development of the infant and will dramatically influence the baby's future.

- Discuss the importance of healthful eating with breastfeeding mothers. Servings from each of the four food groups are essential, and breastfeeding mothers will need to increase their caloric intake.

- Advise the breastfeeding mother not to smoke, drink, or use illicit drugs since these will likely pass to her baby and harm the child.

- Remind mothers that although breastfeeding typically suppresses ovulation, it is not considered a reliable form of birth control. The patient should discuss birth control options with her partner and her doctor or nurse practitioner.

EXAM QUESTIONS

CHAPTER 10
Questions 76–84

76. The female breast is partly formed from which type of tissue?

    a. glandular

    b. nervous

    c. muscle

    d. granular

77. The hormone primarily responsible for lactation is

    a. estradiol.

    b. progesterone.

    c. estrogen.

    d. prolactin.

78. How many lobes are generally found in each breast?

    a. 20

    b. 10

    c. 5

    d. 50

79. An antibody-rich yellow fluid secreted from the female breasts after childbirth is

    a. breast milk.

    b. lochia.

    c. serosanguineous fluid.

    d. colostrum.

80. By the end of the first week postpartum, the average amount of breast milk produced by the mother per day will be

    a. 50–100 ml.

    b. 200–300 ml.

    c. 400–600 ml.

    d. 750–900 ml.

81. Suckling of the infant causes the pituitary to release which hormone?

    a. Oxytocin

    b. FSH

    c. Estrogen

    d. Progesterone

82. Which of the following measures help hasten uterine involution?

    a.   application of a tight abdominal binder

    b.   frequent uterine massage

    c.   fundal massage and breastfeeding

    d.   warm compresses to the abdomen

83. Lactation is *most* effectively suppressed by:

    a.   Binding the breasts.

    b.   Avoidance of suckling.

    c.   Application of ice.

    d.   Injection of prolactin.

84. Lactation, the result of complex neurohormonal events, is primarily mediated by which gland?

    a.   Mammary

    b.   Ovary

    c.   Pituitary

    d.   Adrenal

CHAPTER 11

THE NEWBORN

CHAPTER OBJECTIVE

After studying this chapter, the reader will be able to identify normal and abnormal characteristics of the newborn and specify nursing measures for assessment of the newborn, integration into the family, and discharge planning.

LEARNING OBJECTIVES

After studying this chapter, the student will be able to

1. Identify normal characteristics of the newborn.

2. Recognize complications that may occur during a pregnancy or delivery that can have deleterious effects on the fetus.

3. Identify physiological changes that must occur for the newborn to adapt to extrauterine life.

4. Differentiate pathology in the newborn and select sources for referral and consultation.

5. Select elements of newborn care and discharge planning.

6. Choose assessment strategies of the newborn, including Apgar scoring.

7. Recognize basic infant nutritional facts.

INTRODUCTION

This chapter serves as a review of the fundamental facts of newborn life and the basic care of the newborn. A review of the normal newborn and the changes each infant undergoes at birth are presented. Assessment of the well baby is discussed. Complications that may arise during pregnancy and delivery and their effect on the infant are examined. Another section helps the nurse differentiate common pathologies in infants and guides the nurse to the appropriate resources for obtaining help for the infant. The chapter includes a summary of nutrition and discharge planning and concludes with a list of specific nursing strategies that may be useful when caring for the newborn.

THE TRANSITION FROM FETUS TO NEWBORN

The transition from intrauterine to extrauterine life presents a number of challenges to the fetus. To leave the nurturing environment of the mother's womb, it must endure intense contractions of the uterus and pass through the birth canal or the mother's abdomen to the waiting world. Upon birth, the newborn's body must establish circulation, initiate respirations, and maintain its own metabolism—all tasks previously managed by the mother through the placenta. Incredible and formidable as all these tasks are, most newborns sail through this transition smoothly. Yet, when difficulty is encountered, an astute nurse is often the first to note the signs and alert the pediatrician or nurse practitioner so prompt intervention can begin.

Caring for newborns requires a knowledge of the transition from fetus to newborn. The major events involved in making the transition from intrauterine to extrauterine life are reviewed below.

Respiration

As described in Chapter 7, the mother's body assumes the role of gas exchange for the fetus. This is accomplished through the placental and fetal circulation, which delivers oxygenated blood to the fetus and removes carbon dioxide to the mother for excretion. This gas exchange occurs in a liquid, the blood. But when the fetus becomes a newborn, the gas exchange is between a liquid (the blood in the alveolar capillaries) and a gas (the oxygen in environmental air). If this transition is to support extrauterine life, according to Korones (1986) four requirements must be satisfied:

- Respiratory movements must be initiated.

- Entry of air must overcome opposing forces if the lungs are to expand.

- Some air must remain in the alveoli at the end of expiration so that the lungs do not collapse (establishment of functional residual capacity).

- Pulmonary blood flow must be increased, and cardiac output must be redistributed.

The fetal lungs are normally quiescent during pregnancy, but fetuses often make movements that simulate breathing, especially toward the end of pregnancy. It is within seconds after delivery that the newborn should take his or her first breath. Many experts believe the stimulus for the first breath is a combination of the sudden change in temperature as the infant is propelled from the mother's warm body into the colder environment of the delivery room, the acid-base changes and

asphyxia that occur as the fetus survives labor, and the rubbing or touching most newborns receive immediately at birth.

The infant's first inspiration pulls the diaphragm down, causing air to flow into the lungs due to the negative pressure gradient generated by the lungs' expansion. Fluid that filled the lungs in utero is then removed by circulation, drainage, swallowing, and evaporation (Reeder & Martin, 1987). A regular breathing pattern should soon emerge in the normal infant.

Circulation

With the initiation of respiration, the fetal circulation undergoes changes that allow the newborn to sustain extrauterine existence. These begin with the clamping of the umbilical cord and the first breath taken by the newborn. Korones (1986) identifies five attributes of fetal circulation that must be altered for the infant to make the switch from fetal to mature circulation:

- Closure of the foramen ovale.

- Closure of the ductus arteriosus.

- Closure of the ductus venosus.

- Decreased pulmonary vascular resistance.

- Increased aortic blood pressure.

These changes are generally complete after a period of several hours or during the first day or so of life.

Other Systems

The newborn must begin to manufacture, break down, and excrete substances on its own. Disorders of metabolism such as hypocalcemia or hypoglycemia may result if the newborn is not up to the challenge. The neurologic system must begin the functions that protect and preserve life. The urinary system must be patent and excrete urine, and the gastrointestinal system must become functional.

ASSESSMENT OF THE NEWBORN

The newborn period refers to the first 28 days of life. During the early hours of life, the newborn should receive a complete assessment. According to Phibbs in Rudolph (1982), there are three general goals when assessing the newborn:

- To detect significant medical problems so they can be treated appropriately.

- To protect the newborn from harmful processes such as chilling or nosocomial infections.

- To promote good health by facilitating the normal adaptations to extrauterine life.

Parents will also want assurances that their infant is healthy and normal. And when an infant is not normal, the nurse must have an understanding of the pathology, since parents commonly turn to the nurse for information, support, and guidance. It is frequently the nurse who first notices something is amiss with an infant, so nurses need a working knowledge of how to assess a newborn. This section reviews newborn assessment in the delivery suite, including Apgar scoring, then describes the more in-depth examination of the newborn that should take place later in the first days of life.

Apgar Scoring

A brief assessment of the newborn must be undertaken immediately after birth. As described in detail in Chapter 8, the five signs of the Apgar are assessed and scored at one and five minutes of life. At delivery and before the initial assessment takes place, some obstetricians or nurse midwives elect to place the apparently normal infant on the mother's abdomen where she and the child glimpse each other for the first time; others immediately hand the infant to the obstetric or neonatal nurse for assessment and care. In either case, after the mother (if she is awake) has seen the infant, the nurse places it on a warming bed in the delivery suite, briefly examines it, suctions the mouth/nose if necessary, obtains footprints, applies identifying bands to the extremities, cleans it superficially, and returns it to its mother.

Physical Assessment of the Newborn

Much of the infant's physical exam can be conducted without awakening it, although it must be fully exposed at intervals for a complete and accurate examination. Recover the infant as soon as possible after the exam to avoid chilling. Scrupulous handwashing is essential before touching the infant to avoid transferring microorganisms.

General: When assessing a newborn, always take a few moments to get an overview of the infant in his or her environment. Note overall appearance, and when possible, the mother's interaction with the child. Significant information can be obtained simply by looking and listening at this point. The sleeping newborn typically assumes a symmetrical position at rest; if he does not, pathology (typically a neurologic or orthopedic injury) may be present. Note the shape and size of the body, and the proportions of its different areas. Assess the skin color. Note the infant's predicted gestational age according to the mother's due date. More accurate estimates of gestational age can be determined by special assessments of the infant, but the most important concept here is to determine whether the infant appears of normal size and development for the estimated gestational age. From there, many examiners take a head-to-toe or systems approach to the exam.

The pre-term infant. Pre-term infants are generally considered to be those born before 37 weeks gestation. Advances in modern medicine mean that resuscitation and salvage attempts are started at an earlier gestational age nearly every year, sometimes as early as 22–24 weeks of gestation. Obviously, this is a topic laden with volatile ethical and emotional issues.

Some extremely pre-term infants survive and thrive; others live only a short while or are tragically impaired when they do survive. It is important, though, not to be blinded by numbers such as the infant's weight or due dates. *Figure 11-1* reveals just how deceptive the newborn's size can be in relation to the gestational age. Obviously, the more advanced the gestational age, the greater the chance of survival in most cases. Survival is greater in advanced neonatal intensive care units where the staff are specially trained to deal with the pre-term infant, although not every pre-term infant will require intensive care.

The post-term infant. The post-term infant is one who is delivered after the 42nd week of gestation. These infants may suffer hypoxia and stress during labor; 75% to 85% of all deaths among postmature babies occur during labor (Korones, 1986).

Skin: The normal fullterm newborn is covered with a cheesy material called vernix caseosa, which helps protect the skin in utero. Premature infants will not have vernix, and post-term infants may only have vernix in skin folds. After it is wiped away and the infant is bathed, the skin should be soft like velvet. Premature infants are covered with a downy hair called lanugo, but very premature infants will have gelatinous skin that almost seems transparent. Grasping a fold of skin over the abdomen will give the nurse an idea of the tissue turgor; the skin should snap back into place when released. If it does not, the infant may be suffering from dehydration. Note the color of the skin, including any alterations in color, lesions, or discolorations. Wrinkled, peeling skin is common in post-term infants. Wrinkles on the soles of the feet are less prominent in pre-term infants.

FIGURE 11-1

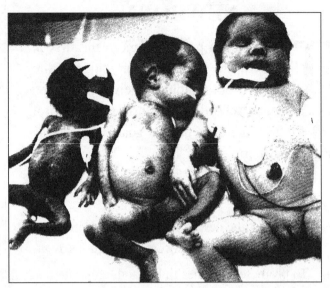

Source: *High-Risk Newborn Infants, The basis for intensive nursing care,* Korones, S. B. & Lancaster, J. C., V. Mosby Co., 1986

Head and Neck: The bones of the newborn's skull are not as rigid as an adult's. These bones are joined by connective tissues referred to as sutures; the areas where the sutures meet are called fontanels. The fontanels are often referred to as "soft spots;" they may not be palpable in all infants because of the overlapping of the cranial bones. If the fontanels are palpable, they should be soft and never bulging or tense; bulging could indicate increased intracranial pressure.

A prolonged labor and slow passage through the birth canal can cause extreme molding of the head, which can be quite alarming to the parents. Assure them it will resolve spontaneously as the swelling and edema of the scalp subside. Bruising of the scalp or face may occur as a result of birth trauma or forceps delivery. The head should be palpated for obvious deformities, since skull fractures may occur in infants delivered with forceps. The head of the infant is normally quite large compared to the rest of the body, which eventually catches up. The circumference of the head should be recorded and tracked as the infant grows to detect any changes that might indicate pathology. The newborn neck is rather short and should be free of masses or lesions.

Observe the infant's facial structure, since abnormalities may be most obvious here. Palpate the bones of the face and note any disruptions or crepitation that might indicate fractures sustained during birth.

Caucasian newborns generally have blue eyes at birth, changing to the final color by the end of the first year of life. The eyes may have minor drainage after the prophylactic eye treatment is performed. Look for any clouding that might indicate cataracts, and any disruptions in the corneal surface. Remember that the alert, wide-eyed baby who appears to be sucking may be suffering the effects of intrauterine hypoxia (Korones, 1986).

The ears of the term infant are well formed. Pre-term infants lack cartilage and their ears are very soft and flexible. Low-set ears are often associated with a number of congenital anomaly syndromes. The awake baby should turn toward, blink, or react with a startle to a sudden noise; if not, a hearing disorder may be suspected.

Newborns breathe through the nose. Any flaring of the nostrils may indicate respiratory distress.

A finger run over the surfaces of the newborn's mouth will help identify any lesions or abnormalities, such as precocious teeth that may be loose or need to be removed to facilitate breast-feeding and prevent aspiration. Epstein's pearls are tiny projections on the hard palate that disappear spontaneously. Some newborns will exhibit circumoral cyanosis, a bluish tinge of the lips in the first hours after birth; it usually resolves quickly.

Chest: The newborn has a barrel-shaped chest; the circumference should be measured and recorded. After the first period of reactivity, respirations should be quiet and free of adventitious sounds like rales or rhonchi. Both sides of the chest should expand equally with inspiration. A grunting sound on expiration or a gasping, shrill sound on inspiration indicates respiratory distress and should be called to a pediatrician's attention immediately. If the sternum appears to be pulled back toward the spine on inspiration, retractions associated with respiratory distress have developed and the physician should be notified immediately. The clavicles should be palpated, since either or both may have been fractured during delivery, sometimes deliberately to facilitate passage of a particularly large baby through the birth canal in an emergency. Feel the breasts for engorgement and check for the presence of nipples. Extra (supernumerary) nipples are not uncommon and generally are not significant.

Abdomen: The infant's abdomen should be soft and may be protuberant or flat. The umbilical cord stump should be inspected for the presence of two arteries and one vein; if three vessels are not noted the possibility of congenital malformations should be investigated. There should be no drainage from the cord, which will usually dry and fall away 7–10 days after birth. The abdomen should be palpated for masses and the pediatrician notified if any abnormal masses are felt. Bowel sounds are generally active.

Genitals: The genitals of the fullterm newborn should appear to be normally formed. In the male, the foreskin will cover the glans; an orifice should be present at the tip. The testes can usually be palpated in the scrotum. In the female, the labia minora can be prominent but should be covered by the labia majora. Some vaginal discharge in response to maternal hormones is normal and clears spontaneously. The anus can be evaluated for patency during rectal temperature measurement, but the area should still be inspected for presence of a fistula. In the breech infant, the genitals may be edematous and discolored from passage through the vagina.

The Back: Hold the infant prone and evaluate the spine. It should not have abnormal curvatures or lesions. Investigate any dimples, indentions, and tufts of hair that may indicate fistula formation.

The Lower Extremities: Check the legs for symmetry, range of motion, and proportion to the rest of the body; note the structure and number of digits. With the infant supine, flex the legs, then abduct the legs bilaterally until they touch the table surface. Note any clicking or popping sounds and notify the pediatrician or nurse practitioner immediately if they are present, as this can indicate a dislocated hip. The soles of the fullterm infant are normally wrinkled; because wrinkling increases with gestational age, wrinkles may be absent in the pre-term infant. Acrocyanosis, a blue color of the hands and feet, is common immediately after birth, but generally disappears within hours. Palpate along the surfaces of the bones in order to detect fractures. Any spasticity or flaccidity of the upper or lower extremities should be immediately reported to the pediatrician or nurse practitioner, since this may indicate a neurologic injury.

The Upper Extremities: Again, note the proportion to the rest of the body, the symmetry, and spontaneous movement of the arms and hands. Full range of motion should be present, and the extremities should be palpated for any disruptions that might indicate fractures. Newborns typically hold their hands in fists and will normally grasp fingers or objects placed in their hands. Long fingernails are associated with the pre-term infant. The palms of the hands may reveal the presence of abnormal simian creases that are associated with certain conditions like Down's syndrome.

Neurologic: The normal newborn exhibits the following reflexes: the Moro (startle) reflex; the tonic neck reflex; the stepping reflex; the grasp reflex; and the rooting/sucking reflex. The newborn who appears jittery or exhibits jerky movements of the extremities may suffer from low blood sugar, disturbances of calcium metabolism, or may in fact be having seizures.

Cardiovascular: After quieting the child with a pacifier or finger, auscultate the heart sounds and feel for pulses in the upper and lower extremities. Although cardiac murmurs are not uncommon as the newborn makes the transition from intrauterine to extrauterine life, they should be documented and the pediatrician or nurse practitioner routinely informed. Congenital heart defects may or may not be obvious in the first days of life.

WHEN COMPLICATIONS ARISE

The transition from intrauterine to extrauterine life ordinarily proceeds smoothly, but unfortunately there are times when just the opposite is true. With good prenatal care, a number of complications can be foreseen and either prevented or detected in time for preparations to be made to meet the challenge. Korones (1986) summarizes it well: "The events that follow birth have their origins in those that preceded it." It is therefore critical that the nurse be aware of the mother's prenatal course and labor history, to understand what has happened and prepare for what is to come.

The neonatal mortality rate in the early 90's was 5.6 per 1,000 live births, down dramatically from 15.1 in 1970. The leading causes of neonatal mortality are premature births and resulting low birth weight (Neff, 1996).

There are a multitude of clinical situations that can cause concern in the intrapartum or neonatal period; a full discussion would be beyond the scope of this review. Some of the more common occurrences and their outcomes are reviewed below.

The Severely Depressed Infant

Fetal distress may cause the infant to be born hypoxic and flaccid. This is most often in response to asphyxia, and the source can be traced to inadequate circulation to the fetus or inadequate oxygen in the blood circulated to the fetus. Other factors include maternal medication such as narcotics, and congenital anomalies. In any event, the depressed infant with low Apgar scores (<3 or 4 at 1 minute) requires immediate intervention. A skilled neonatal resuscitation team should be summoned if one is available. In the absence of such support, the obstetrician, anesthetist (if present), or nurse may assume management of the depressed newborn. Treatment involves opening the airway, delivering oxygen to the lungs, supporting the breathing, and maintaining the circulation.

Respiratory Distress

This is a common term used to describe a number of different clinical syndromes. Respiratory distress has many causes, and may be due to prematurity, infection, congenital malformations, heart disease, and meconium aspiration, among others. Some of the more common types are reviewed briefly below.

Meconium aspiration: Meconium is a thick, sticky green or black substance found in the large intestine of the fetus. It may be passed in utero, generally in response to asphyxia.

When meconium is present in the amniotic fluid, there can be some presumption of fetal distress. Upon breathing for the first time, the meconium can be inhaled into the lungs, causing a chemical pneumonitis. Alternatively, an overzealous healthcare provider can blow meconium down into the lungs by positive pressure from a manual ventilating bag.

When an apneic baby is born with meconium staining, it is imperative that the meconium be suctioned from the oropharynx and trachea before artificial ventilation begins. Treatment depends on severity of the aspiration, but generally includes oxygen administration and antibiotics along with circulatory and ventilatory support where indicated. Meconium aspiration can prove fatal. It is seldom seen in pre-term infants.

Hyaline membrane disease: Surfactant is a phospholipid which decreases the surface tension of the alveolar sacs. This allows them to fill with air and prevents them from collapsing upon expiration. Sufficient amounts of surfactant are usually not present in the fetus until the 36th week of gestation. In the pre-term infant, the administration of artificial surfactant via an endotracheal tube helps decrease the surface tension until the infant is able to produce sufficient amounts of his/her own.

Congenital Anomalies

Just as giving birth can be one of the most exhilarating and critical events in a woman's life, the birth of an infant with congenital anomalies or malformations can be devastating. This is a time when the utmost sensitivity and support from the nurse is essential. Some congenital anomalies such as cleft palate, while distressing, are not life-threatening. Others, such as heart defects, can swiftly fell the infant. A discussion of all congenital anomalies is of course beyond the scope of this chapter. Common syndromes are reviewed below. In general, though, the astute nurse will search for additional congenital deformities in the patient who has one congenital deformity, because where there is one, there may be more.

Trisomy syndromes: Usually, the cells contain chromosomes or genes that are paired, but in some circumstances there may be a third chromosome present. This is referred to as a trisomy syndrome. The infant born with a trisomy syndrome generally exhibits a pattern of distinguishing clinical features, such as the familiar Down's syndrome. Depending on the degree and severity of the clinical features, the infant may or may not require immediate care in the delivery room.

Heart defects: There are a multitude of heart defects, some of which are associated with genetic syndromes. A number of heart defects can be detected before delivery if the mother has had an ultrasound of the fetus. In that case, she can be referred to a high-risk women's hospital where a skilled team will stand by to manage her baby. In other cases, signs and symptoms of the defect may not emerge for days or even years. This is a situation where good prenatal care can prevent or lessen tragedy. The nurse should note that not all heart defects involve cyanosis.

Fetal alcohol syndrome: Since alcohol is the most abused substance in America, it is no surprise that an alarming number of infants are born with fetal alcohol syndrome. During pregnancy, alcohol ingestion can cause malformation; after birth the infant may suffer withdrawal symptoms. In general, the infant with fetal alcohol syndrome can have alterations in the head (mental retardation, an abnormal face), the heart (congenital defects), and the hands (abnormal palmar creases).

Diaphragmatic hernia: In some cases, the diaphragm fails to close completely and the abdominal contents may slip up into the thoracic cavity. The newborn develops respiratory distress soon after birth and bowel sounds may be heard in the chest. The diagnosis is usually obvious on radiograph. Surgery is indicated to correct the deformity; the mortality rate can be quite high.

Cleft lip is a congenital anomaly of one or more clefts in the upper lip which results from incomplete fusion of the oral cavity. The size of the cleft ranges from a small dimple or larger clefts which can extend up into the nose. Surgical repair generally occurs between 1–2 months, depending upon the cleft's extent and the infant's general condition. This condition, which occurs more often in boys, affects approximately 1;1,000 births.

Cleft palate is a congenital anomaly which occurs either in isolation or in conjunction with a cleft lip. The severity of the condition ranges from a cleft only involving the soft palate to extensive openings in the hard palate and portion of the maxilla. Depending upon the extent of the cleft, the infant may have difficulty sucking and formula may come out through the nose. These infants are at increased risk for frequent otitis media. Surgical correction is generally performed between 6–18 months and may require several surgical procedures to complete. Early correction is recommended in order to promote normal development of the infant's speech pattern. cleft palates occur more frequently in girls and occurs in approximately 1:2500 births.

Other: There are numerous other types of congenital defects; many involve a failure during the embryonic period of development. Conditions include defects in the abdominal wall so that intestines are outside the body, or conditions where the spinal cord is not properly enclosed. Digits may be malformed or missing, genitals may be ambiguous, or the anus may be imperforate. The trachea and/or esophagus may be malformed. All require careful assessment and evaluation by a pediatric specialist.

Rh sensitization is an antigen-antibody immunologic reaction within the body which occurs when an Rh negative woman carries an Rh positive fetus. If fetal red blood cells enter the maternal circulation, the "different" Rh factor stimulates the production of Rh antibodies. In subsequent pregnancies,if the fetus is Rh+, these antibodies will cross the placenta, enter the fetal circulation and lead to erythroblastosis. Although there is no direct connection between the maternal and fetal circulation, small leakage can occur following invasive procedures such as amniocentesis, abortion/miscarriage, percutaneous umbilical blood sampling (PUBS), and trauma. In order to prevent the formation of antibodies, all Rh- women must receive an intramuscular injection of Rhogam following any invasive procedure during pregnancy and again within 72 hours of delivery, if lab tests indicate the infant is Rh+.

ABO incompatibility, which is generally less severe than Rh sensitization, usually involves a blood type O mother (either Rh+ or -) whose infant is either type A, B, or AB. Anti-A and anti-B antibodies in the mother's blood will destroy the red blood cells of the infant with either type A, B, or AB blood. This RBC destruction releases bilirubin which can lead to jaundice. Phototherapy is the usual treatment of choice with careful monitoring of bilirubin levels via heel stick. Unlike Rh sensitiza-

tion which does not occur during the first pregnancy prior to antibody formation, ABO incompatibility can affect the woman's first pregnancy.

Infection

Neonatal infections can be fatal if not noted and treated in time. Some, such as syphilis, AIDS, or herpes, are acquired from the mother. Others are nosocomial and passed to the infant by healthcare providers, indicating once again the importance of handwashing before touching the newborn. Septicemia caused by group B streptococci takes a swift toll on the newborn and is frequently fatal. Antibiotics and supportive care are indicated for the infected newborn.

Group B strep (GBS) is the leading cause of perinatal bacterial infections in the United States. Approximately 15–40% of pregnant women are asymptomatic carriers of GBS. Risk factors which have been identified for selection of patients most likely to benefit from intrapartum antibiotic chemoprophylaxis include maternal colonization with GBS PLUS:

* pre-term labor or
* pre-term, premature rupture of membranes, or
* prolonged rupture of membranes (>18 hours) or
* sibling affected by symptomatic GBS infection, or
* maternal fever during labor.

Treatment of choice for symptomatic GBS infection of mother or baby is penicillin or ampicillin. Mothers who are allergic to these medications may receive Erythromycin or Clindamycin instead. Selective intrapartum chemoprophylaxis can prevent GBS early-onset neonatal disease and reduce maternal puerperal morbidity. There does not appear to be an effect on late-onset neonatal disease.

Hepatitis vaccine: For newborns whose mothers test negative for hepatitis B surface antigen (HBSAg), the recommended hepatitis B immunization schedule is for the infant to receive the first dose during the first 2 days of life, the second at 1–2 months and the third at 6–18 months. If the mother is HGSAg+, the schedule is for the infant to receive the first dose as soon as possible after birth, the second at 1 months and the third at 6 months.

Metabolic

Newborns may fall victim to a number of metabolic disorders, some of which may be genetic. These disorders, such as sickle cell anemia, are frequently detected if the infant is screened before leaving the hospital. three other common metabolic disorders are discussed below.

Hyperbilirubinemia: When hemoglobin is broken down, bilirubin results, and it is excreted through the feces. When the newborn's liver is unable to process excessive amounts of bilirubin, jaundice, or a yellowing of the skin, may result. This situation can be dangerous: High levels of bilirubin in the blood can cause kernicterus or a bilirubin encephalopathy that may lead to brain damage or death. (See Appendix for the Normal Neonatal Lab Values.) Treatment of hyperbilirubinemia generally includes phototherapy. This involves exposing the skin to special blue fluorescent lights that enhance the breakdown of bilirubin so it can be excreted. The lights are often set on top of an incubator in which the nude infant is placed. The infant's eyes should be protected by a mask or eye patches during phototherapy. Another option is an exchange transfusion, where the infant's blood is withdrawn in increments and replaced with donated blood.

Hypoglycemia: Birth abruptly halts the source of maternal glucose flowing to the child, but when the infant is put to the breast or bottle fed, the serum glucose will generally stabilize. (See Appendix for Normal Neonatal Lab Values.) However, the infant of a diabetic mother or of a mother who received glucose containing infusions during labor is most susceptible to a rebound hypoglycemia. Seizures and brain damage may result. Treatment includes administration of glucose-containing solutions to increase the serum glucose to normal levels. Monitoring of blood glucose in infants is usually performed by placing a drop of blood from a heel stick on a blood glucose reagent strip.

Phenylketonuria: Phenylketonuria (PKU) is an inborn error of metabolism that results in high blood levels of the enzyme phenylalanine. If left untreated, this can lead to brain damage and mental retardation. Most states require newborns to be screened 24–48 hours after birth. Treatment involves limiting dietary intake of the amino acid phenylalanine. As an infant, an enzymatic hydrolysate of casein, (i.e., Lofenalac or Progestimil powder) is substituted for milk. Dietary restrictions generally continue throughout the child's life.

Birth Trauma

The number of injuries infants can sustain during the birth process is nearly infinite. Suffice it to say that every newborn should receive a complete physical assessment to search for fractures, abrasions, and other injuries that may be due to forceps, force, or instruments used during delivery. The most common birth trauma is a fractured clavicle.

Hypothermia

Newborns are prone to chilling, and hypothermia in infants sets off a chain of events that can culminate in death. Infants, especially post-term ones, have limited thermoregulation capacity, so it is essential that the nurse protect the newborn from chilling.

Fluid Imbalance

Prevention and treatment of fluid imbalance in the sick or compromised neonate is imperative. It requires careful monitoring of early signs of dehydration or overhydration. Keeping the infant in a neutral thermal environment can prevent insensible fluid loss. Calculating fluid intake and losses can alert the nurse to early shifts in fluid balance (May & Mahlmeister, 1994).

NUTRITION AND THE NEWBORN

Chapter 10 recommends breast milk as the best choice for healthful nutrition in the newborn and offers further information on infant nutrition. Yet sometimes the mother may elect not to breastfeed her baby and choose instead to use a commercially prepared formula. In either case, the nurse should be supportive and nonjudgmental about the mother's decision. The nurse should be sensitive to the mother's personal situation when it comes to feeding her infant, and offer referrals to social programs that will help her obtain formula if she is not able to purchase it. Most infants are fed *ad lib,* or as desired, and this usually results in normal growth. Encourage all mothers to follow up with regular health screenings as their infant grows. This will help ensure that any nutritional deficits are identified early.

DISCHARGE PLANNING AND ASSESSMENT

Most institutions have a discharge planning checklist that must be completed before the infant is released for discharge. The nurse should review that checklist carefully, because in most cases it has been carefully designed to ensure a safe discharge and pre-vent tragedy. The goals of discharge planning include the following:

- Safe transfer of the infant and mother to their home. Parents should possess and use an approved infant car seat when leaving the hospital in a private car. The nurse must also check identification bands and then double-check to ensure that the correct baby is being released.

- Parental mastery of the skills involved in feeding, diapering, bathing, dressing, and providing a safe environment for the baby. The nurse should observe the caregivers carrying out basic care before discharging the infant.

- Parental ability to identify when to seek help with their infant and who to call for that help, including the number of their pediatrician, pediatric nurse practitioner, or local health clinic. Parents should also demonstrate an understanding of the importance of well-baby checkups and immunizations.

- Parental knowledge of the date and times of follow-up appointments for both mother and child.

Going home is traditionally a big moment for the family, and supportive nursing care can help ensure that the bliss of this moment is not marred by tragedy.

NURSING STRATEGIES FOR THE CARE OF THE NEWBORN

The nursing goal in caring for the newborn is to ensure that the infant makes a safe transition from the mother's uterus to her arms, bonds with the family or caregivers, receives essential care, and goes home in good condition with the family. Below are nursing strategies and interventions that the nurse may find useful when caring for newborns and their families. In clinical practice, specific nursing actions should be within the scope of the institution's practice guidelines and the state Nurse Practice Act, commensurate with the nurse's skills and training, and appropriate to the clinical situation at hand.

- Note the interaction between the mother and her new baby. Use of information gathered during this observation guides the nurse in determining if bonding is adequate or intervention is indicated. If a high-risk parenting situation exists, a referral to a social worker for further evaluation should be made.

- Don't give a bottle to the baby of the mother who wishes to breastfeed without first offering her the opportunity to put the infant to the breast, because that could reduce her chances of success with breastfeeding.

- Do not turn away from an infant who is on the examining table. A second of inattention can spell tragedy if the infant falls from the table.

- Remember to support the head and neck of the newborn because the infant will not have adequate head control. Not providing support could cause harm to the infant.

- Always wash hands before touching the infant. Many neonatal infections are transferred to the infant by healthcare providers, and good hand-washing techniques will reduce the transmission of disease.

- Remind the new mother and family to wash their hands before touching the newborn in the hospital, since this can reduce the incidence of disease transmission.

- Do a complete examination of the body surface of the infant born by Cesarean section. The infant may have been nicked or cut by the surgeon's scalpel, and early detection will allow prompt treatment.

- Protect the newborn from chilling by placing it under a radiant warmer or by wrapping it in warm blankets and covering the head with a snug cap (most heat is lost through the head). Hypothermia in the newborn infant can cause serious complications, including metabolic disturbances that lead to death.

- Suspect and search for additional anomalies when one anomaly is found in the newborn. Infants with one obvious congenital anomaly often have more that are not so obvious.

- Be aware of and advise the new mother of parenting classes offered in her community. Many hospitals, social organizations and churches offer parenting classes at little or no cost. These can help her gain valuable parenting skills. Refer the mother of a sick newborn to a support group that can help her develop coping skills and provide her with empathy and compassion during this difficult time.

- Since a newborn could inadvertently be infected, do not work in a nursery when running a fever, carrying a communicable disease, or when suffering from any infectious process or lesion. The consequences could be disastrous.

- Use Standard Precautions

- Wear gloves and consider protective eyewear when handling the newborn who has not been cleaned. Some maternal diseases can be transmitted to the infant, who in turn could infect the healthcare provider.

EXAM QUESTIONS

CHAPTER 11
Questions 85–100

85. The newborn period refers to the first
    a. 2 hours of life.
    b. 28 days of life.
    c. year of life.
    d. 24 hours of life.

86. The downy hair that covers the body of the fetus is called
    a. lanugo.
    b. surfactant.
    c. meconium.
    d. vernix caseosa.

87. The bones of the newborn's head are joined by connective tissue called
    a. fontanels.
    b. sutures.
    c. ligaments.
    d. surfactant.

88. Tiny projections on the hard palate of the newborn are usually
    a. thrush.
    b. milia.
    c. precocious teeth.
    d. Epstein's pearls.

89. A bluish, cyanotic tinge of the lips is called
    a. circumoral cyanosis.
    b. acrocyanosis.
    c. hypoxic cyanosis.
    d. oral cyanosis.

90. The condition in which the infant's sternum appears to pull back toward the spine is
    a. grunting.
    b. flaring.
    c. hypoxia.
    d. retractions.

91. With regard to vernix caseosa the full term infant will
    a. not have any.
    b. be covered with it.
    c. have it only in the skin folds.
    d. have it only on the scalp.

92. The infant's Apgar score must be assessed at____and____minutes of life.
    a. 2, 5
    b. 1, 5
    c. 2, 7
    d. 1, 3

93. A condition where bowel sounds can be heard in the chest is

    a. fetal alcohol syndrome.

    b. omphalocele.

    c. cystic fibrosis.

    d. diaphragmatic hernia.

94. Infants with fetal alcohol syndrome generally exhibit malformations of the

    a. face and heart.

    b. head and intestines.

    c. legs and lungs.

    d. hands and extremities.

95. A thick, sticky green or black substance found in the large intestine of the full-term infant is

    a. surfactant.

    b. meconium.

    c. vernix caseosa.

    d. lanugo.

96. The *first* action when caring for a baby born with meconium staining is

    a. suctioning.

    b. applying oxygen.

    c. ventilating the lungs with positive pressure.

    d. bathing.

97. Hyaline membrane disease involves a deficiency of

    a. meconium.

    b. vernix caseosa.

    c. surfactant.

    d. lanugo.

98. The first treatment for hyperbilirubinemia is often

    a. exchange transfusion.

    b. calcium infusion.

    c. phototherapy.

    d. isolation.

99. Hyperbilirubinemia can lead to

    a. respiratory distress.

    b. encephalopathy.

    c. meconium aspiration.

    d. hypoglycemia.

100. Hypoglycemia in the infant can lead to

    a. seizures.

    b. aspiration.

    c. kernicterus.

    d. phenylketonuria.

CHAPTER 12

IMPLEMENTING THE NURSING PROCESS IN MATERNAL-CHILD CARE

OBJECTIVE

After studying this chapter, the reader will be able to identify the five components of the nursing process and utilize the information presented in the previous eleven chapters to specify appropriate nursing care interventions in the following case presentations.

LEARNING OBJECTIVES

After reading this chapter, the student will be able to

1. Specify the rationale for using the nursing process.

2. Define the five phases of the nursing process.

3. Indicate appropriate nursing diagnoses and nursing interventions in the case presentation.

THE NURSING PROCESS

The foundation for the practice of nursing depends upon the utilization of the nursing process in all aspects of patient care. The nursing process provides an organized and comprehensive framework for directing nursing activities; it is based upon the scientific method for problem-solving and includes five distinct, yet interrelated, components. These components are assessment, diagnosis, planning, implementation, and evaluation (Christensen & Kenney, 1990). To help define nursing practice more clearly, the nursing process should be used within the context of a nursing model. It is a nursing model that provides the structure to collect and analyze patient assessment data, as well as serve as a guide for nursing interventions. Each component of the nursing process will now be discussed individually and illustrated within a case presentation.

Assessment

The first and most important step in the nursing process is that of data collection; the nurse identifies and collects information about the patient, family, and environment that is relevant, thorough, and accurate so that an appropriate plan of care can be devised. The focus of the assessment is to determine the patient's response to her health concerns and problems; nursing models provide unique definitions of nursing, the patient, environment and health/illness and can structure the data collection phase within its holistic framework. Standardized nursing assessment tools are now more readily available to perinatal nurses to help streamline the process and to ensure its completeness. The information to be collected for maternity patients from the initial antepartum visit, admission to, and discharge from the birthing unit has been presented in the previous chapters. Identification of sociocultural factors that can influence teaching and learning, for example, is important information that is needed to plan effective care.

There are five methods for collecting assessment data: (1) interview to complete a history and to determine how the patient and significant others are responding to current and past events, such as health, illness, psychosocial events; (2) physical examination, laboratory testing; (3) review of records and diagnostic reports (i.e., prenatal records, previous hospital admissions); (4) observation; and, (5) collaboration with colleagues (Carpenito, 1993). A prerequisite to collecting the data, however, is the nurse's ability to observe, communicate and interpret the data accurately and effectively. Knowledge of and experience with therapeutic communication skills and human interaction patterns are important. Interpreting the data involves an ability to draw inferences or conclusions from certain cues (e.g., signs, symptoms, "red flags") ascertained from the data. An example of this would be the nurse's skill and experience in interpreting information from the fetal heart rate monitor or cardiac monitor.

Nursing Diagnosis

From the collected assessment data, the nurse then draws conclusions or clinical judgments about the patient's needs and problems. In 1990, the North American Nursing Diagnosis Association (NANDA) approved an official definition of nursing diagnosis as "a clinical judgment about individual, family, or community responses to actual or potential health problems" (Carpenito, 1993). Nursing diagnosis directs appropriate nursing interventions to resolve the identified needs. They should be written clearly and concisely as descriptive and etiological statements. There are nursing diagnoses that are particularly applicable to maternity and newborn patients *(see table 12-1).*

Planning

Before nursing interventions are carried out, a comprehensive plan of care is devised. The first step in the planning phase is to set priorities and determine which of the nursing diagnoses should

be addressed first. Next, long-term goals are identified and then specific, measurable, and patient-centered objectives to achieve the goals are written with input from the patient. The objectives are short-term descriptions of what is expected from the patient after the nursing interventions are performed (Christensen & Kenney, 1990). Nursing standard care plans, as well as procedures and protocol, are available to use in planning strategies and specifying nursing orders for each intervention. Strategies may include teaching/learning, problem solving, behavior modification, caring, therapeutic use of self, contracting, group process, and stress management (Christensen & Kenney, 1990). The teaching/learning strategy is used extensively in maternity nursing and is often based on adult learning theory; anticipatory guidance and discharge teaching for self care, for example, are high priorities for new parents and require detailed planning.

Implementation

Implementation is the carrying out of the nursing care plan by the patient, nurse, and other specified health team members. In order to execute the planned activities, the nurse must have the required interpersonal, intellectual, and technical skills to accomplish the objectives. The implementation phase includes preparation. implementation, then post implementation. In the preparation stage, the plan of care is validated with the patient, family, and other involved health team members. Next, the patient and family are carefully instructed about what will occur as the plan is carried out. The delivery of care should be safe, outcome oriented, and consistent with the written objectives. After the care plan is executed, the postimplementation stage begins. This is when the nurse summarizes and clarifies the intervention(s) and plans for follow-up. The nurse also observes and documents the patient's response to the activities. It is important to note that the other phases of the nursing process

TABLE 12-1
Nursing Diagnoses Related to the Childbearing Family

NURSING DIAGNOSIS	SPECIFIC EXAMPLE IN PERINATAL CARE
Anxiety	Anxiety related to pregnancy changes
Impaired Adjustment	Impaired Adjustment related to inadequate support system during early parenting
Hypothermia	Hypothermia related to physiologic immaturity of the new born
Effective Breastfeeding	Effective Breastfeeding
Ineffective Breastfeeding	Ineffective Breastfeeding related to mastitis and maternal pain
	Ineffective Breastfeeding related to poor sucking reflex and neonatal immaturity
Constipation	Constipation related to physiologic changes of pregnancy and iron supplementation
Decisional Conflict	Decisional Conflict related to desire to maintain pregnancy and worsening maternal physiologic condition
Compromised Family Coping	Compromised Family Coping related to multiple strains of high-risk pregnancy treatment
Ineffective Family Coping	Ineffective Family Coping related to parental role overload in caring for triplets
Family Coping: Potential for Growth	Family Coping: Potential for Growth related to additional source of support
Altered Family Processes	Altered Family Processes related to birth of a neonate with a defect
Fatigue	Fatigue related to first trimester of pregnancy
Fear	Fear related to threatened loss of mate from pregnancy complication
Altered Health Maintenance	Altered Health Maintenance related to disruption of routines in early parenthood
Ineffective Infant Feeding Pattern	Ineffective Infant Feeding Pattern related to poverty
High Risk for Infection	High Risk for Infection related to unprotected intercourse with multiple partners
Knowledge Deficit	Knowledge Deficit related to lack of experience in caring for a newborn
Altered Nutrition: Less than Body Requirements	Altered Nutrition (Less than Body Requirements) related to nausea and vomiting in pregnancy
Altered Nutrition: More than Body Requirements	Altered Nutrition (More than Body Requirements) related to cultural beliefs regarding food intake during pregnancy
Pain	Pain related to persistent occiput posterior presentation of fetus during labor
High Risk for Altered Parenting	High Risk for Altered Parenting related to adolescent parenthood and inadequate social support
Altered Role Performance	Altered Role Performance related to demands of new parenthood
Altered Sexuality Patterns	Altered Sexuality Patterns related to physical or psychological changes during pregnancy
Altered Urinary Elimination	Altered Urinary Elimination related to physiologic changes of pregnancy

From North American Nursing Diagnosis Association, (1993). Classification of nursing diagnoses: Proceedings of the tenth conference. Philadelphia, J. B. Lippincott.

(i.e., assessment and planning) continue while the plans are being implemented.

Evaluation

The purpose of the evaluation phase is to determine if the patient was able to meet the specific goals and objectives. Evaluation involves deliberation about the structure, process and outcome of the implementation. Structure refers to the facilities, equipment, and qualifications of the staff; process denotes appraisal of the efficiency, effectiveness, appropriateness, and the adequacy of the nurse's implementation activities; and, outcome determines if the patient's behavior has changed as desired (Christensen & Kenney, 1990). Based upon the results of the evaluation, the plan of care is revised if necessary, or if there is success in resolving the problem, that portion of the care plan is completed.

APPLICATION OF THE NURSING PROCESS

Case Presentation

Mrs. Carolyn Andros is a 26-year-old, married, gravida 2, para 0 who is admitted to the hospital labor suite for pre-term labor. She is accompanied by her husband, Ted. Carolyn is 30⁴/₇ weeks gestation. She was previously admitted at 27 weeks gestation for pre-term labor, which was suppressed at home with subcutaneous then oral terbutaline sulfate. She was able to discontinue the tocolytic agent at 29 weeks gestation but maintained limited activity at home. Her first pregnancy approximately one year ago ended at 12 weeks gestation with a spontaneous abortion.

Assessment: She has been having irregular, mild uterine contractions every 10 minutes for the past two and a half hours. A sterile speculum exam revealed a cervical dilatation of 2 centimeters, effacement 50%, and presenting part

not engaged. Leopold maneuvers reveal a single fetus, vertex presentation, LOA position. The test for ferning is negative, and there has been no vaginal bleeding. Fetal heart rate is regular at 156 bpm. Maternal vital signs are normal. She is started on bedrest in left lateral position. The continuous fetal heart rate monitor has been applied and intravenous magnesium sulfate therapy initiated. She expresses fear that she will deliver a sick baby and is having difficulty resting.

Nursing Diagnosis: Several problems can be identified when a woman experiences pre-term labor and undergoes tocolytic therapy. Based on the above assessment data, the nursing diagnoses that take priority are:

- Fear related to diagnosis of pre-term labor and possibility of pre-term delivery.

- Knowledge Deficit related to the effects of her condition on her fetus.

- Potential for Maternal Injury related to side effects of tocolytic therapy.

Planning: Based on the assessment data and the three nursing diagnoses, the nurse and Mrs. Andros mutually agreed upon the following three outcome objectives:

1. Carolyn will be able to continually express confidence in the plan of care.

2. Carolyn will verbalize correct understanding of the purpose of her tocolytic therapy and its side effects and possible adverse reactions to herself and her baby within 48 hours of therapy initiation.

3. Carolyn will continually have no complications from the tocolytic drugs.

Implementation: Several nursing activities to help achieve each of the expected outcomes include

1. a. Encourage the patient and family to verbalize fears, anxiety, and concerns.

    b. Assess her support and coping systems and

include them in her care.

 c. Establish a trusting patient/nurse relationship.

 d. Explain all procedures, equipment, and pertinent policies affecting her care.

 e. Make referrals as appropriate to social services, and/or clergy.

 f. Keep communication lines open between staff, patient, family, and physicians.

2. a. Discuss possible neonatal complications.

 b. Teach Carolyn and her family about the effects of pre-term labor and pre-term birth.

 c. Reassure the patient and her family.

 d. Arrange for a tour of the neonatal intensive care nursery, or consultation with the NICU staff.

3. a. Assess per protocol fetal well-being (e.g., electronic fetal heart rate monitoring, fetal movement activity).

 b. Assess per protocol deep tendon reflexes, pulse oximetry, intake and output, uterine contraction pattern, vital signs (especially, cardiorespiratory functioning).

 c. Monitor serum magnesium levels.

 d. Keep 10% calcium gluconate at the bedside.

 e. Check that resuscitative equipment is functioning properly and is readily available.

 f. Observe patient frequently for signs and symptoms of allergic reactions, and drug toxicity.

 g. Maintain a quiet environment.

Evaluation: There were three attempts over the next few days to wean Mrs. Andros off of magnesium sulfate so that she could go home on oral terbutaline, but all failed. She continued to have uterine contractions when the magnesium doses were decreased. She remained free of signs of magnesium toxicity; there were also no signs of fetal stress or distress. She and her family stated that they felt more reassured about the baby's health and care after delivery. She talked with the Neonatal Clinical Nurse Specialist and her childbirth educator. She also was visited by a mother who had experienced post-term labor and birth.

On day 7 of hospitalization, her bag of waters ruptured. Fetal lung maturity was determined with presence of phosphatidylglycerol (PG). Tocolytic therapy was discontinued and labor progressed without complications. Carolyn delivered vaginally a 5 lb. 3 oz baby girl eight hours later using epidural anesthesia. The baby's apgar was 7 at one minute and 9 at five minutes. Postpartum recovery was uneventful. The baby was admitted to the intermediate nursery for assessment and stabilization. The baby was brought to the breast about 1½ hours after delivery but was not able to latch on and nurse. Carolyn expressed frustration, but agreed to try again in one hour with assistance from the lactation consultant. The baby still appeared sleepy and disinterested.

Questions

1. If you were the lactation consultant, what additional assessment data would you need to identify Carolyn's and the baby's needs? (Refer to Chapter 10.)

2. Identify two needs that take priority. How would you state these needs as nursing diagnoses (*see Table 12-1*).

3. What interventions should the nurse take to help ensure maintenance of adequate milk supply since the baby has not yet established an effective nursing pattern? (Refer to Chapter 10.)

4. How would you evaluate the effectiveness of your interventions?

SUMMARY

Utilizing the nursing process helps define and explain the unique practice of nursing. Its use encourages creative, comprehensive, systematic, and patient-oriented care that is more easily communicated to all health care team members. Its five phases—assessment, nursing diagnosis, planning, and evaluation—are founded in a scientific problem-solving method that can be utilized in all settings where nurses practice. To supplement and guide the nursing process, a nursing model should be selected. Nursing organizations and health care institutions have developed standardized nursing care plans, nursing diagnoses, and policies, procedures and protocols to define and promote quality patient health care. Knowledge of and adherence to these standards and guidelines are the responsibilities of each practicing nurse.

APPENDIX

THE PREGNANT PATIENT'S BILL OF RIGHTS

American parents are becoming increasingly aware that well-intentioned health professionals do not always have scientific data to support common American obstetrical practices and that many of these practices are carried out primarily because they are part of medical and hospital tradition. In the last forty years many artificial practices have been introduced which have changed childbirth from a physiological event to a very complicated medical procedure in which all kinds of drugs are used and procedures carried out, sometimes unnecessarily, and many of them potentially damaging for the baby and even for the mother. A growing body of research makes it alarmingly clear that every aspect of traditional American hospital care during labor and delivery must now be questioned as to its possible effect on the future well-being of both the obstetric patient and her unborn child.

One in every 35 children born in the United States today will eventually be diagnosed as retarded; in 75% of these cases there is no familial or genetic predisposing factor. One in every 10 to 17 children has been found to have some form of brain dysfunction or learning disability requiring special treatment. Such statistics are not confined to the lower socioeconomic group but cut across all segments of American society.

New concerns are being raised by childbearing women because no one knows what degree of oxygen depletion, head compression, or traction by forceps the unborn or newborn infant can tolerate before that child sustains permanent brain damage or dysfunction. The recent findings regarding the cancer-related drug diethylstilbestrol have alerted the public to the fact that neither the approval of a drug by the U.S. Food and Drug Administration nor the fact that a drug is prescribed by a physician serves as a guarantee that a drug or medication is safe for the mother or her unborn child. In fact, the American Academy of Pediatrics' Committee on Drugs has recently stated that there is no drug, whether prescription or over-the-counter remedy, which has been proven safe for the unborn child.

The Pregnant Patient has the right to participate in decisions involving her well-being and that of her unborn child, unless there is a clearcut medical emergency that prevents her participation. In addition to the rights set forth in the American Hospital Association's "Patient's Bill of Rights," (which has also been adopted by the New York City Department of Health) the Pregnant Patient, because she represents TWO patients rather than one, should be recognized as having the additional rights listed below.

1. *The Pregnant Patient has the right,* prior to the administration of any drug or procedure, to be informed by the health professional caring for her of any potential direct or indirect effects, risks or hazards to herself or her unborn or newborn infant which may result from the use of a drug or procedure prescribed for or administered to her during pregnancy, labor, birth or lactation.

2. *The Pregnant Patient has the right,* prior to the proposed therapy, to be informed, not only of the benefits, risks and hazards of the proposed therapy but also of known alternative therapy, such as available childbirth education classes which could help to prepare the Pregnant Patient physically and mentally to cope with the discomfort or stress of pregnancy and the experience of childbirth, thereby reducing or eliminating her

need for drugs and obstetric intervention. She should be offered such information early in her pregnancy in order that she may make an informed decision.

3. *The Pregnant Patient has the right,* prior to the administration of any drug, to be informed by the health professional who is prescribing or administering the drug to her that any drug which she receives during pregnancy, labor and birth, no matter how or when the drug is taken or administered, may adversely affect her unborn baby, directly or indirectly, and that there is no drug or chemical which has been proven safe for the unborn child.

4. *The Pregnant Patient has the right,* if Cesarean birth is anticipated, to be informed prior to the administration of any drug, and preferably prior to her hospitalization, that minimizing her and, in turn, her baby's intake of nonessential pre-operative medicine will benefit her baby.

5. *The Pregnant Patient has the right,* prior to the administration of a drug or procedure, to be informed of the areas of uncertainty if there is NO properly controlled follow-up research which has established the safety of the drug or procedure with regard to its direct and/or indirect effects on the physiological, mental and neurological development of the child exposed, via the mother, to the drug or procedure during pregnancy, labor, birth or lactation—(this would apply to virtually all drugs and the vast majority of obstetric procedures).

6. *The Pregnant Patient has the right,* prior to the administration of any drug, to be informed of the brand name and generic name of the drug in order that she may advise the health professional of any past adverse reaction to the drug.

7. *The Pregnant Patient has the right* to determine for herself, without pressure from her attendant, whether she will accept the risks inherent in the proposed therapy or refuse a drug or procedure.

8. *The Pregnant Patient has the right* to know the name and qualifications of the individual administering a medication or procedure to her during labor or birth.

9. *The Pregnant Patient has the right* to be informed, prior to the administration of any procedure, whether that procedure is being administered to her for her or her baby's benefit (medically indicated) or as an elective procedure (for convenience, teaching purposes or research).

10. *The Pregnant Patient has the right* to be accompanied during the stress of labor and birth by someone she cares for, and to whom she looks for emotional comfort and encouragement.

11. *The Pregnant Patient has the right* after appropriate medical consultation to choose a position for labor and for birth which is least stressful to her baby and to herself.

12. *The Obstetric Patient has the right* to have her baby cared for at her bedside if her baby is normal, and to feed her baby according to her baby's needs rather than according to the hospital regimen.

13. *The Obstetric Patient has the right* to be informed in writing of the name of the person who actually delivered her baby and the professional qualifications of that person. This information should also be on the birth certificate.

14. *The Obstetric Patient has the right* to be informed if there is any known or indicated aspect of her or her baby's care or condition which may cause her or her baby later difficulty or problems.

15. *The Obstetric Patient has the right* to have her and her baby's hospital medical records complete, accurate and legible and to have their records, including Nurses' Notes, retained by the hospital until the child reaches at least the age of majority, or, alternatively, to have the records offered to her before they are destroyed.

16. *The Obstetric Patient,* both during and after her hospital stay, has the right to have access to her complete hospital medical records, including Nurses' Notes, and to receive a copy upon payment of a reasonable fee and without incurring the expense of retaining an attorney.

It is the obstetric patient and her baby, not the health professional, who must sustain any trauma or injury resulting from the use of a drug or obstetric procedure. The observation of the rights listed above will not only permit the obstetric patient to participate in the decisions involving her and her baby's health care, but will help to protect the health professional and the hospital against litigation arising from resentment or misunderstanding on the part of the mother.

Prepared by Doris Haire

Published by International Childbirth Education Association, Inc.

P.O. Box 20048, Minneapolis, Minnesota 55420 U.S.A.

Female Laboratory Values

LAB TEST	PREGNANT	NONPREGNANT
Hemoglobin	11.5–12.3 g/dl	12–16 g/dl
Hematocrit	32%–46%	36%–48%
White blood cells	5,000–18,000/µl	4,000–11,000/µl
Neutrophils	60%± 10	60%
Lymphocytes	34%±10	30%
Platelets	100,000–300,000/µl	Same
Calcium	7.8–9.3 mg/dl	8.4–10.2 mg/dl
Sodium	Increased retention	136–146 mmol/liter
Chloride	Slight elevation	98–106 mmol/liter
Iron	Decreased	40–150 mcg/dl
Fibrinogen	450 mg/dl	200–400 mg/dl

Source: Conrad, L. *Maternal-Neonatal Nursing* 1997 Springhouse: Springhouse Corporation.

Normal Neonatal Laboratory Values

LAB TEST	VALUE
Erythrocytes	5.0–7.5 million/µl at birth 3.0–4.0 million/µl by 8–10 weeks
Hemoglobin	15–20 g/dl at birth 14 g/dl at 1–3 months
Hematocrit	45%–65% at birth
Red blood cells	5.0–7.5 million/µl
White blood cells	9,000–30,000/µl
Eosinophils	2%–3% at birth 4.1% at 1 week 2.8% at 1 month
Neutrophils	40%–80% at birth 34% at 1 week 15%–35% at 1 month
Lymphocytes	30% at birth 41% at 1 week 31%–71% at 1 month
Monocytes	6%–10%
Platelets	150,000–400,000/µl
Reticulocytes	3%–6%
Glucose	35–90 mg/dl at birth
Calcium	9.0–11.5 mg/dl in cord blood 9.0–10.6 mg/dl at 3–24 hrs 7.0–12.0 mg/dl at 24–48 hrs 9.0–10.9 mg/dl at 4–7 days
Sodium	139–146 mmol./liter at birth
Chloride	97–110 mmol/liter at birth
Total protein	4.6–7.4 g/dl at birth
Potassium	3.5–7.0 mEq/liter
Magnesium	1.4–2.2 mEq/liter
Blood urea nitrogen	5–12 mg/dl
Creatinine	0.2–0.4 mg/dl
Bilirubin	<2 mg/dl at birth 2–6 mg/dl at 24 hours 6–7 mg/dl at 48 hrs 4–12 mg/dl at 3–5 days

Source: Conrad, L. *Maternal-Neonatal Nursing* 1997 Springhouse: Springhouse Corporation.

Cervical Dilatation Chart

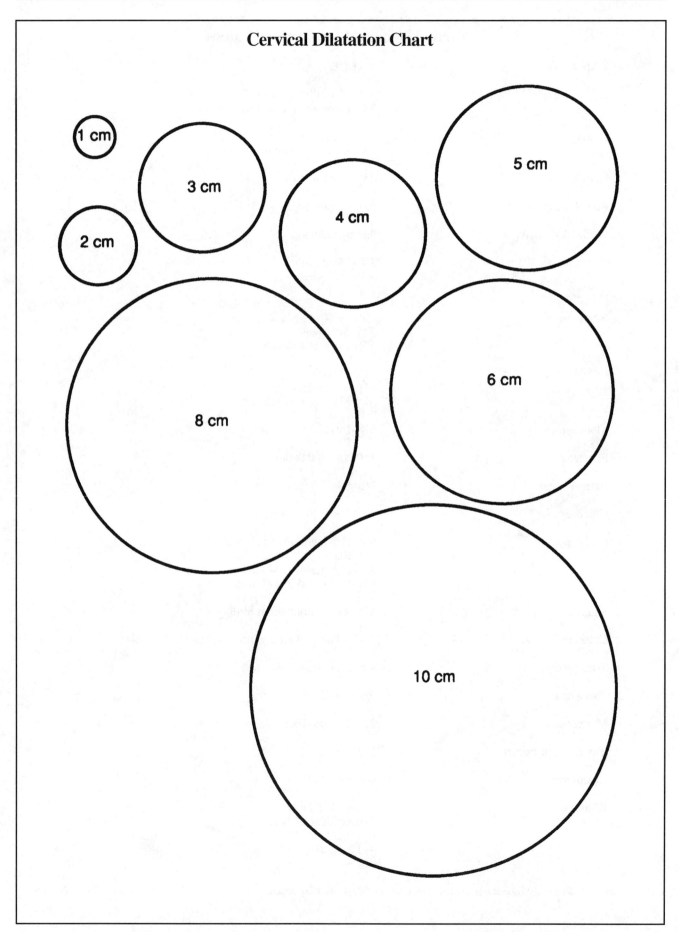

RESOURCES

American Academy of Husband-Coached Childbirth
P.O. Box 5224
Sherman Oaks, CA 91413
(818) 788-6662

American Academy of Pediatrics
Guidelines to Perinatal Care
141 Northwest Point Road
P.O. Box 927
Elk Grove Village, IL 60009-0927

American Diabetes Association
Diabetes Information Service Center
1660 Duke Street
Alexandria, VA 22314
1-800-ADA-DISC

American Society for Psychoprophylaxis in Obstetrics (ASPO)
1840 Wilson Boulevard
Suite 204
Arlington, VA 22201
(703) 524-7802
Publishes *LAMAZE Parents'* Magazine

AWHONN (The Association of Women's Health, Obstetric, and Neonatal Nurses)
Department 3299
Washington, D.C. 20042-3299
1-800-673-8499

Centers for Disease Control
(404) 639-3311

Childbirth Graphics, Ltd.
P.O. Box 20540
Rochester, N.Y. 14602-9938

Child Magazine's Guide to Having a Baby
CHILD Publishing Division of The New York Times Company
110 Fifth Avenue
New York, NY 10011
(212) 463-1000

International Childbirth Education Association (ICEA)
P.O. Box 20048
Milwaukee, WI 55420

March of Dimes National Foundation
1275 Mamaroneck Avenue
White Plains, NY 10605
(914) 428-7100

National AIDS Hotline
1-800-342-2437

National Maternal and Child Health Clearinghouse
3520 Prospect Street, N.W., Ground Floor
Washington, D.C. 20057

GLOSSARY

Abruptio placenta Premature separation or detachment from the wall of the uterus of a normally situated placenta; can be partial or complete separation.

Acceleration Refers to a periodic rise in fetal heart rate from the baseline in response to stress, lowered oxygen availability, or fetal movement.

Acrocyanosis The slightly bluish, grayish discoloration of a newborn's hands and feet within the first 24 hours of birth.

Alphafetoprotein (AFP) A glycoprotein and a major component of fetal blood; small amounts are found in the amniotic fluid of normal fetuses. Elevated levels may indicate neural tube malformations.

Amniocentesis A procedure for removing amniotic fluid from the amniotic sac by inserting a needle through the abdominal wall usually to assess fetal health or maturity.

Amniotomy The artificial rupture of amniotic membranes when an amnihook or other rupturing device is introduced into the vagina and a small tear is made in the membrane.

Anencephaly A congenital anomaly in which part of the brain and spinal cord is missing.

Antepartum period The period of time from conception to before labor begins.

Anterior fontanel Diamond shaped fontanel located at the juncture of the coronal, frontal, and sagittal sutures.

Apgar A five part scoring system to assess newborns at one minute and five minutes after birth regarding heart rate, respiratory effort, muscle tone, reflex irritability, and color.

Appropriate gestational age (AGA) When a newborn's birth weight is within the 10th to 90th percentile expected for that length gestation.

Asphyxia A decrease in the amount of oxygen and an increased amount of carbon dioxide in the body as a result of some interference with respiration.

Attachment The establishment of a reciprocal relationship between the parents and the newborn after a period of bonding; development of a deeper intimacy which grows over time.

Baby Blues A common transient mild depression or emotional disturbance affecting the mother after delivery due to hormonal changes, sleep deprivation, emotional letdown.

Ballottement When palpated, the fetus floats away, then returns to touch the examiner's fingers.

Biofeedback Process of detecting physiological actions within the body by the brain to help change the physiological response or behavior.

Bishop's Score A prelabor scoring system with five components (cervical dilatation, effacement, consistency, position, and fetal station) to help determine if induction of labor will be effective.

Bloody Show Rupture of the small cervical capillaries when the cervix begins to dilate and efface; when the mucus plug is lost the resultant cervical drainage is pink-tinged.

Bonding The initial attraction and period of exploration between the parents and newborn; becoming acquainted.

Braxton Hicks The intermittent, irregular painless uterine contractions which occur during pregnancy; they do not dilate and efface the cervix. (*See* True labor.)

Breech presentation When the buttocks or the feet of the fetus is delivered first, rather than the head (vertex).

BUBBLE An acronym standing for important assessment areas of a postpartum woman: breasts, uterus, bowels, bladder, lochia, episiotomy, and extremities.

Caput Succedaneum Localized edema occurring just under the presenting part of the fetal scalp during labor; disappears within a few days to one week.

Cardinal movements The predictable sequence of movements through the birth canal that the fetus will go through during labor and birth: descent, flexion, internal rotation, extension, external rotation, and expulsion.

Case Management Controls the process of health care activities for individual patients through the coordinating efforts of a case manager.

Cephalhematoma A collection of blood between the newborn's skull bone and periosteum resulting from pressure or trauma during labor or delivery; does not cross suture lines.

Cephalic presentation When the head of the fetus is the presenting part; may be vertex, face, sinciputal, or brow presentations.

Cervical Dilatation The opening or enlargement of the external cervical Os from a few mm to 10 centimeters when completely dilated.

Cervical effacement The thinning or shortening of the cervix during labor from 0% to 100% when completely effaced.

Cesarean Delivery Delivery of the fetus either through a transverse or low vertical abdominal incision.

Chadwick's sign The bluish or purple coloration of the vagina and cervix when pregnancy is presumed.

Chorionic Villus Sampling A procedure to obtain a sample of the chorionic villi from the placenta via aspiration; tests for chromosomal and biochemical disorders during early pregnancy.

Coach A person who assumes the role of advocate and support person for the laboring woman; assists with conditioned techniques for relaxation and breathing.

Contraction Stress Test (CST) A procedure to help measure fetal well-being by stimulating the uterus to contract with oxytocin administration or nipple stimulation and measuring the response of the fetus to the contractions; can be interpreted as positive, negative, or equivocal (suspicions). (*See* also Oxytocin challenge test.)

Colostrum The first secretion of human milk; high in protein and low in fat.

Couplet Care A system in which one nurse cares for the postpartum mother and her newborn as a single unit; also known as mother-baby dyad.

Curandero Term for "healer" in the Mexican-American culture.

Diaphragmatic hernia A condition when the diaphragm does not close completely and the abdominal contents slip into the thoracic cavity; causes respiratory distress in the newborn.

Doppler monitor Uses ultrasound to detect audible fetal heart rate sounds; an intermittent, and simple monitoring technique.

Ductus arteriosus A connection between the main pulmonary artery and the aorta of the fetus; closes after birth and becomes a ligament.

Dysfunctional Labor Occurs when there is a problem with the frequency, duration, and intensity of uterine contractions, and/or the resting tone of the uterus between contractions.

Dyspnea Air hunger resulting in labored or difficult breathing usually accompanied by pain.

Dystocia Difficult labor due to mechanical factors or inadequate muscular problems with the passenger (fetus) or the passage (the pelvis of the mother).

Early deceleration A transitory decrease in the fetal heart rate caused by head compression, which stimulates the vagus nerve to slow down the heart rate.

Early Discharge Discharge from the hospital usually within the first 24 hours after childbirth.

Eclampsia A pregnancy-induced hypertensive disease associated with hypertension, proteinuria, edema, tonic and clonic seizures, and coma.

Electronic Fetal Monitoring A type of monitoring in which information about the fetal heart rate and the laboring woman's uterine contraction pattern is continually assessed; can be either direct (invasive or internal) or indirect (noninvasive or external).

Encephalocele Protrusion of the brain through a cranial fissure generally in the occipital area.

Engagement Also referred to as lightening; when the fetal presenting part moves downward into the mother's pelvic cavity.

Engorgement The swelling and distention of the breasts, usually during the early days of initiation of lactation, due to vascular dilatation as well as the arrival of the early milk.

Epidural Block A type of regional anesthesia used to produce relief from pain during labor and delivery.

Episiotomy An incision in the perineum to facilitate delivery.

Expected Date of Confinement (EDC) The estimated date of delivery based on Naegle's rule or ultrasound.

Expected Date of Delivery (EDD) The estimated date of delivery based on Naegle's rule or ultrasound.

False Labor Characterized by irregular Braxton-Hicks contractions which do not change the cervix and do not increase in intensity, duration, or frequency. (*See also* True labor.)

Family Centered Care The maternity delivery system that emphasizes professional quality health care of the total family unit; utilizes a combined nursery and postpartum nursing staff to form one mother-baby dyad. (*See* Couplet care.)

Fetal attitude The relationship of the fetal parts to each other; flexion and extension.

Fetal bradycardia When the fetal heart rate is less than 120 beats/minute during at least a 10 minute period of continuous monitoring.

Fetal distress A compromise in fetal well-being; can be either acute or chronic.

Fetal lie The relationship of the body of the fetus to the body of the mother, is either longitudinal or transverse.

Fetal position The relationship of the landmark on the presenting fetal part to the front, sides, or back of the maternal pelvis.

Fetal presentation The lowest part of the fetus that comes first through the maternal pelvis and birth canal: either vertex (cephalic), shoulders, breech.

Fetal station Refers to the relationship of the fetus's presenting part to an imaginary line drawn between the maternal ischial spines and the pelvic outlet.

Fetal surveillance Methods to assess and monitor the well-being of the fetus during pregnancy, labor, and birth; includes fetal biophysical profile, biochemical assessments, amniocentesis, genetic studies, antenatal testing, fetal movement counting, non-stress testing, contraction stress testing, and clinical assessments.

Fetal tachycardia When the fetal heart rate is greater than 160 beats/minute during at least a 10 minute period of continuous monitoring.

"Floating" When the presenting part is entirely out of the maternal pelvis and can be moved by the examiner not engaged.

Foramen ovale The septal opening between the atria of the fetal heart which closes soon after birth.

Four P's The four forces of labor including passage, passenger, power, and psyche.

Freidman curve A method of evaluating the relationship of three factors to help determine normal or abnormal labor patterns over time; these three factors are uterine activity, cervical dilatation, and fetal descent; can be plotted on a graph.

Gestational age The number of complete weeks of fetal development, calculated from the first day of the last menstrual cycle.

Gestational Diabetes Mellitus (GDM) Glucose or carbohydrate intolerance of variable severity which develops or is discovered during the present pregnancy; the condition subsides at the completion of the pregnancy.

Grandmultiparity Used to describe the woman who has five or more live births.

Gravida A pregnant woman.

Gravidity Refers to the total number of a woman's pregnancies regardless of their duration.

Grunting Audible sound made by the newborn on expiration often indicating respiratory distress.

Heger's sign Softening of the lower segments of the uterus during the 2nd and 3rd month of pregnancy.

HELLP This syndrome refers to a severe, and potentially fatal complication of pregnancy-induced hypertension involving hemolysis of red blood cells, elevated liver enzyme levels, and a low platelet count.

Hematoma Occurs when blood escapes into the connective tissue of a traumatized area; can be life-threatening; may or may not cause severe pain.

Hemorrhage Blood volume loss of more than 500cc or blood loss of more than 15% of the total estimated blood volume.

Homan's sign A method for detecting thrombophlebitis in which the leg is held straight and the foot flexed back; if the maneuver produces pain upon dorsiflexion of the foot, the test is positive and thrombophlebitis should be suspected.

Hydrocephalus The increased accumulation of cerebrospinal fluid within the ventricles of the brain; may result from congenital anomalies, infection, injury, or brain tumor

Hyperbilirubinemia A condition when there is an excessive amount of bilirubin in the blood; excessive levels can lead to brain damage.

Hypertonic Labor Occurs when uterine contractions are of poor quality and ineffectual in dilating the cervix.

Hypertonic Uterus Labor contractions lasting longer than 90 seconds, caused by too much stimulation of the uterus.

Hypotonic Labor Occurs during the active phase of labor causing ineffectual contractions and a lack of progression of labor.

Involution The reduction in size of the uterus following delivery.

Intrapartum period The time from the onset of labor to the delivery of the newborn and the placenta.

Labor A process that involves a series of integrated uterine contractions that occur over time, and work to propel the fetus from the birth canal; relies on the uterine muscles and cervical compliance.

Labor Delivery Recovery and Postpartum Care (LDRP) A system of health care delivery in which a woman labors, delivers, recovers, and is discharged home from the same room and cared for by a primary care nurse; is home-like environment within a hospital setting. (*See also* Single room maternity care.)

Lactation The process of preparing for and maintaining the production and secretion of milk including mammogenesis, lactogenesis, and galactopoiesis.

Lamaze method An approach to childbirth emphasizing relaxation and breathing techniques to allow for a "painless childbirth;" also known as psychoprophylaxis method.

Lanugo A fine, downy hair covering the fetus between the 17th week gestation and soon after birth.

Late deceleration A periodic decrease in the fetal heart rate below baseline occurring after the peak of the contraction; due to uteroplacental insufficiency and a sign of fetal distress.

Leopold maneuvers A system of evaluating the position and presentation of the fetus by palpating the maternal abdomen in four distinct locations.

Lightening The movement of the fetus and uterus downward into the pelvic cavity; an early sign of impending labor. (*See also* Engagement.)

Lochia The discharge of blood, mucus, and tissue from the uterus during the postpartum period; changes from rubra, to serosa, to alba.

Low Birth Weight (LBW) Infant weighing less than 2500 grams.

Macrosomia large body size; newborn at term weighing more than 4000 grams or large for gestational age.

Managed Care A system of health care delivery in which prescribed patient care activities are coordinated in a timely and cost-efficient manner from the initiation of care to its completion.

Managed Care Path A written plan of care which specifies the expected progress and outcome criteria for an individual patient.

Mastitis Breast infection as a result of milk in the ducts.

Maternity care Complete care of the pregnant, laboring, and newly delivered woman and her newborn; also includes pre-pregnancy counseling, infertility counseling, and parenting education.

Meconium The first stool passed by the newborn; dark green or black material passed from the large intestine from the term or near-term fetus.

Molding Normal overlapping of the skull bones of the baby to allow the fetal head to fit through the pelvis during labor.

Multigravida A woman who has been pregnant 2 or more times.

Multipara A woman who has had two or more pregnancies that terminated at the stage when the newborns were viable.

Multiple gestation Pregnancy with more than one fetus, e.g., twins.

Naegle's rule Used to determine the estimated date of confinement (EDC) or delivery date by subtracting 3 months from the first day of the last menstrual period, then adding 7 days.

Newborn period From birth through the first 28 days of life.

Nonstress test (NST) A noninvasive test used to determine fetal well-being; involves external fetal monitoring of the fetal heart rate and observing the response of the heart rate to fetal movement; interpreted as reactive or non-reactive.

Nuchal cord The presence of one or more loops of the umbilical cord around the neck of the newborn.

Nulliparous A woman who has never given birth to a child.

Opthalmia neonatorum Severe purulent conjunctivitis in the newborn.

Ortaloni's sign A technique for determining the presence of a congenital dislocation of the hip; performed as part of the newborn exam.

Oxytocin challenge test (OCT) A test to assess fetal well-being by administering oxytocin via intravenous infusion to induce uterine contractions and assessing the fetus's response; can be interpreted as positive (abnormal), negative (normal), or suspicious (inconclusive). (*See also* Contraction stress test.)

Parity Refers to the number of past pregnancies that have gone to viability and have been delivered, regardless of the number of children involved (e.g., the birth of triplets increases the parity by only one).

Parturient A woman in labor.

Perinatal Denotes a time period between 20 weeks of gestational age to 28 days after birth.

Placenta The oval or discoid spongy structure attached to the uterus through which the fetus derives its nourishment and through which waste products from the fetus pass into the mother's blood.

Placenta previa Placenta which is abnormally implanted in the lower uterine segment.

Polyhydramnios Excessive volume of amniotic fluid usually greater than 1.2 liters.

Postpartum depression Delayed emotional disturbance affecting the new mother sometimes one to three weeks postpartum; less commonly experienced; more intense and serious than the postpartum "baby blues."

Postpartum period Period of time after a woman gives birth until her recovery 6 weeks later; when all of the reproductive changes which occur over a 9 month pregnancy return to the pre-pregnant state.

Postterm pregnancy When the pregnancy continues past 42 weeks gestation.

Precipitate delivery When labor lasts for less than 3 hours before spontaneous delivery; unexpected, sudden, and often unattended.

Preeclampsia Also referred to as toxemia or PIH; a hypertensive disorder of pregnancy usually occurring after the 20th week gestation; characterized by high blood pressure, proteinuria, and edema. (*See also* Eclampsia.)

Pregnancy Induced Hypertension (PIH) A hypertensive disorder during pregnancy including conditions preeclampsia and eclampsia; characterized by hypertension, proteinuria, and edema. (*See also* Eclampsia and preeclampsia.)

pre-term labor When labor begins before the 37th completed weeks of gestation from the first day of the last menstrual period.

Primigravida A woman who is pregnant for the first time.

Primipara A woman who has delivered one pregnancy in which the fetus has reached viability, without regard to the child's being born alive or dead at the time of birth. Some authors consider that the designation of primipara includes women in the process of giving birth to their first child.

Prolapsed cord An emergent event, when the umbilical cord slips in front of the presenting part and protrudes from the cervix into the vagina; the presenting part may press the against the mother's pelvis cutting off the blood and oxygen to the fetus.

Prolonged labor When the latent phase of labor lasts longer than 24 hours without spontaneous delivery.

Psychoprophylaxis Term first applied to the Lamaze childbirth method which emphasizes relaxation, breathing, and positioning to help obtain a "painless childbirth." (*See also* Lamaze.)

Quickening Sensation of fetal movement usually felt around the 16th week of pregnancy; a presumptive sign of pregnancy.

Regional anesthesia A nerve block with an anesthetic agent which ranges from local infiltration to spinal block anesthesia; the most commonly used regional anesthesia used in childbirth is the epidural.

Relaxin A polypeptide hormone secreted in the corpus luteum during pergnancy.

Rooming-in concept First practiced in the 1940s when healthy newborns were allowed to stay in their mothers' room where they were cared for instead of remaining in the nursery; a nursery nurse and a postpartum nurse still cared for the mother and baby separately.

Rupture of the membranes (ROM) Refers to the breaking of the amniotic membranes and the leaking of the amniotic fluid; may be done spontaneously as an early sign of the onset of labor, or artificially ruptured with a device. (*See* Amniotomy.)

Single room maternity care A system of caring for a woman and family during labor, delivery, and recovery in one room from her admission to the hospital until her discharge home. (*See also* LDRP.)

Small for gestational age (SGA) A classification for infants based on weight and gestational age at birth; refers to an infant whose birth weight is below the 10th percentile expected for that length gestation.

Striae gravidarum The bluish or pink streaks occurring on the abdomen during pregnancy due to the stretching of the abdomen as the uterus grows.

Thermoregulation The regulation of body temperature; prevention of heat loss by regulating the newborn's environment.

Tocodynamometer Device for estimating force of contractions of the uterus during labor.

Tocolytic therapy Medication to quiet or inhibit the smooth muscle activity of the contracting uterus.

TORCH syndrome Acronym for a group of infections which are particularly damaging to the fetus or newborn; includes toxoplasmosis, rubella, cytomegalovirus, and herpesvirus type 2.

True labor When uterine contractions are regular with increasing intensity and occur with greater frequency; contractions effect a change in the dilatation and effacement of the cervix. (*See also* False labor.)

Ultrasound Also called sonogram; used to visualize the uterine environment by using sound waves that pass through soft tissue until an interface between the structures of different tissue densities is reached. When this occurs, some of the energy is reflected back to the transducer, which creates an image on the screen.

Vacuum extraction Used to assist in the delivery of the infant instead of applying forceps; after a vacuum cup is applied to the fetal scalp, a negative pressure is exerted to help draw the fetus's head through the birth canal.

Vaginal, Birth After Cesarean (VBAC) Permits patients the opportunity of a trial of labor and a vaginal delivery after previously delivering by cesarean section.

Variability The change in the baseline fetal heart rate caused by the interplay of the sympathetic and parasympathetic nervous systems; may vary from 5–10 beats/minute with contractions and fetal or maternal movement.

Variable deceleration A periodic slowing of the fetal heart rate either with a contraction or between contractions; due to umbilical cord compression; variable in duration, intensity and timing of the deceleration.

Vernix caseosa A protective cheese-like substance found on the newborn to protect the skin from the drying effect of the amniotic fluid.

Vertex presentation The fetal head or cranium is the presenting part with the head flexed on the chest and the chin in contact with the thorax; also called cephalic presentation.

Very low birth weight infant (VLBW) When an infant weighs between 500 –1499 grams.

BIBLIOGRAPHY

ACOG *Technical Bulletin #96.* (September, 1986). Drug Abuse and Pregnancy, Washington, D.C.

ACOG *Technical Bulletin #217.* (December 1995). Induction of Labor.

ACOG *Technical Bulletin #218.* (December 1995). Dystocia and the Augmentation of Labor.

ACOG *Technical Bulletin #219.* (January, 1996). Hypertension in Pregnancy.

Aftrait, C. (1989). *Electronic fetal monitoring.* Rockville, MD: Aspen.

American Diabetes Association, Inc. (1993). *Medical management of pregnancy complicated by diabetes.* Alexandria, VA: American Diabetes Association, Inc.

American Heart Association and the American Academy of Pediatrics (1994). *Textbook of neonatal resuscitation.* IL.

American Society for Phychoprophylaxis in Obstetrics. (1987). *Guidelines for developing a teaching plan, ASPO/Lamaze teacher certification program for childbirth educators.* Washington, DC.

Associated Press. (2/23/95). U.S. urges AIDS testing of pregnant women. *The San Diego Union-Tribune,* A-5.

Auerback, K. (1990). The effect of nipple shields on maternal milk volume. *Journal of Obstetric, Gynecologic, and Neonatal Nursing, 19*(5), 419.

Avant, K. C. (May/June 1988). Stressors on the childbearing family, *JOGNN.*

Bartholomew, S. (September 1992). You first, mom. *Diabetes Forecast,* 67–71.

Bland, R. (1995). *Biomedical Policy.* Chicago, IL: Nelson-Hall Publisher.

Bloom, R. & Cropley, C. (1995). *Textbook of neonatal resuscitation.* American Academy of Pediatrics.

Bobak, I. & Jensen, M. (1993). *Maternity & gynecologic care: The nurse and the family* (5th ed.). St. Louis: C.V. Mosby.

Campbel, A. & Worthington, E. (1982). Teaching expectant fathers how to be better labor coaches. *MCN: The American Journal of Maternal-Child Nursing, 7*(28).

Canick, J. & Knight, G. (April 1992). Multiple-marker screening for fetal Down syndrome, *Contemporary OB/GYN.*

Carpenito, L. (1993). *Nursing diagnosis: Application to clinical practice* (5th ed.). Philadelphia: J. B. Lippincott.

Childbrith Graphics Ltd. (1980, 1985, 1990).

Christensen, P., & Kenny, J. (1990). *Nursing process: Application of conceptual models* (3rd ed.). St. Louis: C. V. Mosby.

Cohen, S., Kenner, C., & Hollingsworth, A. (1991). *Maternal, neonatal, and women 's health nursing.* Springhouse, PA: Springhouse Corporation.

Conrad, Lynne H. (1997). *Maternal-neonatal nursing,* (3rd ed.). Springhouse, PA: Springhouse Corporation.

De Santo, P. & Hassid, P. (1983). Evaluating exercises, childbirth educator, *American Baby.*

Dorhmann, K. R., & Lederman, S. A. (Nov./Dec. 1986). Weight gain in pregnancy. *JOGNN.*

Esposito, C. (Spring 1993). Abuse: breaking the cycle of violence: the victim's perspective, *Trends in Health Care, Law and Ethics, 8*(2).

Flamm, B., & Goings, J. (1989). Vaginal birth after Cesarean sections: Is suspected fetal macrosomia a contradiction? *Obstetrics and Gynecology, 74* (5).

Flamm, B., Newman, L., Thomas, S., Fallon, D., & Yoshida, M. (1990). Vaginal birth after Cesarean delivery: Results of a 5 year multicenter collaborative study. *Obstetrics and Gynecology, 76* (5).

Folsom, M. (March/April 1997). Amnioinfusion for meconium staining: does it help, *The American Journal of Maternal/Child Nursing, 22,* 74–79.

Forfar, J. O. (2nd ed.) *Drug effects on the fetus and newborn,* Oradell, NJ: Medical Economics Books.

Galvan, B., & Broekhuizen, F. (1987). Obstetric vacuum extraction, *JOGNN, 13*(3).

Gibbs, C. (June 1985). Planned vaginal delivery following Cesarean section. *Clinical Obstetrics and Gynecology, 23.*

Gilbert, E. & Harmon, J. (1993). *Manual of High Risk Pregnancy & Delivery.* Philadelphia: Mosby.

Hilton, A. S. (1986). *Protocol of care for the battered woman.* New York: March of Dimes Birth Defects Foundation.

Honig, J. C. (Jan/Feb 1986). Preparing preschool-aged children to be siblings. *MCN 11.*

International Childbirth Education Association, Inc. (1986). *ICEA position paper: The role of the childbirth educator and the scope of childbirth education.* Minneapolis, MN.

Jiminez, S. L. M. (Mar/Apr 1980). Education for the childbearing year. *JOGNN.*

Johnston, M. (Jan/Feb 1980). Cultural variations in professional and parenting patterns. *JOGNN.*

Johnson, S. H. (1979). *High-risk parenting: Nursing assessment and strategies for the family at risk.* Philadelphia: J. B. Lippincott.

Korones, S. B. (1986). *High-risk newborn infants: The basis for intensive nursing care.* St. Louis: C. V. Mosby.

Ladewig, P. W., London, M. L., & Olds, S. B. (1990). *Essentials of maternal-newborn nursing.* New York: Addison-Wesley.

Ladewig, P. W., London, M. L., & Olds, S. B. (1998). *Maternal newborn nursing care,* (4th ed). New York: Addison-Wesley, Longman, Inc..

Lindberh, C. (July/August 1995). Perinatal transmission of HIV: how to counsel women, *The American Journal of Maternal/Child Nursing, 20,* 207–212.

Luegenbiehl, D., et al. (1990). Standardized assessment of blood loss. *MCN: American Journal of Maternal Child Nursing, 15*(4), 241.

Maloni, J. (1991). Physical and psychological effects of antepartum hospital bedrest: A review of the literature. *Image, 23*(3).

Mandeville, L. & Troiano, N. (1992). *High-Risk Intrapartum Nursing.* Philadelphia: Lippincott.

Martin, E. (Ed.). (1990). Intrapartum management modules. Baltimore: Williams & Wilkins.

May, K., & Mahlmeister, L. (1994). *Maternal and neonatal nursing* (3rd ed.). Philadelphia: J.B. Lippincott.

McKenzie, C. A. M. & Vestal, K. W. (1983). Predictions, implications, and planning for high risk perinatal care. *High risk perinatal nursing.* St. Louis, MO: W.B. Saunders.

Metzger, B. & the Organizing Committee (1992). Summary and recommendations of the third international workshop-conference on gestational diabetes mellitus. *Diabetes Spectrum, 5*(1), 22–25.

Michels, V. (October 1, 1992). *Nursing management of the first and second stages of labor: Nursing assessments and challenges.* Presented at the National Conference of Obstetric Nursing, Chicago, IL.

Mohrbacher, N. & Stock, J. (1997). *LaLeche League International: The Breastfeeding Answer Book.* Illinois: La Leche League International.

Murray, M. (1988). *Essentials of electronic fetal monitoring: Antepartum and intrapartum fetal monitoring.* Washington, D. C.: NAACOG.

NAACOG OGN Nursing Practice Resource. (1989). *Mother-baby Care.*

NAACOG. *Nursing responsibilities in implementing intrapartum heart rate monitoring: Position statement.* AWHONN (1992, reaffirmed 1994) Washington, D. C.

NAACOG. (1990). *OGN Nursing Practice Resource: Fetal heart rate auscultation.* Washington, D. C.

NAACOG Electronic fetal monitoring: Joint *ACOG/NAACOG* statement. Washington, D. C.

Neeson, J. D. (1987). *Clinical manual of maternity nursing.* Philadelphia, PA: J.B. Lippincott.

Neff, M. & Spray, M. (1996). *Introduction to Maternal and Child Health Nursing.* Philadelphia, PA: Lippincott Publishers.

Nichols, F. & Humenick, S. S. (1988). *Childbirth education: Practice, research, and theory,* chapter 27. Philadelphia, PA: W.B. Saunders.

Niswander, K. R. (1981). *Obstetrics,* (2nd ed.). Boston, MA: Little, Brown.

Olds, S., London, M. & Ladewig, P. (1988). *Maternal newborn nursing,* (3rd ed.). New York, NY: Addison Wesley.

Oxorn, H. (1986). *Human labor & birth,* (5th ed.). New York, NY: Appleton-Century-Crofts.

Perez, P. (August, 1988). The emotional work of pregnancy. *International Journal of Childbirth Education.*

Pillitteri, A. (1995). *Maternal & Child Health Nursing: Care of the Childbearing and Childrearing Family.* Philadelphia, PA: J.B. Lippincott.

Pohodich, J., Ramer, L. & Sasmor, J. L. (1981). Psychosocial aspects of childbearing. March of Dimes Birth Defects Foundation, Series 2, Module 4, *Prenatal Care.*

Raff, B. & Freisner, A. (1989). *Quick Reference to maternity nursing.* Rockville, MD: Aspen Publishers.

Reeder, S. J. & Martin, L. L. (1987). *Maternity nursing,* (16th ed.). Philadelphia, PA: J.B. Lippincott.

Reproductive Health Hazards, NAACOG (1985), Washington D. C.: *Nursing Practice Resource.*

Rhodes, A. M. (1986). "Baby Doe" rules: Implications for nurses. *MCN, 10.*

Rhodes, A. M. (1986). Maternal versus fetal rights: implications for nurses. *MCN, 11.*

Ross Laboratories. (1980, 1987, 1989). Ohio.

Snydal, S. (1988). Methods of fetal heart rate monitoring during labor. *Journal of Nurse-Midwifery, 33* (1), 4–14.

Spong, C. Amnioinfusion; indications and controversies. *Contemporary OB/GYN, 42*(8) 138–139, 143–144, 149, 153–154, 156, 159.

Styles, M. M. (1990). Challenges for nursing in this new decade. *MCN, 15.*

Taylor, Burr, & Bartelli, Editors. (May 1996). *Perinatal Transmission of HIV: A Guide for Providers.* Columbia School of Public Health, National Pediatric and Family HIV Resource Center and the New Jersey AIDS Education and Training Center.

Thompson, J. (September 30, 1992). *Access to care: Perinatal outcomes as a barometer of the nation's health.* Presented at the National Conference of Obstetric Nursing, Chicago, IL.

Tucker, S. (1988). *Pocket guide to fetal monitoring.* St. Louis: Mosby.

U. S. Department of Agriculture. *Nutrition and your health: Dietary guidelines for Americans.* (1990). Home and Garden Bulletin No. 232. Washington, D.C.

White, A. (February, 1992). Staying fit during pregnancy. *Diabetes Forecast,* 45–46.

Wilkerson, N. N. & Barrows, T. L. (1988). Synchronizing care with mother-baby rhythms. *MCN,* 13.

INDEX

PRETEST KEY

1.	B	Chapter 1
2.	C	Chapter 1
3.	A	Chapter 2
4.	A	Chapter 2
5.	D	Chapter 3
6.	D	Chapter 3
7.	B	Chapter 4
8.	B	Chapter 4
9.	C	Chapter 5
10.	C	Chapter 5
11.	A	Chapter 6
12.	A	Chapter 6
13.	C	Chapter 7
14.	B	Chapter 7
15.	D	Chapter 8
16.	C	Chapter 8
17.	C	Chapter 9
18.	A	Chapter 9
19.	D	Chapter 9
20.	D	Chapter 10
21.	B	Chapter 10
22.	C	Chapter 10
23.	B	Chapter 11
24.	A	Chapter 11
25.	B	Chapter 11

Notes

Notes

Notes

Notes

Notes

Notes